THE BOOK OF
GINSENG

THE BOOK OF
GINSENG

AND OTHER CHINESE HERBS
FOR VITALITY

STEPHEN FULDER, PH.D.

Healing Arts Press
Rochester, Vermont

Healing Arts Press
One Park Street
Rochester, Vermont 05767
Web Site: http://www.gotoit.com

Note to the reader: This book is intended as an informational guide. The remedies, approaches, and techniques described herein are meant to supplement, and not to be a substitute for, professional medical care or treatment. They should not be used to treat a serious ailment without prior consultation with a qualified healthcare professional.

Library of Congress Cataloging-in-Publication Data

Fulder, Stephen.
[Tao of medicine]
The book of ginseng: and other Chinese herbs for vitality / Stephen Fulder.
    p.   cm.
Originally published: The tao of medicine. Rochester, Vt. : Healing Arts Press. c1990.
Includes bibliographical references and index.
ISBN 0-89281-491-8
1. Ginseng—Therapeutic use. 2. Medicine, Chinese. I. Title.
[RM666.G49F84   1993]
615'.321–dc20   93-14-095
                                                                                CIP

Printed and bound in the United States.

10 9 8 7 6 5 4 3

Healing Arts Press is a division of Inner Traditions International

Distributed to the book trade in Canada by Publishers Group West (PGW), Toronto, Ontario

Distributed to the health food trade in Canada by Alive Books, Toronto and Vancouver

Distributed to the book trade in the United Kingdom by Deep Books, London

Distributed to the book trade in Australia by Millennium Books, Newtown, N.S.W.

Distributed to the book trade in New Zealand by Tandem Press, Auckland

Distributed to the book trade in South Africa by Alternative Books, Randburg

This book is dedicated to
Joseph Needham, F R S, 'a sage who,
while clad in homespun, conceals on
his person a priceless piece
of jade'

Contents

Olympic athletes take somatensic drugs; Somatensic drugs in war: Genghis Khan and the Vietcong; Ginseng in space: NASA's problems

PART 4: CONCLUSIONS

Acknowledgments

I would like to acknowledge the great help of the late John Blackwood, as well as Imogen Dawes and my sister Adele Moss, for reading and commenting on the manuscript. I would like to thank Professor Michael Ginsberg, Professor E. Shellard, Alan Barnett, John Bagwell, Mick Plewman, and Deepak Shori for discussions, and my wife, Rachel, for constant encouragement. I would also like to thank Lee Harris for first awakening my interest in ginseng and keeping the ginseng kettle bubbling thereafter. I acknowledge the many scientists and friends, especially Dr. Hyo Won Bae of the Korea Ginseng Research Institute, who supplied me with useful information.

Preface

At first sight this book may seem rather large for a book about ginseng, which many may already believe to be some kind of Oriental panacea. Is there really all that much to say about a single herb, even a famous one? This question is partly a challenge to myself, and the obvious response is to invite the reader to turn to any page to see whether it consists of lengthy, boring, irrelevant "ginseniana." The reader might be surprised to come across botany, mythology, drug studies, thoughts on the Taoist perception of the world, clinical tests, health advice, chemistry, Oriental medicine, and perhaps something that blends all these disparate topics together.

For the book is not just about ginseng. It is not a drug cookbook. It is an analysis of a whole system of remedies. Outrageous claims have been made for ginseng—claims surviving on the general ignorance of the true nature of the root. Far from making further claims and encouraging false hopes, one of my purposes here is to lay down the basis for the realistic use of such substances. If ginseng and related Oriental medicines can be put into wider therapeutic perspective, it will become possible for the first time to put honest labels on the bottles.

But there is more to my endeavors than that. The book is also about the world that ginseng belongs to: the rich world of Oriental wisdom on health and well-being. Ginseng is the vehicle that carries us on a journey into that world. Like many travellers, we find ourselves constantly shopping. We will discover, of course, many new and unfamiliar remedies with remarkable properties. In doing so we can bring back a completely new understanding of health and well-being, of energy and longevity and human performance. This practical wisdom has been under development for thousands of years in China but has been sadly neglected in the West, especially since the dominance of the mechanistic world view and its resulting disease-oriented medical orthodoxy. The journey is clearly a long one, and even this large book can only scratch the surface.

In trying to understand the ideas and remedies of Oriental medicine we take a Western point of view and use science as a central analytical tool. This helps us to see how Oriental medicine can be used within a Western context and to deal with everyday concerns in the modern world. For example, I develop in the book certain models and theories about how Oriental herbs, as well as other health practices, can improve vitality by making the body's hormone control systems more efficient. This approach may be very helpful in grasping the whole field of Taoist or Oriental self-care practices. However, it has obviously the limitations arising from transplantation across cultures and across languages. To gain a truly full knowledge of these practices, we must suspend Western concepts and language, at least temporarily, and plunge into the Oriental field of awareness in its own terms—for example, by studying at one of the colleges of Oriental medicine in the West or the East.

When this book was first written, ginseng couldn't be found in health food stores. It was a somewhat mysterious Oriental potion enjoyed by the cognoscenti. Today, ginseng is everywhere. It has become a household word. Does this book still have the same value? Could it be said, perhaps, that this book, along with others, has already done its job in introducing ginseng into the modern world? In fact, as I read it again today, I am quite sure that this book is even more relevant than when it first came out, because—although ginseng is everwhere—people understand very little of its powers and potentials. There is little understanding of how to use it properly, what it should be used for, and what its true nature is. In other words, this book is needed today more than ever because of the widespread use, misuse, and ignorance about one of the most valuable and interesting things to emerge from the Orient since the bamboo curtain was lifted.

The same could be said of Oriental medicine in general. When the book first came out, Chinese medicine was believed in the West to be a form of witchcraft, and investigation and use of it was a kind of heresy. My experiences as a heretic are recounted in the first chapter. Today there are acupuncturists on every street corner. For example, in Oxford, England, my hometown, there are more acupuncturists within the city limits than doctors practicing conventional medicine. Nevertheless, there is a great misunderstanding and ignorance of what Oriental medicine really is. The reason is partly that Oriental practitioners diagnose using pulse, tongue, observation, and other means unfamiliar to us. They treat people using needles, moxa, or herbs. But both patient and the general public have little idea of what is going on in terms that we understand from growing up in the postindustrial West. Who can really describe a meridian, say what the pulses actually measure, or define "shen" or even "kidney" in a meaningful yet modern way? Insofar as this book attempts to make Oriental herbal medicine meaningful to Westerners, it is needed even more today than when so few people were interested in Oriental medicine that it was dismissed by society as a giant placebo effect.

So the book is not just about ginseng. It uses ginseng as a tool or vehicle to help us understand the way Oriental medicine and the Oriental view of the world actually work. Ginseng is a substance that you can actually hold in your hand. You can swallow it, and certain changes will happen to you that you can easily notice. In a sense, then, it is much easier to use as an aid to understanding Oriental medicine than, for example, a meridian, which is so subtle that you can neither feel it readily nor easily research it scientifically. Since ginseng can be tested in the laboratory, and yet is a pure Oriental health discovery with no connection to the Western view of drugs, it provides a wonderful opportunity for opening up Oriental medicine and Oriental thinking to our Western eyes. The tool is science. Hundreds of studies are quoted in this book, because science is our most respected form of inquiry in the West. But the goal is not to reduce Oriental medicine to science. It is to enrich us with a vast and deep alternative wisdom.

ing on the general ignorance of the true nature of the root. Far from making further claims, and encouraging false hopes or false despair, my intention is to lay down the basis for the realistic use of such medicines. If ginseng and related Oriental remedies can be put into a therapeutic perspective, it will become possible for the first time to put some honest labels on the bottles.

PART 1
Background

I

The Root with Two Faces

PANACEA OR PANEGYRIC?

I first came across ginseng in two utterly different settings.

It happened like this. One winter night in 1972, I was sitting in the library of the National Institute for Medical Research, in London. During a routine survey of scientific journals in my field of research, I found an article elaborately titled: 'Testing of Compounds for Capacity to Prolong Post-mitotic Lifespan of Cultured Human Amnion Cells: Effects of Hydrocortisone and *Panax ginseng*'.[1] This described the discovery that an Oriental plant, when added to human cells that were growing in the laboratory, could preserve them and prolong their life.

This intrigued me, for I was involved with research into the ageing process. I also happened to be growing human cells in the laboratory at the time, to study how they aged. I knew that certain substances can be added to cells to prolong their life. Yet none of these chemicals could even remotely qualify as an 'elixir of life' since they happened to be harmful when given to people. Now here was a plant which I had never heard of before, which could not only prolong the life of cells, but was apparently used, according to the authors of the paper, as 'a tonic and preventative of old age debility'.

I hardly had time to digest this, when I ran into ginseng again. This time its surroundings were more alchemical than biochemical.

It was shown to me reverently by a long-lost friend of mine. He was now trading in herbs, knick-knacks and strange discoveries. Ginseng was his prize find. At the back of his shop, amid the old sweet jars full of aromatic herbs, was a balsa-wood box containing the ginseng. It was a root; maroon, gnarled and crusty, as if aged by the elements. Yet it was also crystalline and peculiarly translucent. I could even see light through it when I held it up to the lightbulb. I tasted some. It was extremely hard and its flavour evoked the sweetness of liquorice, the bitterness of orange peel . . . and the dryness of dust.

My friend bubbled with enthusiasm about it:

'It is quite unique. The potion of the Emperors. The Chinese take it whenever they can, especially the old people. They say that it gives them strength and energy, you know, to keep them going, and that it is useful against impotence too. I take it every morning with my tea. It makes me feel buoyant, almost sparkling, very positive. But it is also mysterious. It doesn't work in the same way for everybody. The Chinese say that its effect is related to your inner state. Why not do some research on it?'

I thought about it. How odd that I had never heard of it before. Why was this material not assiduously studied by scientists and taken avidly by old people around the world? It occurred to me that if it had been a newly synthesized chemical, there would have been trumpetings from laboratory rooftops. As it was a Chinese plant, it was left to hide in the dusty corners of the scientific literature or the backstreet Chinese shops. Or had it already been studied, and rejected? Or maybe it was commonly known under another name?

So I returned to the library. The *British Pharmacopoeia*: no mention of it. The *British Pharmaceutical Codex*: no mention. The *American Pharmacopoeia*: nothing. The *US National Formulary*: nothing. The medical dictionaries: no mention. The trade indexes of drugs: no mention. *Martindales Extra Pharmacopoeia*: ah! there was something, but only a disappointing item on the root's appearance and a sentence that it was reputed to be a restorative, having a 'sedative effect on the cerebrum and mildly stimulating action on vital centres. . . .' *Index Medicus* had one or two obscure and irrelevant references and was little help. *Index Nominem*: nothing. No synonyms, no traces. It was a puzzle. I left it. But it didn't leave me. Panax ginseng stayed with me like a knot in my handkerchief.

As the weeks went by I kept an eagle's (and sometimes a night owl's) eye open for information. The puzzle became an enigma. *Encyclopaedia Britannica* informed me that ginseng '. . . was a worthless plant. Any action of the drug appears to be entirely psychic,' while in a later edition of the same encyclopaedia I found it quoted as an example of one of the only true aphrodisiacs in existence! Marco Polo extolled it as an elixir and so did many other travellers to China; Sir Richard Burton ascribed the health and vitality of the elderly wealthy Chinese to ginseng alone. It was the most expensive plant in the world. One record from 1904 noted, 'There are 400 million Chinese and all to some extent use ginseng. A curious fact is that the Chinese highly prize certain shapes among the roots, especially those resembling the human form. For such they gladly pay fabulous prices, sometimes 600 times its weight in silver.' Nevertheless, the US National Formulary had dropped ginseng in 1937, noting that 'the extraordinary properties and medical virtues formerly ascribed to ginseng had no other existence than in the minds of the Chinese'.

I did find it mentioned in the pharmacopoeiae of Asian countries. The Pharmacographica Indica intoned that 'Ginseng enjoys in its native country the reputation of a panacea, and especially of being aphrodisiac. The affections for the cure of which it is most esteemed are such as are usually treated by aromatic stimulants, including dyspepsia, vomiting and nervous affections.' The Japanese and Soviet pharmacopoeiae all gave detailed accounts of how to recognize ginseng, but said little concerning its effects other than a cryptic 'tonic'. At the other extreme, I found tales and myths of ginseng in which its virtues were worshipped – how it was the ultimate panacea, how it was the spirit of man taken root in the earth, how it could bring the dead to life or could prolong life by many years, how it constituted the beneficial agencies of nature coalesced together into a root which was the zenith of concentrated potency, and how life-preserving radiations were emitted from it. The poetry made the problem worse, not better, and for every enthusiastic account there was a dismissive one.

Ant-like, I carried on steadily gathering data. Computers searched through their memories for the key word: ginseng. Libraries provided me with obscure Asian journals. I found that certain scientists were working on it in Russia, Bulgaria and in the Far East. A flood of letters went out to Russian scientists who were delighted to cooperate, to the Japanese who showed boundless courtesy and to the Koreans who had the will but not the language to reply. An odd collection of research results emerged: that ginseng could apparently increase the stamina of mice, that it could both increase and decrease blood pressure, that it could prevent rats from dying as a result of poisons, cold or heat or radiation, that it could excite the brain; again there were the persistent reports of its use by old people in China. These papers were a bane, for I couldn't honestly believe them all. They seemed too good to be true, somewhat like the ancient myths of ginseng rephrased in the language of science. And it was quite clear that no one else in the West believed them either, or even knew of them, otherwise I wouldn't have encountered a vacuum when first looking for information.

In that case was the West's disregard trusty and reliable, the Eastern science overenthusiastic, if not downright fraudulent? Did the myths relate to nothing more than the crock of gold at the end of the rainbow? After all, who dares to talk seriously of panaceas?

Or had the Chinese discovered something extraordinary which we were as yet too myopic to appreciate?

DIPPING A FINGER

Compelled by this question, I took a long-delayed trip down to the Chinese shops in Soho. My eyes wandered along the shelves, taking in the exotica of Oriental medicine: tonic wines with various herbs emblazoned on the labels, little silver pills, large black round speckled pills, pills containing seahorse tails, Royal Jelly ampoules, or Royal Jelly with chameleon extract, numerous packets of dried herbs or bits of root and wooden boxes covered in Chinese ideograms. Fascinating but, as the current dogma goes, how can chameleon extract provide anything more than frogs' legs can? Why should there be anything special in herb wines when even chartreuse, a distillation of over a hundred alpine herbs, was not a medicine, and how could there be some hidden healing property in seahorse tails that didn't exist in shrimps? No, it was preposterous to imagine that all these things were effective as medicines. But I wasn't *really* sure. Would we know it if they were effective? Maybe we don't know how to look or what to look for?

I bought a red crystalline ginseng root from a smiling Chinese girl, who brought it out from behind the counter like something precious or illegal. I took it home for a further step in my investigations: to eat it myself. This is an obvious and natural part of the exploration of drugs, but fallen somewhat out of fashion these days. Pharmacologists now prefer to give rats the first try, although there are still a surprising number of pharmaceutical chemists who quietly dip their fingers in their products. I read about the Chinese use of ginseng: how it was boiled all night in special silver kettles, how it was to be taken daily for a month set aside for this purpose, during which it was important to rest, eat moderately, avoid stimulants and remain celibate.

I took ginseng for a month – a month which, despite my intentions, turned out to be no more temperate than usual. Yet something definitely happened. I felt infused with a particular positivity and energy. Tedious tasks were transformed by a relaxed enthusiasm. I got up earlier, needed less sleep, and above all was never tired during the day. The annual round of colds and flu seemed to pass me by. My steps seemed lighter and my mind more crystalline. There was no doubt that the plant had some kind of stimulatory effect. It seemed to be so specific and unexpected that I was personally satisfied it wasn't simply self-hypnosis which was making me feel so effervescent. After a month I stopped taking it regularly, but kept some by for when I was tired or run down. At those times it didn't produce the agitated jittery kind of wide-eyed alertness which comes from too much coffee or strong stimulants. It simply made me forget that I was tired. Nor did it prevent my sleeping when I laid my head down.

I gave it to colleagues and relatives, friends young and old, healthy and unhealthy. I gave it to a relative dying of cancer. I gave it to people who asked about it. The responses were most encouraging. Some people were amazed at how good they felt. One scientist went so far as to describe her 'euphoria' at initially taking ginseng; it settled down after a while to a sense of energy and integration. Others kept asking me for ginseng and I was pleased to note that any left lying around would rapidly disappear. Many people also took it and felt nothing, but these were often people who were anyway highly energetic. There seemed to be a general pattern that the worse people felt, the more noticeable the improvement. Professor Edward Shellard, head of the Department of Pharmacognoscy at

Chelsea College, and himself an expert on the constituents of ginseng and many other plants, stated, 'I used to get very tired at night – and now I don't – and all I can say is that the only difference between me now and then is the ginseng.'

The letters came. 'I felt I must write and tell you of the wonderful effect the ginseng tablets have had on me,' wrote one woman. 'I have just passed my eightieth birthday and it is many, many years since I have felt so full of vitality and fitness as I have in the last few weeks. It was by coincidence that I was introduced to ginseng. I was going through a patch of weakness . . . my youngest sister asked me to try ginseng. . . . Usually I am sceptical of taking tablets recommended by other people because of unknown side-effects, but there seemed no possible risk of this. I have been simply amazed at the improvement, not only in my physical condition, but also the effect it has had on my mental alertness. Even the younger members of my family have been convinced of its efficacy.' The same lady wrote to me eighteen months later to thank me when I sent her some information, reiterating that 'I really do find ginseng a great help'.

Testimonials, comments and personal experiences have relevance to discovery but not to proof. They are subjective experiences. The story of one man and his drug has no general validity; anecdotes will not convince scientists. But my own consumption of ginseng and observations on others gave me a personal conviction that there was something of great interest in the root. It added impetus to the quest to understand its mystery. However, the puzzle was still very great, although I now had a lot more pieces.

One morning my colleagues were surprised to find me arriving at the laboratory clutching an armful of white Korean ginseng roots, gnarled and crusty. I began grinding, churning, extracting, filtering and freeze-drying like a veritable Wizard of Oz. Eventually I ended up with a thick dark brown goo which contained, I hoped, all the good things for which people gave their life-savings. I made a sterile preparation, and added it in varying amounts to little dishes containing human cells. Over the next few days I kept an eye on the progress of the cells, putting them under the microscope to watch for any changes. Slowly but surely, those cells receiving specific small amounts of ginseng did change in comparison to the others.

They grew faster, they were more compact in shape and, as I had read in the first paper, they seemed more resistant, staying alive for longer in adverse circumstances.[2] Now I had confirmed, at least to my own satisfaction, that ginseng actually did something. It was a far cry from the Chinese elixir, far from the solution to the many mysteries. Nor did I know what was in this murky material that invigorated my cells. But it was a start.

THE BAMBOO CURTAIN

The log jam began to move when it became clear that the problem was not only scientific but also cultural and political. Science could be used alone in understanding the specific properties of the root, but not in guiding the search. In order to cut through the knots of claim and counterclaim concerning ginseng, there was no alternative but to make a thorough examination of its use and history in China, while at the same time gathering all possible scientific material. By homing in on it from both East and West, I felt that it might be possible to meet somewhere in the middle and distinguish the fact from the fancy.

With this in mind, I went to Cambridge and there sought the help of Joseph Needham, a man whose life had been spent in the fusion of East and West, an historian, a biochemist and the world authority on Chinese culture. Science was not, for Needham, a closed circle which professionals carved into segments. He understood immediately what I was trying to do; the ginseng enigma could only be solved by using every possible avenue into Chinese life: the language, the medicine, the science, the religious life and the deep-seated view of nature and its products. In a gentle but persistent manner, Needham offered suggestions and unravelled mistranslations. The Chinese language was a serious and subtle barrier to understanding. It uses signs, not letters, and thus gives figurative names to things which on translation turn into poetic and gross overstatements. The Chinese term for Librium is 'a pill that profits the eyes to rest'. Many of the names of ginseng functioned more like trade marks than words: the 'constellation of Orion', the 'wonder of the world', the 'regenerative elixir which removes wrinkles from the face' and, above all, the codes for man/spirit/earth/essence which appeared in various kaleidoscopic combinations.

In the medical books from China was a wealth of information on the use and purpose of ginseng and how it fitted into a structured but extraordinary therapeutic framework. Slowly the realization dawned that once the layers of poetry and dreams concerning ginseng were stripped away, underneath was revealed an ancient core of knowledge and experience which is rational and consistent. Moreover, ginseng was not alone: it had a range of relatives, all of whom have connected medicinal uses and effects. These first brief explorations at Cambridge laid the groundwork for the discussion of Chinese medicine in Chapter 3.

Needham, respected by the Chinese above any Westerner living, one of the last of the great encyclopaedists, is a man of great humility and spirit. My book is dedicated to him, as he dedicates his work to his ancestors in the Taoist tradition. Before my departure from Cambridge he turned to me and said: 'You are studying ageing. Well, I would ask you one thing. Find something for me which will keep me going just long enough to finish my fifth volume.' I left with the distinct impression that such things were more likely to be found in his own rich library of ancient Chinese sources than in my laboratory.

THE GINSENG INDUSTRY

These enquiries were upstaged by a new turn of events. By the spring of 1972 ginseng was fashionable. It had moved from its ancestral home among the Chinese and become a popular pick-me-up of the alternative society. Two books on plant drugs generated a wide interest.[3] One was Margaret Kreig's *Green Medicine,* which colourfully pointed out how many drugs in our pharmacies were first discovered by talking to witch-doctors and traditional healers. The other, *Nature's Medicines* by Richard Lucas,[4] reported the history of ginseng, 'the man-root', and included some incredible stories of its healing abilities, proclaiming that it could revive those near death. It also related Lucas's first-hand knowledge of the use of ginseng in Manchuria to cure impotence. This book, in particular, was quoted and misquoted remorselessly. Ginseng, expensive and exotic, appeared on the shelves of all the high street health food shops, and became a household word. Newspapers chattered about ginseng as the source of Chairman Mao's longevity and, as the *Daily Mail* mentioned, 'The secret of Henry Kissinger's bustling energy as he flies on his so far vain peace missions can be revealed – I have traced it down to a Russian potion . . . twenty-four bottles of ginseng. . . . The aromatic elixir has found favour, I hear, with both Henry and Nancy. . . .'

In America ginseng became a vogue and a big export market as the 6000 health food shops there began furiously selling it. Korean exports of cultivated root grew and grew, reaching $70 million in 1978. It was packaged and consumed in many forms from sweets to shampoo. More and more people acknowledged that they used it. At one official gathering in Seoul related to ginseng, I heard a Saudi Arabian dignitary announce to the assembly that he wanted to let everyone know how highly ginseng was regarded. 'Indeed,' he said, 'it is now used in the highest household of the land.'

Firms found themselves in competition to catch hold of a lucrative market. Small specialist herbalists were elbowed out by larger concerns who broadcast their new product as a longevity drug and a panacea in the best soapbox tradition, while sex shops turned it into a sex drug. Advertisers were extreme, leapfrogging over each other to make further claims and retell legends already told. This led to an eventual crackdown by the UK Advertising Standards Authority in a unique recommendation that no claims whatsoever be allowed for ginseng. But there are many ways to sell, and the root that is sacred to the Chinese found itself offered to chemists together with free pandas. Even more strange and disturbing were the stories concerning a Reverend Sun Myng Moon, a Korean millionaire and head of the Unification Church. Questions were asked about this in the Houses of Parliament: 'It was concluded in a most objective study that in many ways the cult was reminiscent of the Ku Klux Klan and of the Cagoule in France. . . . One of the sales gimmicks that my hon. friend will be concerned with . . . is ginseng tea. One Church brochure . . . was investigated by the advertising standards authority . . . it still claims properties which relieve the symptoms of about twenty different maladies.'[5] The United States

Food and Drug Administration followed suit in banning claims, with the result that in 1978 six million Americans bought over two hundred million doses of this substance without any official or commercial information about what it actually does.

Unscrupulous sales of ginseng caused irreparable damage to the reputation of the root. For while in the early days ginseng might have been a curio worth exploring, it then became a touted nostrum which no one in the medical world would wish to be associated with. It nauseated doctors who at best spurned it and at worst scorned it. The attitudes of some colleagues and contacts changed from a healthy scepticism to a rather unhealthy cynicism. I was continually placed in the uncomfortable position of defending ginseng as a possible new medicine while attacking the claims widely made for it.

There was a steady gentle pressure on me to drop my work. Funds were unobtainable. Occasionally there would be real stumbling-blocks. For example, I managed to set up a pilot study, with others, of the effects of ginseng on nurses doing night duty at a London Hospital. However, the chief pharmacist stubbornly refused to make up dummy capsules for the trial when he was told what was being tested. As recently as November 1978, we received from a worried official a letter concerning the same study, which said that '. . . an additional source of anxiety, however, was some recent publicity which seems to associate the use of ginseng tea with certain pseudo-religious cults. . . .'

At the same time there were signs of the growth of a more enlightened interest in Chinese medicine. China opened its doors to Western specialists. Acupuncture, once denigrated as the province of quackery, appeared in London teaching hospitals and is now used in clinics all over America. Pharmacologists went to China and looked for new drugs; the United States National Institute of Health began a succession of exploratory visits to China and medical texts, including the *Barefoot Doctor's Manual*, were translated.

The American Journal of Chinese Medicine began publication, and other journals on acupuncture appeared. Even the normally restrained World Health Organization began a new chapter by performing a *volte face* on traditional medicine and actively seeking to support and encourage the indigenous medical systems of Asia. Of course, the concepts of Chinese medicine were so alien and deep-rooted that it would take a lot more than a few teams of sharp-eyed observers to penetrate through to them. But a psychological barrier was starting to crumble, assisted by the growing numbers of people in the West who were involved with Eastern psychophysiological practices such as yoga and tai ch'i.

Questions took on a new urgency as ginseng and acupuncture became household words without any Western framework to put them in. What was locked up inside the hard material of this strange root? Was it utterly new to Western science or had it turned up before in a different guise? How did it work, and for whom? Was there a whole spectrum of these remedies hidden within the lost kingdom of Taoist and Chinese medicine? Was it possible for Westerners to find and understand them?

Research continued. I took the most ancient and bedraggled mice which still hung on in odd corners of the animal house at my lab. I wanted to see if ginseng affected the health, behaviour and lifespan of this hoary band of rodents. They were tended for months; half of them were fortunate enough (at least I hoped they were fortunate) to get ginseng every day. Then disaster struck. A technician, thinking them so old they were past medical investigation, disposed of the lot! Later I managed to start again at Chelsea College. This time 270 mice were successfully studied in the same way from birth to death. I encouraged others to explore ginseng. It was given to sea creatures in tanks to study their growth, to tissues before bombardment with X-rays, and to rats to study how it worked in the body. I devoted a lot of energy to preparing a large and carefully controlled study with people, which has still not begun. More than that, a pattern, a structure was forming in my mind, concerning the true nature of the root and its meaning to us. In Korea, as I walked through the fields of rich loam, watching acres of ginseng growing, and later under the shadow of Mount Shoji where collectors still hunt for the fabled wild root, I felt the structure had reached a stage of completion and that it could be communicated.

It was necessary to build a house with material which clamoured to be incorporated into a castle. Every item of information, scientific or ethnic, seemed to be claiming something big for itself. The house was built as much by elimination as by construction. When I stood back and saw the result, I was astonished. For the house had indeed become a castle. The simple stones of my ideas concerning certain Chinese medicines had transformed themselves into a much larger conception. It was clear that I was not dealing just with new drugs, however interesting they may be from a therapeutic point of view. It was a whole way of thinking about drugs, about medicine, nature and life itself.

The root has two faces. An Eastern face, familiar and cherished for thousands of years. A Western face, enigmatic and impenetrable. I looked at both faces with a combination of Eastern and scientific points of view. This told me why Eastern medicine can discover and use such remedies, and how Western medicine is bound to miss their possible benefit. As I began to understand the two faces I saw how they could be turned towards each other. Ginseng has the potential ability to bridge the medical systems of East and West. Understanding the faces of ginseng generates a whole range of ideas and practices which are a challenge and a stimulus to our mode of healing.

This instils a sense of importance into the confrontation between the drugs of the East and those of the West. This makes the story one of real concern, not just to a few scientists at tea-time conferences, not even to all those people who are particularly involved with drugs – from the members of the marijuana subculture to the tranquillizer-takers – not even to the millions of people who are currently taking ginseng. The story is relevant to our total understanding of health and our medical system derived from it. It is relevant to all of us, for we are all afflicted by the failures of our body and our medical system. Indeed, it is a matter of urgency. Western medicine has reached a critical point. Progress has ground to a halt in the face of the all-but-incurable diseases of later life such as cancer, heart disease and arthritis. These conditions have reached epidemic proportions in the industrial nations, while the doctor is reduced to fighting a rearguard action with drugs which are relatively poisonous.

In contrast to the prevailing gloomy view of the future of technological therapeutics in the West, Chinese plant medicines give grounds for optimism. Chinese traditional medicine can claim to be one of the most sophisticated medical systems known to man. The Chinese methods of treating the healthy to prevent sickness and of treating the sick to establish their health, and their extraordinary skill in the use of subtle therapeutic techniques are so precisely those needed by us at this time that, whether we like it or not, they must gradually alter the face of medicine in the West.

I invite readers to join me on a journey. We start with an appraisal of our origins, asking first what point there is in the journey, what are the drugs we already have, and what is wrong with them and the medical system which generated them. If we are satisfied that new ideas are necessary, we embark on our trip and explore what China has to offer. We witness the incredible experiment of Chinese traditional medicine, with its centipedes and bat-droppings, attempting to fuse with modern medicine with its X-rays and insulin. Then we continue into ginseng territory and the curious undergrowth of medicinal plants. We start to explore what we have found, to question what these medicines are, what they contain, how they work and how they relate to the drugs which we already know. In order to answer these questions we spread far and wide, making merry in the laboratories of Russia, Japan, Korea, Bulgaria and Western countries.

We then bring our discoveries back on the return journey. What uses can we imagine for these kinds of health tools? Who are they for – the sick, the healthy or even the superhealthy? Finally, we ask if the answers are of real importance to our health and the medical system which looks after it, or if it is all a case of holding a candle in the sunshine. Have we brought back medicines and concepts of a past age or of the new age?

2
Medicine in a Cul-de-sac

THE SYMPTOMS OF OUR TIMES

Why do we need to go on this difficult trek to the land of chameleon medicines? Why do we meet *en route* so many people who have fled the medical system which nurtured them and are seeking all manner of alternatives? After all, modern medicine seems immensely successful. Have not remedies been produced which control or eliminate thousands of diseases and irritations? Less than a century ago one child in five would never survive beyond infancy and many more would experience scarlet fever, diphtheria, poliomyelitis, whooping cough and pneumonia, and festering sores, abscesses and infections. Diseases such as leprosy, bubonic plague, typhus, diphtheria, poliomyelitis, scarlet fever, smallpox, tuberculosis and malaria have been effectively squeezed out of modern industrial society. The average expectation of life in the UK was forty-four years at the beginning of the century, and has now moved up to seventy-one years. For the first time we have a culture in which almost everyone will, barring accidents and suicide, arrive at maturity and beyond. Indeed, man now regards it as his right to live into old age. Do we want to return to the days of the plague?

But when we examine modern medicine dispassionately, the situation does not look so rosy. For one thing, the evidence shows that many diseases, epidemics and infections were almost eliminated before the introduction of modern medicine.[1] Antibiotics were first used just before the Second World War, by which time the expectation of life was already twice that of a century before. The death rate from childhood diseases such as scarlet fever and diphtheria was already a tenth that of the mid-nineteenth century. The victory over

tuberculosis is the oft-quoted example of the progress in
health. In 1812 it was the major city disease, killing 700 out of
every 10,000 people in a place such as New York. But before
antibiotics were used on a regular basis, this figure was down
to 48. 'Cholera, dysentery and typhoid similarly peaked and
dwindled outside the physician's control. . . . During the last
century doctors have affected epidemics no more profoundly
than did priests in earlier times.'[2] Deaths were reduced primarily by '(a) a rising standard of living . . . (responsible mainly
for the decline of tuberculosis and . . . typhus) (b) hygienic
changes, particularly improved water supplies and sewage
disposal . . . (the typhoid and cholera groups) and (c) a
favourable trend in the relationship between infectious agent
and human host. . . . The influence of specific prevention or
treatment of disease in the individual was limited to smallpox
and made little contribution [in the West] to the total reduction
of the death rate.'[3] In poorer countries, where the standard of
living is low, different kinds of infections, digestive complaints and bronchial problems occur more frequently and are
more serious, whatever the quality of the local medical services.

Naturally there are certain areas, such as surgery, treatment
of infections, wounds, accidents, diabetes and many serious
diseases, where our medicine is unexcelled and saves lives
every day. If all doctors went home and became carpenters, a
wave of sickness would certainly affect the modern world.
Minor infections might cause deaths, inflamed appendices
would be lethal and there would be more infant mortality.
Antibiotics have genuine value in diseases such as pneumonia.
Cortisone has undoubtedly helped rheumatics, and many of
the modern drugs are extremely effective in limited fields. But
it must be remembered that these ailments were always
among the easier ones to cure, by traditional methods. It is
probable that most people would live to old age if they had an
adequate standard of living and some help to overcome
injuries and passing infections. We know, for example, that in
the Renaissance the privileged sector lived to a very ripe and
healthy old age.

Modern health care, a runaway monster, is now the largest
industry in the United States, costing some $190 billion which
is an enormous 9 per cent of the Gross National Product.

This is *fifteen times* the cost in 1950, although it supplies only 43 per cent more people.[4] Medical costs are still rising faster than inflation and insurance costs are crippling. Meanwhile, an important study has indicated that neither increasing nor decreasing the expenditure on health will have any further impact on how long we can expect to live.[5]

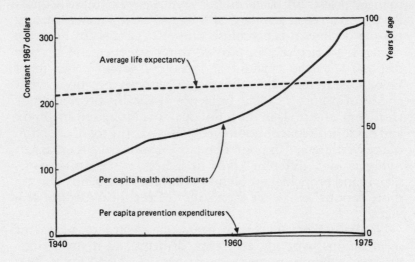

Figure 1   This figure shows how the expectation of life has remained the same despite rocketing costs of health care. The expenditure on disease prevention is minimal. (Redrawn from Gori, M., *Science*, Vol 200, p 1126, (1978).)

Yet despite the massive resources of modern medicine, man is not healthy. Many diseases have been removed but have not been replaced by health. Our modern adult is continually complaining of tiredness, minor virus infections, allergies, chest diseases and a host of minor ailments even before the diseases of later life set in. In one typical industrialized country, Scotland, people are off sick for 10 per cent of the working year by the time they reach middle age. Visits to the doctor approach one per month, and bronchitis, influenza, arthritis and rheumatism, heart disease, back pain, digestive troubles, accidents, neurosis, high blood pressure and alcoholism are common in the adult population.[1] Roughly half the people in England and America take a medically prescribed drug every day. Modern man is 'fat, toothless and constipated', according to the *British Medical Journal*. Is this health?

Meanwhile, what is our medicine doing? It is fiddling with fancy equipment of unproven effectiveness. Is it cranky Luddites who say such things?

Most of the world's medical schools prepare doctors, not to take care of the health of the people, but instead of a medical practice that is blind to anything but disease and the technology for dealing with it; a technology involving astronomical and ever-increasing prices directed towards fewer and fewer people who are often selected not so much by social class or wealth as by medical technology itself, and frequently focused on persons in the final stages of life. . . . The medical empire and its closely related aggressive industry of diagnostic and therapeutic weapons sometimes appears more of a threat than a contribution to health . . . the very attempt to diagnose and treat one ill may produce another, be it through side effects or iatrogenesis. . . .[6]

This is Dr Mahler talking, the Director General of the World Health Organization.

OUR FAVOURITE DISEASES

The real bane of our times are the degenerative chronic diseases. They arise from long-term deteriorations which are occurring continuously in the body, so that by the time we reach maturity our health is noticeably impaired and sooner or later they kill us. These go by the names of cardiovascular disease (diseases of the heart and the blood vessels), cancer, certain renal diseases (kidney diseases), and crippling diseases such as arthritis. These diseases are so common that they have been described as pandemics to rival and exceed any of the special delicacies that existed in plague-ridden history. Circulatory diseases are the single largest cause of death in industrial nations. The heart and blood vessels are the weakest link of modern man. Some 15 per cent of American adults suffer from high blood pressure, and half a million death certificates a year have 'atherosclerosis' written on them. Indeed, most people suppose that just as they have a natural right to old age, the natural way of dying is from degenerative diseases. But this is not so. The diseases existed in earlier times and exist in other cultures but were and are far rarer, even in the very old. Indeed, some primitive cultures look on modern man as peculiarly sick and weak, and cancer and heart attacks as a kind of punishment for his unwise life-style. Cancer is almost unknown in many cultures and when it occurs it is regarded as a terrible and rare visitation. Heart diseases are also unknown in most simple communities and in earlier times were thought to be dangerous only for those given to excesses of rage and passion.

René Dubos, one of the greatest biologists of modern times, has summed up medical surveys of primitive tribes in the last two decades and found these folk to be 'essentially free from dental caries, high blood pressure, cancer and other degenerative diseases so common in civilized, prosperous cultures'. They do of course suffer from infections and epidemics, especially when their established patterns of social life suffer from pressures or upheavals. Man has, by means of public health and social change, ensured his survival to an old age which is laden with degeneration and sickness. Medicine does not understand such diseases at all well. They do not fit into our standard models of disease, and little success has been accomplished in curing them.

The cardiac ambulances, heart pacemakers, digitalis, and the panoply of modern surgery – valve replacement, bypasses, heart transplantation – may seem theatrical lifesavers. But the sirens of the cardiac ambulance in reality signal treatment that is far too late, too elaborate, too insensitive and too ineffective. A relaxed rest cure may be as effective after a heart attack as the stresses of high technology healing.[7] 'The slight decline in heart disease mortality rates which began in 1968 may be due at least in part to changes in adult smoking habits and other primary prevention developments rather than to increased spending on medical care.'[4]

The same goes for cancer. Every day we read of the successful war against malignancy. A child with leukaemia used to be given six months to live but now nearly all cases live for longer. Ninety-five per cent of patients with early skin cancer survive five years after surgery. But lucky a man will be if it is one of those cancers which affect him, for the cancers which have been successfully treated are the rare ones. Survival rates for 90 per cent of cases of cancer have not changed substantially in twenty-five years. In fact, if the figures are probed with great care, much of our vaunted progress disappears. For example despite the success of therapy for some forms of leukaemia, the disease itself is becoming more fatal so that the net result is no change. The best analysis of the change in the chances of long-term survival for *all cancers put together* since 1950 is very· clear: zero.[8] Meanwhile, 'doctors involved in treating cancer too often employ Draconian techniques. They poison their patients with drugs and rays, and mutilate them with the scalpel, in a desperate attempt to treat the untreatable'.[9]

HOMO LIBRIUM

Drugs are medicine in action. If we now focus on drugs to see whether the problems that have arisen with our medicine are reflected in our drugs, a hauntingly similar pattern emerges. After a time of great progress, of considerable excitement and speedy discoveries, of successful new miracle cures and wonder drugs, has come the crunch. The drugs we now use have been found to be generally harmful and in many cases of questionable benefit. There are tens of thousands of different drugs on the market now, such a confusing plethora that the World Health Organization recently prepared a model list of essential drugs for Third World countries, and found that only 2 per cent of the total of drugs sold were really necessary. 'There has been a tremendous increase in the number of pharmaceutical products marketed,' complains the World Health Organization; 'however there has not been a proportionate improvement in health.'[10] A recent Wall Street survey showed that less than 1 per cent of the drugs which were currently on trial promised important therapeutic gains.[11] Even the new therapeutic advances are often so specialized that they leave the health of the majority of people untouched. Instead of concentrating on the discovery of useful new drugs, companies spend an excessive amount of their resources on a gross and aggressive promotion, trying to carve out bigger slices of established markets. The doctors seem befuddled by ever more pressure. 'Doctors are pushed around and bullied and bribed by the drug industry. They have undoubtedly lost

control of their own profession and must consequently be held
responsible for all the disasters and errors which bad prescrib-
ing produces.'[12]

This frantic flea-market of unnecessary drugs is a sequel to a
more subtle problem. It is becoming much more difficult and
expensive to find new drugs. It now costs some $50 million to
develop a new drug and more to manufacture and sell it. Only
twenty-five companies around the world can afford this type
of investment, and the expense is squeezing drug companies
into a land of diminishing returns. One reason for this is that
health authorities are exerting much more stringent controls
on safety and effectiveness. More science needs to be presented
before a drug can be licensed. One company mentioned that it
presented 300 volumes of evidence on a single drug to the
authorities of a single country. This is the drug companies'
own fault, to some extent, for they have consistently sold
medicines which have later proved harmful. So tight controls
are an inevitable sequel. Another important reason for the
decline in new drugs is scientific exhaustion. More and more
effort is being directed towards fewer and fewer ideas. The
pace of invention is slowing down. Where is the next generation of drugs to come from?

The problem is made much more acute by the innate
harmfulness of many modern drugs. The extent to which the
health of man is compromised by drugs is never fully appreciated. The care of patients suffering from the harmful effect of
drugs is now put at around 3000 million dollars annually in the
United States alone. One study calculated that some 15 per
cent of old people are admitted to hospital as a direct result of
the consumption of drugs. We hear of the most dramatic cases
such as thalidomide, the sleeping pill which caused foetal
deformities. But this is the tip of the iceberg. Depression, for
example, is a form of drug side-effect that is produced by
almost every kind of drug known. Yet it is ignored by doctors
and tolerated by the patients themselves, or countered by
other drugs which have alternative side-effects. Many people
are resigned to drug side-effects as a necessary part of the
treatment. The people who take drugs against high blood
pressure put up with impotence and lethargy because they feel
they have no choice.

Salicylic acid was one of the first pure chemicals to be

isolated and taken medicinally. Now acetyl salicylic acid, or aspirin, is the most widely used drug in the world. Fifteen thousand million tablets were consumed in 1976 in the United States. Yet evidence is only now emerging of gastric damage and possible infertility as a result of aspirin use. Pregnant women taking aspirin may have smaller babies, more complications and stillbirths, and their babies' health may be affected.[13] In many cases, drug side-effects only appear after years of use and what was once an ultra-safe drug turns into a gradually damaging one.

Although man has always used psychotropic drugs, the practice is taking a nasty turn. There is a tendency to make a helpless pilgrim's progress through life which starts at the age of twenty or thirty with stimulants, continues at forty or fifty with tranquillizers, moves pitifully into the sixties with pain-killers and mindlessly into the seventies with incurable dementia, in which state man then presents himself to his maker.

When 15 per cent of the population of Europe takes tranquillizers, the true end-point of modern drug use seems to be a human race as dependent upon drugs as it is upon the vitamins our bodies need.

If we look at medical progress during this century, we see heady growth followed by retrenchment and disenchantment. Our medicine is now giving diminishing returns, running faster and faster and eating up more and more of our resources just to stand still. The life-span has not increased in recent years. The degenerative diseases sound the death knell of our current approach to medicine and health. The attempt to cure them imposes such an intolerable burden on society, provides so little benefit to the people who need treatment, and causes so much extra pain and degradation to them in the process, that our society can no longer put up with it. Medicine has after years of great success at last run itself into a cul-de-sac.

How did this happen? Where did it lose its way?

HOMO EQUILIBRIUM

In order to understand our current predicament, we need to go right back to the beginning. The roots of medicine in the West go deep into Egyptian and Greek culture. Medical prescriptions 6000 years old have been found in Egypt. One papyrus, the Ebers papyrus, contained 700 medicines, many of which we are familiar with today. Aesculapius, the son of Apollo, is the legendary father of Greek medicine. Medicine was practised in Aesculapian temples where priests diagnosed, massaged, mixed medicine and offered musical and spiritual assistance to the body and mind. The ascetic Pythagorean brotherhood introduced certain fundamental concepts into Greek medicine. The most important was the doctrine of *physiological harmony*. The body was regarded as undifferentiated from the environment, and there was a flux between them. The body, like the rest of the universe, was composed of fundamental elements described metaphorically as earth, air, fire and water, together with affinities between these elements. Disease arose, according to Alcmaeon, from a preponderance of one or other of the fiery (hot), watery (fluid), earthy (solid) or airy (diffuse) elements. Medicines possessed within them corrective powers to make adjustments to the internal balance. Some might restore the fire or the dryness to the body, others drain the moisture.

This is a fundamental world view. The elements permeate other ancient cultures, such as the Chinese or Indian:

> Earth, my own mother; father Air; and Fire
> My friend; and Water, well-beloved cousin;
> And Ether, brother mine: to all of you this
> Is my last farewell. I give you thanks
> For all the benefits you have conferred
> During my stay with you.[14]

The four elements were later taken up by Aristotle, and through him transmitted to Europe where they were a central dogma in life and medicine until the Renaissance. Even after that time the doctrine of equilibrium between elements lived on, although fire, earth, air and water were abandoned as its constituents. These elements are now regarded askance by science. They are thought to be the epitome of arcane rubbish. It is commonly held today that it was the doctrine of the four elements which led European culture into the pit and blocked real progress for many centuries.

It is, of course, very hard to see the elements as a useful way of looking at the world. How can such a primitive, mystical conception as the four elements generate any kind of basis for

action, let alone a healing system? If we take it seriously are we
not undoing the tightly rolled skein of progress and landing
ourselves back in the Dark Ages?

Yet if we approach the concept with an open mind we
should first of all ask what a modern scientist would use to
replace earth, fire, air and water as basic qualities of the
universe. For example, if we asked a biochemist what muscle
is composed of, he would answer that it contained substances
like actin, creatinine, enzymes, nucleic acids and so on. But he
would at the same time admit that these words are actually
codes or ciphers to describe particular kinds of molecular
structures. Each type of molecule is detected by its qualities
such as mass, energy, electrostatic charge, cohesiveness and so
on. These are the properties which in the end distinguish
'stone' from 'muscle'.

The four elements are also metaphors to describe qualities of
the world and, surprisingly, these qualities are almost identical
to those used by the modern physicist. The Buddhists, for
example, maintain that earth means the quality of mass or
solidity, air means motion, fire means energy and water means
the binding quality. They all move in space, or ether, sometimes called the fifth element. They are not useless mumbo-
jumbo, but a primitive kind of symbolism with which to deal
with the world, a poetry which is the distant ancestor of the
equations of the modern physicist.

The symbols are tools. If an ancient Greek or Indian practitioner determines that an organ is too 'earthy', he may be
saying that it is too dense and compact for its own good. He
was able to use this language to describe the way the body
reacted to the elements outside itself; the heat of the season
generated 'heat' diseases, heavy foods generated 'solid' diseases. The physician applied these terms to help him understand the causes of disease and the right methods for healing.

The four elements are important for our purpose since they
are typical of a philosophy which produced healing systems
utterly different from our own, yet which were its precursors.
The core of these systems was that health was automatic
provided man, an aggregate of elements, maintained an
equilibrium with nature, which consisted of all the other
aggregates of the same elements.

Have we lost something vital in uprooting ourselves so

violently from these origins? Let us continue through history with this question in mind.

Hippocrates, to whom lip-service is paid as the father of Western medicine, criticized the Pythagorean four elements as insufficient: 'Did he who turned wheat into bread remove from it the hot, cold, dry or moist?' Instead he introduced the concept of 'humours' or fluid qualities of the body which again needed to be in equilibrium – 'crasis' – for proper health. Every person had a natural dominance of certain humours constituting his individuality. Disease arose when the humours were pushed or strayed out of phase with a person's natural dispensation. In so far as the body was the cause of its own diseases, it could also heal itself by an inner restorative process, the *vis medicatrix naturae*. Hippocrates always attempted to encourage self-healing by designing a health regimen for a diseased person involving diet, exercise, relaxation and other methods. These were supplemented by various drugs which were administered in order to correct those imbalances in the bodily secretions which produced the weakness and susceptibility to disease.

With the appearance of a conglomerate Greek empire under Alexander, intellectual and medical life developed towards specialization and analysis. Medicine became orientated towards pathology and anatomy, with a decidedly mechanical bent. The body was seen as a plumbing system, with nerve, blood and air (more accurately the pneuma, the breath of life) circulating around the body. The circulation was balanced in health and upset in disease. However, this theory did not generate effective medicines, and it was soon overturned by an empirical school which said, bluntly, that for every disease there are symptons and for every symptom there is a cure: 'Diseases are cured, not by argument but by medicines.'[15]

These theories are the bones of Western medicine. One aggressive physician put sufficient flesh on these bones to ensure their survival for two millennia. This man was Galen, born in Pergamum in AD 130, the son of Nicon the engineer. In his fiery mission to bring reason, logos, to bear upon medicine he threw out the concept that disease arose either from God or from poor plumbing, and restored the importance of the humours and the Hippocratic physis as a life force. The life force manifested itself in the organism as various powers such as ingestion, expulsion and so on. These balanced the humours, which Galen also saw as the arbiters of internal equilibrium, much as we see hormones functioning in today's physiology. Drugs could restore the inner balance by regulating those self-same body powers. This would, according to the Galenic system, restore the physis and the body would then throw off disease by itself. Galen prepared many effective plant drugs and made the first attempts at standardization of doses and of botanical sources. The systems of Galen and Dioscorides, a compiler of plant medicines, together with a smattering of Hippocratic naturalism, were the legacy of Greek medicine. This was preserved in a circuitous manner by the Arabs, spiced by the return of some occult law. However, the early Middle Ages appear to be a low point in medical finesse. Medical remedies, many of which were grown in monastery herb gardens, were combined with much sorcery and mumbo-jumbo: 'Against dysentery: a bramble of which both ends are in the earth, take the nether root, delve it up, cut nine chips with the left hand and sing three times the Miserere Mei Deus and nine times the Pater Noster . . . boil in milk. . . .' Much of the theory was derived from Galen 1500 years before, but was distorted and ossified. The four elements lost their symbolic value. New principles appeared, including the infamous Doctrine of Signatures. Formally advanced by Paracelsus, this states that divine design had made physical resemblances between a medicinal plant and the disease or organ that the plant could cure.

THE RISE OF SCIENTIFIC MEDICINE

Actually Paracelsus has a greater importance for current therapeutics than as the elaborator of cosmic doctrines. He was the first to combine medicine with chemistry. As an alchemist his method was the purification of the impure. If compounds could be purified in the crucibles of the laboratory, then perhaps disease was also an impure state and could be cleaned up by the action of purified substances, namely chemicals prepared in his alchemical furnaces. He rejected the four humours and the plant concoctions of Galen, introducing instead poisons as medicines, compounds made of antimony, lead and mercury.

Against the background of the Renaissance, the Paracelsan school fought hard for scientific or chemical medicine. But they were regarded as unorthodox and heretical, and did not get very far. The medical establishment was universally Galenicist and hounded the chemists as poisoners; the chemists fought back by describing the Galenicists as purveyors of 'filth, spittle, urine, flyes and the ashes of an owles head'. However, gradually there came the recognition that chemicals did sometimes work, and efforts were made to control rather than attack the chemists. The next three centuries saw more and more specific drugs introduced by the chemists.

The transformation to modern therapeutics occurred gradually during the course of the nineteenth century. In the early years, the doctors and their patients shared a common system of medicine and health still recognizably based on Galen and Hippocrates. The life-style and diet of a person, the seasons and climate, interacted continually with the organism to prop up or undermine health. Equilibrium was synonymous with health and a distortion of the processes of flow of materials through the body was an invitation to disease. 'The body could be seen as a kind of stew pot, or chemico-vital reaction, proceeding calmly only if all its elements remained appropriately balanced.'[16] The physician regulated the secretions, giving drugs, extracting blood and influencing perspiration and urination, in order to restore equilibrium according to well established theories. However, these theorists were being pressurized by a more aggressive empiricism. New substances were continually being isolated and proving immensely effective without any theoretical basis at all. Quinine did cause fevers to plummet, morphine did kill pain; strychnine, brucine, atropine, codein, picrotoxine and other compounds isolated from the old vegetable drugs could be seen to work. They were strong. A spoonful of crystals had such a massively amplified effect that it placed traditional doctors in the shadows, mouthing their Galenic principles to a fast disappearing audience.

Scientific medicine also gathered strength from the permission of the Church to study and dissect the body (provided the soul was left to the scalpels of the clergy), from the artifice of the chemists, and from the materialistic quantitative mode of thought of industrial man. It became a body of knowledge, with principles akin to those of the Empiricists of ancient

Greece. Each disease arose from a specific cause, and was a discrete entity that could be cured by drugs which were applied only to that pathological condition. It was not necessary to cure the patient, but the disease itself must be the focus of medical attention with the patient as a kind of inert carrier of his condition. The doctor was not interested in equilibrium. He was at war. Medicines were discovered by observation and experiment, and they had to be tested in an objective manner to ascertain if they actually worked. The centre of therapeutics became the laboratory, with assessment based on weight of numbers, not weight of impressions. The science of drugs, called pharmacology, arose because the effective new drugs needed to be understood. The equation, 'specific disease + corrective chemical = normality', was amenable to experimental analysis, even if all the terms in the equation had to be simplified in the process.

Scientific medicine horrified its critics because of its apparent lack of system. 'Out of the false pride of the laboratory . . . has arisen the worst evil of therapeutic nihilism.'[16] But as the years went by, humours, secretions, vital energy, internal balance left medical jargon, never to return. They could only be found in ancient books, old herbalists' manuals and the archaic language of a few senile European physicians. The nihilistic therapeutics became a rational system in its own right. Whereas in the middle of the nineteenth century those who proclaimed that specific drugs existed to cure specific diseases were called quacks, a century later it was the traditionalists who were the quacks. Whereas in the seventeenth century the chemists were persecuted by the Galenicists because of their poisonous distillations, it is now the herbalists who are persecuted by the chemists. And while in the mid-nineteenth century the new scientific medicine was thought irrational and irresponsible, so in the mid-twentieth century science regards the few traditionalists as irrational and romantic ostriches in a world of successful progress.

THE SEE-SAW

Scientific medicine has arrived at an invidious position. It now imagines that it is the only medical system in existence. Modern medical principles have turned from a theory to a dogma, and those who wonder what has been left behind are branded as heretics. Galen has been forgotten. Hippocrates is, apart from his oath, utterly abandoned, like the Red Queen's Cheshire cat that vanished apart from its grin. A modern pharmacology text states, 'thus emanating from a background of mystery and magic, from folklore and empiricism, the medical science pharmacology emerged coincidentally with the turn of the century'. We can now see how erroneous and insular is this view. It is designed only to bolster the illusion of progress. What actually happened was the opposite. Modern medicine itself was founded on pure empiricism and it arrived as the latest in a succession of medical (not magical) systems going back a very long time. It is the latest, and presumably not the last. Each system makes assumptions as to the nature of health and disease, according to the world view of the society and epoch to which it belongs.

Reviewing all these systems, we find two opposing ways of thinking. On the one hand we have a more naturalistic medicine in which the concept of harmony is most important. Diseases arise through imbalances, health through equilibrium, and medicine and its drugs are essentially adjustive and restorative. On the other side is the reductionist view that disease is a specific physical spanner in the works, arising from a certain cause and curable by attacking the origin of the disease. It *replaces harmony by specificity*. These two views have been see-sawing their way through history. In the Greek period the see-saw rocked violently as Empiricists contended with Hippocratics. In the seventeenth and eighteenth centuries the struggle was refought as the chemists contended with the Galenicists, and in the nineteenth the see-saw began to fall towards the specificity side as scientific medicine overcame the humoralist school. Now the see-saw is so firmly grounded on that side that the harmony end does not appear to exist. This is what we have lost. Can we trace our current impasse back to this lopsidedness? Is it not time to rock the see-saw back a little?

SACRIFICING LONG-TERM HEALTH FOR SHORT-TERM SURVIVAL

How is it that the loss of these fundamental principles has had such disastrous consequences? One reason is that it has deprived us of an adequate understanding of the meaning of 'health'.

Are you sick or are you healthy? How difficult it is to give an honest answer. As difficult as the answer to the question – are you happy? For it is our personal experience that there is no such thing as health or sickness but a spectrum of states, ranging from very fit to fit to healthy to a bit off colour to partly sick to sick and so on. Historically the Greek, Arab and Renaissance physicians recognized this and argued only over how many stages there actually were between the extremes. Medicine has now lost interest in states of health, retaining only a rough series of adjectives for states of illness, such as 'minor', 'recovering' and 'critical'. A man may be affected by subtle damage brewing inside him – a cancer or clogged arteries – and still be called healthy. He may be decrepit, debilitated, lethargic, incapable, doped, with chronic aches, irritations, infections and itches; he would still be classed as 'not ill' by his doctor. As Professor Chapman notes, 'There hardly exists a vocabulary, other than in the humanities, to deal with ideas of health.'[17]

What makes this serious is that the major Western afflictions are all the result of subtle and insidiously accumulated ill-health which only reveals itself to the man or his doctor when it is too late to do anything about it. While Western medicine can provide many cures for obvious disease, it is incompetent in dealing with these states of chronic sub-health. This is the practical consequence of defining health as the absence of sickness, producing . . . *absence of illness but not presence of health*. Therefore the first step is to revise our attitude to health, to add more subtle concepts of health to the already advanced concepts of disease.

With this in mind, we might consider as a useful minimal definition of health that put forward by the World Health Organization: 'Health is a state of complete mental, physical and social wellbeing and not merely the absence of disease.' However, you cannot call a man healthy unless he is capable of fulfilling some of the potential of Homo sapiens. Therefore one could improve the definition by adding something about capacity. One could improve it even more by adding something about longevity. For health is substantial if it can lead to resistance to the greatest pathogen of them all: *time*.

Excellent! We now have a wonderful utopian definition of health which is no more effective than a shout in a gale. Doctors have been quick to point out the irrelevance of the WHO definition. No one can use it since it does not fit into the 'specificity' framework, the working philosophy of Western medicine, which buys immediate survival at the cost of long-term health.

This also undermines the current efforts at disease prevention. Most experts recognize that the most important modern chronic diseases are caused largely by environment and life-style. This has led a vociferous group of health and community medicine workers to put forward programmes of preventative measures as solutions to the ills of modern man. They propose more instruction on diet, cigarette smoking, blood pressure and physical fitness. People would be tested for risk factors at regular intervals and legislation introduced to reduce environmental contamination and improve foods. Health maintenance organizations would be set up and the population would also be continuously screened to detect diseases early. These health care efforts would go side by side with improvements in clinical medicine and each would be given a more appropriate slice of the cake.[4]

Such measures are steps in the right direction, but the whole problem will then only be postponed for some time until the health burden builds up again to the same levels. They do not get to the root of the problem. Prevention is essential, but it must be tied to a more enlightened view of health, otherwise preventive measures will be like trying to dam a river with sand. Cancer, heart and circulatory diseases are primarily a long slow drift from harmony in the workings of the body, aided and abetted by environmental stresses. The details are not at all understood at present. Despite the application of colossal resources to the problem, it is only possible to state that the causes are so subtle and diverse that none of the programmes currently recommended will make more than a minor dent in the mortality data. To stop smoking and reduce consumption of cholesterol will only, so to speak, cream off the top of the chronic disease figures, but not bring them down to the level of simple agricultural communities. It will extend the life-span, but only a little. It will relieve the health services, a little. It will improve the health of those surviving to old age, a little. If we want to achieve very much more than that, the subtle development of the degenerative diseases needs to be dealt with by subtle measures, and these are only to be found way outside our present paradigm.

THE DRUGS WE GET ARE THE DRUGS WE DESERVE

The problems with modern drugs are also an inevitable result of the way our culture thinks about the nature of health and disease. For this determines the way drugs are discovered, tested and selected. Let us look at how modern drugs reach us and we will get some idea of how our outmoded biomedical model manifests in practice.

In 1932 Hildegarde Domagle pricked her finger with a knitting needle. She developed septicaemia and would have succumbed but for the good fortune of having a father who worked for a German chemical company. He gave his daughter one of his company's red dyes called Prontisol and his daughter recovered. The dye was found to contain sulphanilamide. This was the first of the antibiotics and soon a multitude more were developed by industry. Many new drugs were found in this way. Often they were found by chemists who sought new uses for ranges of chemicals which they had made for other purposes. This was particularly true of dyestuffs. The biggest drug companies in the world, Ciba, Geigy, Hoffman-La Roche and Sandoz, started to make dyes for the Swiss textile industry and then turned to drugs. Laboratory research has produced other drugs, such as Fleming's discovery of penicillin through the accidental contamination of a bacterial culture with spores of the bread mould. Another source of material is still, though more rarely, the plant and animal kingdom. Plants may be selected because of their use in traditional medicine or because it is known that certain classes of plants make certain kinds of chemicals. Famous twentieth-century examples are ephedrine, derived from a Chinese medicinal plant, which revolutionized the treatment of bronchial complaints, and reserpine, which revolutionized the treatment of mental illness and comes from a plant used in India for thousands of years against insanity.

A compound which is known to be effective is analysed

chemically and a range of slightly different derivatives is made. This produces families of remedies with connected but different pharmacological actions. Many new drugs such as antibiotics and anaesthetics are produced in this way. It is usually the case that the mother compound of this family is discovered from natural sources or by lucky strikes in the lab. It is also common that scientists pull drugs out of the top hat of biochemical theory. When it is felt that a certain chemical might produce an effect on a known biochemical reaction, chemists are directed to go out and make the key that fits the lock.

Whatever kind of substances are discovered, they must go through a number of screens or filters to weed out the harmful or ineffective remedies. They will be tested in the laboratory to see whether they have an effect first in the test-tube, then on animals, such as mice, rabbits or guinea pigs. For example, a new stimulant will be tested on groups of mice to see if it reduces their sleeping time, behaviour, ability to learn, metabolism and so on. Tests will also be carried out on the way a drug is absorbed and excreted, on whether it is converted to something else, and what proportion goes where. In the case of our stimulant, particular attention would be paid to the brain to see how much of it ended up there, and which sections of the brain were affected. Of 5000 chemicals at the start, perhaps only half a dozen will pass all the tests. These are given to human volunteers to try, and perhaps only one will be left as safe and marketable. This is submitted to the health authorities and permission is requested to carry out a study of the effects of the drug on patients, the clinical trial.

The clinical trial judges the effect of the drug on people in a controlled situation, and compares its effect to that of a completely inert substance that appears the same. Why is an inert pill used? Because of the well-known psychological effect of drugs, the so-called placebo effect. An individual's expectations and attitudes can supersede the effects of a drug. Someone taking a completely inert pill may have all sorts of drug effects, while someone taking a drug may have none and can be convinced that it was useless. For example, dummy pills, or *placebos,* can change states of mind, such as anxiety, and might even assist in diseases such as asthma, coughing, diabetes, angina, seasickness or arthritis.[18] The clinical trial is intended to sort out the real from such imagined effects of a drug.

If a drug gets through the clinical trial and is shown to be safe and effective, a licence is applied for. The licensing authorities will normally review all the evidence, including the trials, and if they give the green light, the manufacturer can go ahead and make the drug, market it and sell it. The whole process from discovery to the doctor's prescription pad sounds, on the surface, a sensible and reasonable scheme for discovering effective new drugs and getting them to people.

But a major weakness of this system is the type of sieve used to weed the effective drugs from the ineffective, which mostly takes the form of giving drugs to diseased animals to detect any favourable changes. This ensures absolutely that drugs which are strong will be preferred to those that are mild, since they will show up more dramatically in the tests. It also means that drugs which might be taken by people to improve their health and protect themselves against sickness will be severely discriminated against in favour of those which offer instant cure of a specific disease state.

The use of particular animal models of disease as a tool greatly restricts the possibilities open to us for the detection of new drugs. The pace of drug discovery is slowed down to the pace of discovery of new testing situations. A classic pharmacology textbook states it well: 'Once a pharmacologic model has been established for a class of drugs, it is relatively easy to discover new agents that resemble the old, but the discovery of completely novel approaches to treatment is unlikely . . . a truly different type of antianxiety drug probably would not have passed the usual preclinical screening tests.'

The enormous cost of trials also restricts the potential new drugs. So few drugs can be tested in this way that pharmacologists will only risk trying drugs that have a dramatic effect on animals. Gentle remedies are again excluded. The clinical trial itself can be a further blockage to the discovery of radically new drugs. The trial is only designed to ask certain questions, and is also unable to deal with the unexpected. If a pharmacologist decided that the fictional pleasure drug 'soma' of Aldous Huxley's *Brave New World* had promise as a new tranquillizer, he might set up a clinical trial to see if it reduced anxiety. If some people stated that they felt dreamy and erotic this would be marked down as a side-effect, and the true importance of the drug would be missed.

By the same token, the clinical trial has only limited ability to detect side-effects. It is not possible nor even ethical to test drugs in every conceivable circumstance. For example, the side-effect of impotence is unlikely to be noticed in a clinical trial of a new drug with hospital patients. Drugs are rarely tested on the aged or on children, nor can they be tested on pregnant women. Yet subsequently drugs will be taken by all these people.

A fundamental principle of the clinical trial is that a drug can only be seen to work if the person involved doesn't know whether he has taken the drug or not. But in daily life people usually know that they are being treated and this knowledge is often an important part of the therapy. The attempt to neutralize the psychological component in healing through the clinical trial will also eliminate any remedies which may benefit man through the effect of the mind on the body. Any psychosomatic remedies will be turned down as worthless by the clinical trial. It is not as if there are no alternatives to testing drugs under blind conditions. For example, groups of patients can be made aware of what they are taking but given different test doses. Or the doctors testing may be highly trained to notice changes and use patients who themselves are competent in this regard.

Just as the nineteenth-century critics had predicted, the indiscriminate demand for controlled trials has stripped us of whole classes of drugs which fall through the holes in the testing sieve but which have nevertheless not been shown to be ineffective. One clear example is plant remedies. The pharmacopoeia has been systematically weeded of plant preparations and traditional over-the-counter remedies. On what grounds? 'Many of the plants used as medicines can no longer be considered within the pale of rational therapeutics,' explains a textbook.[19] The words are chosen carefully. The older medicines have not been eliminated on the grounds of uselessness, only on the grounds that they don't fit into the system.

It is not only the principles of testing which have thrown out multitudes of safe traditional medicaments. It is also the rise of pharmacology as a branch of chemistry. The chemists contributed to the disregard for plants since they couldn't find any definable active principles in many of them. However, their chemical analyses were, at the time, so crude that they were bound to miss out the active principles in all plants except those which happen to be saturated with some compound. The plants have never come back. The modern paradigm needs to know exactly what a drug consists of in chemical terms. The purpose of this knowledge is to decide accurately on the therapeutic quantities for each disease state. However, this may be a minor gain when balanced by the cost, the increased toxicity, the increased strength leading to overmedication and the increase in intrinsic harmfulness. The baby has been thrown out with the bathwater.

Our drugs do not obey the Hippocratic commandment to 'heal pleasantly and safely', and it is the established methods of finding and using such drugs which are to blame. The greatest tragedy of modern therapeutics is that the models used to detect drugs, and the clinical trials employed to test them, are designed to miss those drugs which have subtle and health-giving properties, and favour the toxic sledgehammer drugs. The new drugs which are so badly needed to cope with the chronic illnesses of today continue to elude us, for the methods of searching are bound to miss them. All these problems derive directly from our way of regarding healing in the scientific mode – as a process of ridding the body of intruding specific disease entities. The drugs are only a product of the philosophy of healing. This in turn is derived from the cultural milieu. It can thus be fairly said that we get the drugs which we deserve.

OVER THE EASTERN WALL

We have been immensely successful in medical progress this century. But something endemic to our approach has made the victory bitter. We have run headlong down the alley of 'specificity', and found ourselves stopped in our tracks by a pandemic of subtle degenerative diseases. The origin of these diseases lies in loss of internal equilibrium and it is the 'harmony' track which we must follow to deal with them.

What is it we are looking for that might help us solve these problems? First, a philosophy which will tell us more about inner balance, disease resistance and vitality. Secondly, a new practical science on how to maintain genuine health and human capacity for as many years as possible. Thirdly, some new tools with which to do it. This means a fusion of ideas on the one hand, and medicines on the other; a marriage of traditional means to maximize health with modern means to minimize disease.

It is, however, hard to grope our way outside our own assumptions. A clear precedent will be of enormous assistance. What is this precedent to be? Are we to go back to the Greeks? To start learning the four elements in our medical schools? Certainly not. However, there are living medical systems which have a knowledge that has not, as in the West, been disintegrated by time. Perhaps the most sophisticated of them all is traditional Chinese medicine. The ideas which we need now have been in daily use in China for 5000 years. The traditional Chinese physician deals with phenomena which dangle elusively beyond our own biomedical consciousness. The maintenance of internal harmony and energy is the special forte of the traditional Chinese doctor. An intriguing experiment is under way in China, not only to preserve the methods of traditional medicine, but to fuse them with modern medicine. Nowhere else in the world has traditional medicine and modern medicine met without a head-on clash in which the former is severely reduced. The results are of considerable importance to us. Perhaps, too, we can find examples of new subtle medicines in China which we can use to overcome our current therapeutic impasse. It seems to me that having raced forward into the cul-de-sac, we need to scale the Eastern wall.

3
The Chinese Alternative

THE ENIGMA

Liang Li-ying, the agricultural worker, fled from the field. He could no longer walk amid the early budding vegetables. He had piles which irritated and disturbed him more every day and now drove him painfully to the health station of his production brigade. There he was seen by two young *chijiao yisheng*, rural health workers. He knew them well.

'What brings you so early from the fields, comrade Liang?' asked little comrade Li.

'Oh, I feel almost guilty to tell you, it seems so unnecessary for a man of my strength. I have painful inflammations.'

'We have a good preparation for that,' she said, and gave him a bottle of dark liquid. 'We made it ourselves last week. It contains hei mu-erh, pei-mu and k'u-shen.'[1]

'What muck is in here?' he asked, 'Haven't you got a pill?'

'Comrade, you forget the value of our traditional remedies. We must always be guided by Chairman Mao's teaching: "Chinese medicine and pharmacology are a great treasure house, and efforts should be made to explore them and raise them to a higher level." We do have some pills for your problem, but we know that they will only help you to live with it for a short time, and soon you will be back here again. Now where is your revolutionary spirit?'

Liang looked even more miserable after this rap over the knuckles from the sprightly young girl in a white coat.

'Anyway,' she continued, 'there may be a much better remedy than this mixture. Go to the commune hospital tomorrow.'

The next day Liang arrived at the hospital. He talked to the health worker at the entrance, who recognized that his condition was one of those for which modern medicine is not so effective. She directed him to a traditional doctor.

The doctor greeted him with a nod, and asked him to relax.

'I am going to try a remedy recently introduced from Hunan. It is based on traditional ideas. Now let me have a look.'

Liang knelt on a bed with his head on a pillow. The doctor brought down a bright light close to Liang's back until he felt its warmth. The doctor searched long and carefully.

'The best doctor is one who is extremely careful,' he said, 'so it may take some time.' Sensing Liang's tension, he continued, 'And the best patient is one who does not have resistance to the treatment. I quote the Yellow Emperor.'

The doctor searched below and to the side of the seventh thoracic vertebra. He eventually gave a small cry.

'Ha! Here it is.'

'What?' asked Liang.

'The haemorrhoid point. It is a tiny red spot protruding just above the skin. A bit difficult to find among the freckles and marks. I think I can see more than one on your back.'

The doctor set to work. He sterilized the skin and using a fine needle pricked at the little spot. He probed deeper until he found some fine glistening fibres. These he broke with the needle. Then he painted the spot with gentian and put on a plaster. Liang felt a little discomfort and strange travelling sensations near his backside. But shortly afterwards the pain went and the piles too slowly disappeared.

This is happening in China today. But to the Western doctor the whole scenario is crazy. What kind of fibres exist under the skin which can have an effect on another part of the body? Have the Chinese, with their strange ways, magicked up new anatomical tissues that all the electron microscopes of the West have missed?

There are a host of other riddles to stump the Western doctor. What is he to make of the universal practice of moxibustion, the burning of little cones of rolled mugwort leaves placed at critical points of the body? What about all the strange remedies: bat-droppings and scorpions for convulsions in children, frogs baked in mud against cancer, tortoise shells and seahorse tails for virility, or a belt braided of daphnia and clematis roots worn on the skin against backache? What about the well-known story that Peking Man was discovered because skeletons were being dug up and their teeth used as medicines? These remedies are by no means obscure peasant concoctions but are present in the official handbook of the Chinese rural health workers, and are administered in modern hospitals specializing in traditional remedies. Indeed, doctors and scientists from the big cities are avidly gathering more of such remedies from the Chinese hinterland.

Until ten years ago, the People's Republic of China was a black hole on the world map. The West was dimly aware of ferment behind impenetrable barriers. Chinese traditional medicine could be ignored or dismissed as quackery or self-hypnosis backed up by an obscure complex of irrelevant philosophies.

But times have changed. We have been allowed to peep through the bamboo curtain and watch the theatre of Chinese daily life. We have been permitted to witness the unparalleled renaissance of Chinese traditional medicine which has been recognized and incorporated into a sophisticated state-wide medical system. Since Western medicine is also used in China, there is the extraordinary spectacle of 'toasted frog' remedies used alongside modern medical equipment and drug cabinets stacked with familiar Western tablets. No one can be quite sure any more that it is all useless. Now that acupuncture is practised in American teaching hospitals, total scepticism has been slowly giving way. In its place has grown total confusion. Chinese medicine seems to have a logic behind it somewhere, but beyond the ken of most Westerners.

Before we search for possible new ideas and special remedies, we need to dispel some of this mystery, otherwise their is no hope of detecting their possible value. Let us start with the genesis of this system.

THE ANCESTRY

Imagine the China of about 5000 years ago, a huge land mass occupied by scattered primitive independent kingdoms. The people were farmers, hunters, craftsmen, soldiers, who owed allegiance to a patriarchal royalty. Their medicine was in the hands of primitive healers, but their health in the lap of the gods. Their inner diseases were the result of manifestations of the spirits and were not, it seems, permitted regions for the healers. These diseases were fought solely with prayer, incantation and ritual. The outer diseases, more obvious on the body frame, were treated by herbs or with probing stone implements. There are inscriptions of the names of diseases of the eyes, ears, nose, mouth, teeth and skin, on oracle bones excavated from that period. The healers knew the art of mending broken bones, and of treating injuries and wounds.[2] The evidence from that period is minimal, yet it appears that medical knowledge in China 5000 years ago was at a stage not unlike that of Egypt at the same time. Egyptian papyri also reveal an abundance of medicaments coupled with magical methods of dealing with the more invisible inner diseases.

The Yellow Emperor's Book of Internal Medicine, the *Nei Ching Su Wen*,[3] is the most important Chinese medical text and the most ancient. It presents a set of principles and guidelines for the practice of medicine as well as a way of life. It marks the transformation from ancient magical healing to a system; from witch-doctors to physicians. The Yellow Emperor, Huang Ti, is suggested to have lived from 2697 to 2597 BC and to have been the first human ruler of China. However, his existence cannot be confirmed, and the book itself is probably a compilation of more ancient oral teachings, set down in about 1000 BC. Since that time the book has been edited and re-edited with the addition of any number of opinions and commentaries. Yet it remains a key text, still consulted by Chinese physicians. It forms the basis of the medical literature of China.

The earliest fundamental understanding of the nature of health and disease, expounded by the *Nei Ching*, would have been forgotten were it not for an element peculiar to Chinese culture: the worship of their ancestors, a practice which runs far deeper than the respect shown for Western patriarchs. It was formalized by the teaching of K'ung-tzu, whose Latinized name is Confucius. He preached a high moral order in which codes of behaviour towards fellow man and the state, and loyalty to the ancients, were essential to health, welfare and the religious experience. At the same time as Confucius taught, an alternative philosophy was spreading among the villages; Taoism. It began shamanistically and became the dominant imperial creed. It was typified by a poem, the *Tao Te Ching*, written by a legendary sage known as Lao Tzu, the Old Master. It also placed the ancients on a pedestal, but for a different reason. They were seen to be giants of quietness, unconditioned by organized social behaviour. They had the wisdom to avoid disease.

After the Yellow Emperor came many key figures in the origin of Chinese medicine who were well known and emulated by traditional physicians. There was Pien Ch'ueh who is credited with founding the art of diagnosis of disease by feeling the pulse. He lived in approximately the fifth century BC, around the time of Hippocrates. A little later lived Chang Chung-ching (Chang Chi for short), a contemporary of Galen in the West. He wrote two books, which are still extant, concerning the details of acupuncture, moxibustion, respiratory therapy, physiotherapy and massage. There are references to these unique Chinese healing skills in earlier works, but this is the first full methodological account. Hua T'o also lived at this time. He pioneered anaesthesia in operations, through the use of a 'bubbling wine' possibly containing opium. He was credited with the ability to perform extraordinary operations including organ transplantation, and he published charts and diagrams of the interior of the human body. One product of his fertile imagination was a series of therapeutic exercises which mimicked the motions of wild animals such as deer, tigers, bears, apes and birds.[4]

These were some of the founding fathers. Their traditional concepts and methods have lasted, with some revisions and additions, up to the present day. Traditional Chinese doctors are alive and well. Let us examine their system.

THE ELEMENTS

A view of health does not arise like Archimedes' principle; an innovator does not jump up with the sudden perception of its meaning. It arises from cultural patterns of living and attendant philosophies. It comes from the attitude of the society to Nature. In China this was heavily influenced by Taoism, and medicine therefore had a Taoist framework. The early Taoists were hermits who practised quietism. Like Heraclitus, they stated: *Everything flows.* This is the Tao. Often it is translated as the flux of life, but it is more than the flux, and even more than the origin of the flux. It is perhaps best left as 'the Way', remembering, however, the first line of the *Tao Te Ching*: 'The Tao that can be conceived is not the Tao.'[5] Life is too great and changing to encompass with the limited human mind, so let the Tao, the flow, take you along. 'As the soft yielding water cleaves obstinate stone, so to yield with life solves the insoluble.'

Man is only a temporary assemblage of parts in a continually changing and interacting universe: a wave in the ocean, with a tendency to feel himself superior to the rest of the water. But the essence of health is to fall in with the patterns of life. To be in harmony with the Tao. Ill health is caused by swimming against the tide, by 'rebellion', as the *Nei Ching* puts it, against the Tao.

Scientists today will support the case of the essential interchangeability of man and nature. All forms of life are composed of cells containing similar basic biological substances, which continually interact with their environment. Not one bit of the body which is there at birth is still there at death. However, science does not have a concept of harmony in this relationship with nature. This was a Taoist speciality. The Taoists discerned that nature consists of fundamental qualities which the Chinese described by a set of symbols or codes. The most important was polarity.

The Chinese believe that the world was created as a result of the interplay of opposites. The two poles are *Yin* and *Yang*. Yin, originally signifying the northern side of the mountains, is the dark, cold, passive, inner, female, negative aspect of things. Yang is the southern side, light, warm, active, expressive, male, positive aspects. 'The principle of Yin and Yang is the basic principle of the entire Universe. . . . Heaven was created by an accumulation of Yang, the element of light, Earth by an accumulation of Yin, the element of darkness.' In the body, 'Yin is active within and acts as a guardian of Yang, Yang is active on the outside, but regulates Yin.' Organs too have a Yin interior and Yang exterior. But solid organs such as liver and heart are more Yin and active secretory organs such as stomach and bladder are more Yang.

The flow of nature, according to traditional Chinese metaphysics, is also split up into five parts, the quinary. These elements are wood, fire, earth, metal and water. This is the

Chinese version of the similar early Greek system. These elements work for or against each other. They are intimately connected with all aspects of perceived reality. Each element corresponds to colour, taste, climate, body organ, and emotion (Table 1).

Table 1: The Quinary

ELEMENTS	wood	fire	earth	metal	water
SENSES	eye	tongue	mouth	nose	ears
CLIMATE	wind	heat	humidity	dryness	cold
SEASONS	spring	summer	late summer	autumn	winter
POINTS	east	south	centre	west	north
EMOTIONS	anger	joy	sympathy	sadness	fear
VISCERA	liver	heart	spleen-pancreas	lungs	kidney-bladder
PLANETS	Jupiter	Mars	Saturn	Venus	Mercury
TASTES	sour	bitter	sweet	sharp	salty

The interplay of these influences creates a vast net of cause and effect. The five elements can strengthen or weaken Yin or Yang. They are increased or decreased by whatever seasons, moods and so on predominate. An undue dominance of one or the other at the wrong time will cause disease. All kinds of relationships were determined concerning the five elements, for example:

The East creates the wind, the wind creates wood, which creates sour flavour, the sour flavour strengthens the liver, the liver nourishes the muscles, the muscles strengthen the heart, and the liver also influences the eyes. The eyes see the mystery of Heaven and discover Tao among mankind.[3]

The traditional Chinese physicians view the body as a set of purely functional processes such as storage, heating, digestion, elimination and energy production. They use the term 'viscera' to describe these functions. They are poor on anatomy, they carry out little dissection and even less surgery. The body is a dynamic whole, a kind of continuous protoplasm, which could not be chopped up into separately working bits or organs. For example, digestion was described in the *Nei Ching* as occurring in the stomach viscus, the essence of the food was transferred to the 'liver', which then passed on its energy to the muscles; the de-energized material reached the heart, its effects appeared in the pulse and the bulk of it was eliminated by the anus.[6] This, though written two millennia ago, is much like a functional description of digestion which we might read in a high school biology book. Yet it is also very different. Viscera may be translated from the Chinese as stomach, liver and kidney, because these are the only words we have to describe the original Chinese ideograms. However, the Chinese mean phenomena, not organs. They are concerned more with the flux of digestion and metabolism. The processes themselves absorbed Yin or Yang from the food and were changed by it, according to their own degrees of Yin and Yang. They could be overloaded with Yin or Yang and their balance destroyed.

If an organ is too Yang, it signifies excessive activity. There is heat, wastage, and a drain on resources. On the other hand, if an organ is too Yin it implies it is sluggish, cold and static. Yin and Yang must be in equilibrium in the viscera as well as between viscera and in relation to the Yin and Yang qualities of the seasons, geography, inheritance and so on. This does not imply a continuous golden mean. It implies a changing flow, allowing Yin or Yang to dominate in response to changes in the environment.

If Yin is not equal to Yang, then the pulse becomes weak and sickly and madness can result. If Yang is not equal to Yin, then the energies which are contained within the five main viscera will conflict with each other and the circulation ceases in the nine openings of the body.[3]

A crucial factor in this picture is that of the 'vital essence' (ch'i). This would correspond to the life force, or stock of vitality which must be maintained to ensure health. It corresponds to the Sanskrit prana, the Greek pneuma or Hebrew ruach. It is an energy which can be gathered and increased by a wise life-style in harmony with the Tao. Ch'i is increased when Yin and Yang are in balance. It can also be augmented by certain psycho-physiological exercises. Since an adequate degree of ch'i is essential in order to resist disease, much effort in healing

the sick is devoted to its preservation. This is also the object of
the instruction given by the physician to the healthy.

The identity of man and the environment in Chinese eyes
implied that man's inner balance was maintained only as a
result of a fine juggling act. To go with the flow of nature, like
a canoeist riding the rapids, required the greatest skill and
wisdom, for disharmony and its consequence, disease, could
arise from any quarter. Each season, each climate, and even
each type of wind had its quota of the five elements and
therefore would create conditions for the corresponding type
of disharmony in the body, i.e. hot, damp, dry or windy
illnesses. Since the five viscera were also connected to the five
seasons, each season would have a particular relationship with
the viscera. Winter related to the kidney, summer was the time
to take care against diseases of the circulation and spring the
time to watch over the liver. Cold windy air, as we know,
aggravates rheumatic conditions. Superimposed on this, like a
continual background music, was the degree of Yin and Yang
in each season and climate.

The moods were related to the five elements. They could
alter the delicate balance of Yin and Yang. Anger affected the
liver, worry the spleen, and fear and shock damaged the blood
vessels, a fact we can now confirm only too well. Even more
critical than moods were foods. Besides the Yin/Yang nature
of the foods, the flavours relate to the five elements. Pungent,
sour, sweet, bitter and salty flavours have respectively dispersing, condensing, retarding, energizing and softening effects on
the system. Some of the disease relationships which they
arrived at are quite familiar to us, for example that sweet
things cause 'painful bones' (arthritis) or salty things cause
'stiff and delicate' blood vessels (high blood pressure).[2] Others
are novel, for example that bitter things cause skin diseases.

A HEALTH WHICH STANDS THE TEST OF TIME

It is not at all easy to see how practical consequences emerged
from the traditional view of the world. The theories of a
cosmological interplay between man and nature are very nice
to contemplate, but how do they lead to the curing of Liang's
piles?

In order to diagnose disease, the doctor worked backwards from the symptoms to the original disharmonies which caused them. His goal was an assessment of the functional state of all the various organ systems, following which he would make an attempt to isolate the factors in the patient's life-style or environment which were causative. The information at his disposal for diagnosis was the manner in which the various energies, qualities and elements appeared on the outside of the body, as if projected on a cinema screen.

The primary source of information was the pulse which, if sensitively read, would give many clues as to the nature of the internal disharmony. The pulse gave an indication of the severity of the disease and the potential for a cure (prognosis). Each of the five viscera produced a kind of pulse beat which was distinguishable, and the disease could thus be located in the relevant system. There were three pulses on each hand and others scattered at various sites on the limbs. The physician had to observe the rhythms, strengths, sounds and patterns of the pulses. The more finely tuned and delicate his perception, the more information he could obtain about the inner state of the patient. The sensitivity required is illustrated by instructions such as: 'When the pulse is slow and quiet, it acts as a protector and guardian. In days of spring the pulse is superficial like wood floating on water. . . . In winter it is like sleepy insects around the bone, quiet and delicate like a nobleman in his mansion.'[3]

The doctor will also derive valuable clues from examining the colour of the skin, the nose, tongue, mouth, teeth and the various colours of the coating of the tongue. He will listen to the breath, the speech and the lungs. He examines and smells the perspiration, urine and faeces. He inquires about the patient and his manner of life in great detail.

The physician must be able to 'see' the functional state of the body with such subtlety and insight that simple people credit him with almost supernormal powers. But the *Nei Ching* is quite clear that magic has nothing to do with the craft of healing, and it states that the continual development of diagnostic methods over centuries explains the extraordinary capacities of the physician . . . although there are some supremely gifted individuals who can 'see without need for symptoms and taste without flavours, who make use of a profound and mysterious knowledge and resemble those who are divinely inspired.'

The physician has made his diagnosis. He has classified the disease as a distortion of one of the various elements: Yin/Yang, Inner/Outer, Solid/Loose, Cold/Hot, and so on. He has assessed the strength and vitality of the patient – his ch'i. He knows which functions are affected. Now he begins the cure. His first concern is to bring the elements in man into harmony with the environment. He increases the solidity of this organ, the Yin or Yang of that one. At the same time, he applies purificatory techniques to remove poisons and the infecting agents. This would be the only part of the healing process which would be familiar to a Western doctor, for it is similar to the use of modern antibiotics and antitoxins. The healer also guides the patient to increase his ch'i, for without a strong central life force the body will not have the power to return to health. In some cases it is the ch'i which is increased first, the disease itself being mopped up at a later stage.

Unlike their Greek contemporaries, Chinese physicians generally do not bother to classify health, aware of the basic impossibility of the task. They recognize only an undivided spectrum running from supervitality to death. That is not to say that they do not measure health. They actually take the most severe of yardsticks with which to assess health: vitality and longevity. Longevity is so severe a yardstick because it implies a health which stands the test of time. The *Nei Ching* opines that good health means living to 100. By that assessment, most of the population of the world today would be regarded as less than healthy.

The ancient medical system built upon the Taoist view of health taught that the primary activity should be to establish harmony so as to avoid disease. Secondarily, diseases can be treated. 'The ancient sages did not treat those who were already ill; they instructed those who were not ill.'[3] The art of disease prevention was consequently developed to an unparalleled degree. Doctors were enjoined to maintain the health of their 'patients' before anything else. This was in fact what they were paid for. If the patient fell ill, it was partly the doctor's fault, so payments would cease. (I wonder what would happen if we reversed the Western system, and began paying doctors only when we were healthy?) 'The inferior physician begins to help when destruction has already begun. Since his help comes when the disease has already developed, it is said of him that he is ignorant.'[3]

The Chinese doctor was and still is an instructor in living, since health and disease arise from an appropriate or inappropriate way of life. The doctor is a sage, the sage a healer, the healer a philosopher. In contrast to the Western doctor, who is skilled at the examination of pathological symptoms, the Oriental practitioner is skilled at appreciating whether the *conditions for disease* are there or not. He investigates causes. His sensibility is tuned to every person's basic make-up and characteristics, since each individual is a walking record of his development. But he must practise what he preaches. For example, in traditional medicine the state of health of an individual can be partly assessed by measuring the rate and manner of breathing in comparison to the rate and manner of heartbeat. However, in olden times there were no watches with which to measure these things. Thus the doctor measured the patient's breathing by comparison with his own. Yet if the doctor himself were less than completely healthy, his own breathing would be inadequate and he would judge the sick to be healthy and the healthy sick.

The traditional doctors clearly have a great responsibility. Time and time again they are warned that a disease that is incompletely cured can easily flare up again or breed a new disease. The cure must be conscientious and total. As the burden of disease threatens to overwhelm Western medical resources, it would be wise to remember the *Nei Ching*:

To administer medicines for diseases which have already developed is comparable to the behaviour of those who begin to dig a well after they have become thirsty, and of those who begin to make weapons after the battle has begun.

It is difficult to estimate the success of this traditional medical approach to health in an objective manner. We know that there were plagues and there were very healthy people, there were many who died in infancy, and there were many who survived to be extremely old. But when traditional medicine was in its heyday there were no statistics. What we do know is that Chinese medicine in its bloom made some remarkable advances: the circulation of the blood, discovered 2000 years before William Harvey; total anaesthesia discovered at the same time; immunization against smallpox by sniffing powder from pustules of cows with cowpox; the filling of teeth with mercury-silver amalgam in the sixth century; and the discovery of hundreds of unique remedies; to name but a few examples. The real success of Chinese traditional medicine lay in its development of many kinds of methods for preserving health for as long as possible, in accordance with its demanding definitions of health. Its failure, like all traditional medicine, was its inability to remove the great risks associated with illness once disease has gained a foothold.

Where Oriental traditional medicine has failed, our medicine has succeeded; where it has succeeded, we have failed. It would be of great interest to see what is happening in China today, when both systems are co-existent.

CHINESE MEDICINE TODAY

Chinese history is like a carpet continually unrolling. Dynasty after dynasty appears on its face and continues the pattern of development. The ancient culture is by and large maintained and developed as the millennia pass by. By contrast, Western development often rolls up the carpet behind it as it goes along. Culture rises in Greece, and is fragmented; in Byzantium, and then dies; in the Arab world; then, already in its death throes, is passed on to Europe. The West has continually lost sight of its roots, and nowhere is this more in evidence than in the development of modern medicine. We are as far away from the teaching of Hippocrates in 1980 as we are from the teachings of the Emperor Huang Ti. In contrast, Chinese traditional medicine today is the result of a continuous skein of evolution with occasional revisions along the way. Traditional doctors still derive inspiration from the most ancient medical texts, particularly the *Nei Ching*, just as we have in this book.

Much of the oddity of the Chinese medicinal mode of thinking is due to this penetration of the past into the present. It allowed medicine to grow organically. New branches were easily incorporated on a solid pre-existing trunk. However, it also led to strange terminology, excessive formalism and some useless vestiges. This was brought to light when the traditional medicine was, perhaps for the first time, shaken to its roots and almost demolished by a competitor: Western medicine.

It entered China mildly enough, brought by European priests in the seventeenth century. The Emperor K'ang Hsi was cured of a bout of malaria with quinine and enjoyed the confrontation between Chinese, Western and Tibetan physicians, as long as it was restricted to entertainment for the imperial intellect. He must have sensed its danger, however, for when a detailed Western anatomy was prepared for publication he confiscated the manuscript and locked it up. Nevertheless, with the foundation of the powerful East India Company, Western medicine flooded into China. The company oversaw the building of missionary hospitals, with schools for nurses and doctors. Surgeons of the British forces taught surgery and vaccination, and medical works were translated into Chinese. Chinese traditional physicians were keen to learn Western ways but found it difficult to reconcile the two systems. Yu Li-ch'u, for example, was confused enough to write that the Chinaman and the European had their heart and liver in different places, and this must have been the origin of their religious differences. It followed that only Chinese with inverted internal organs were susceptible to conversion by Christian missionaries, and he questioned why the missionaries wanted to bother with such freaks![4]

Traditional medicine suffered considerably, sinking in favour steadily as the intelligentsia of the Chinese urban centres were won over by European ways. The traditional doctor was virtually stripped of his status. During the first part of this century there was social disruption and war. Plagues of cholera, typhoid, tuberculosis and other diseases swept the country, a phenomenon that the traditional doctor was unable to cope with. Yet strangely it was war that saved him. For during the turmoil of the Civil War and the Japanese invasion, only traditional methods were consistently available for civilians and soldiers, and their effectiveness, cheapness and simplicity were tested under the most trying conditions. A similar process happened with the Vietnamese during the war with America. As the Director of the Institute of Materia Medica of Hanoi mentioned recently: 'The old remedies to heal wounds proved especially valuable during the many wars of resistance to foreign aggression.'

So after the revolution in China all doctors were urged to study traditional methods and incorporate them into their modern training. Specialist hospitals using traditional methods and universities of traditional medicine were established, as well as experimental institutes on acupuncture and pharmacology. The Central Research Institute of Traditional Medicine in Peking coordinated the revival. Traditional doctors joined with Western-trained doctors in the Chinese medical association, and a flood of old books, new compendia and reference works were published. Traditional physicians were no longer the second-class experts dominated by imported foreign medical techniques. Their procedures were no longer secret. They handed them over to a new generation of professional traditional doctors. The traditional art again became the medicine of the people as it was before the Europeans arrived, although, as we shall see, there have been certain losses on the way.

The serious state of the nation's health after the revolution also fuelled a dramatic and unique reconstruction of Western-type medicine. The few medical centres in the cities began to train doctors who spread into the countryside. Many medical schools were established, especially 'middle' medical schools, based on the Russian model, to train assistant doctors who worked in the communes. Paramedical personnel were recruited and trained, especially after the cultural revolution of 1965–6. These famous 'barefoot doctors' (who were neither barefoot nor doctors) are workers in industry and agriculture who receive a brief but intensive course in health matters from doctors and assistant doctors. A small unit of 200 workers might have two who are concerned with health. Their function is to diagnose and treat simple diseases, advise people on personal hygiene, vaccinate their groups against infectious diseases, work to eliminate pests and control sewage, and administer the birth-control programmes. The barefoot doctors attempt to bring health matters into every household. Health has become everyone's business. There is no élite group of experts to take over responsibility for health from the individual. Health is regarded as part and parcel of revolutionary consciousness.

The success of the overall Chinese strategy cannot be doubted. China had one of the worst mortality rates in the world. In just thirty years health has improved dramatically. The people of Shanghai, for example, now have a life expectancy greater than that in many Western cities, an infant mortality rate less than half that of New Yorkers and a level of health care and preventive medicine that is the envy of the world. The major factor in increased life expectancy was probably not medicines at all but, as in Europe in the last century and the beginning of this century, vastly improved public health measures. The intervention of the rural health worker on the spot in disinfecting, vaccinating, cleaning and teaching is probably responsible for most of the success. A certain part of it, however, is due to the preservation of old and new. Traditional doctors formed a basic health force able to administer cheap and local medicines which did not require a vast industrial infrastructure to manufacture. They were there in the villages. In a sense, these traditional healers were the first barefoot doctors.

There is, however, a real question whether the new barefoot doctor is actually more useful than the old. While his skills at public health and family planning are indubitable, he has only received a scanty training and is then unleashed on the peasantry with a fat handbook. In this handbook are principles for the diagnosis and treatment of every kind of disease, from the very serious, such as tumours and poliomyelitis, to the superficial, such as a sprained ankle. The barefoot doctor is supposed to distinguish between the two and pass on cases he cannot treat.

Part of the problem has been that recent times have demanded a massive effort at repair of the damaged health of the people. First priorities have therefore been curative remedies and immunization. The people needed freedom from epidemics, not longevity, and therefore the traditional system was required to operate in an area in which it is inadequate. It was forced to provide instant curative answers to diseases and symptoms, when it is rather better at health maintenance through the use of subtle, refined and long-term techniques. The ancient system nevertheless rose to meet the challenge and it evolved a new identity in Darwinian fashion. It lost some of its theoretical ramifications, its rich and powerful understanding of natural processes, and its careful and demanding methods of individual treatment. But it also lost its aristocratic flavour as well as many esoteric but useless principles. The basic theoretical elements of the traditional practice, in particular the Yin–Yang, the five elements, the tonification of the organs, the meridians and to some extent the concepts of internal harmony, have survived. They are absolutely necessary for diagnosis and treatment. Even if the official view of Yin–Yang is now 'an original spontaneously dialectical simple materialistic doctrine',[7] it is still used to compound remedies.

We are particularly interested in those methods by which Chinese medicine achieves the goal of a health which stands the test of time; of treatments with which to win wars, not battles. These methods are known. They have been in use since before the Taoist period and refined continuously thereafter. The current disruption is a mere hiccup in their development. They include acupuncture, moxibustion, massage, physical culture and medicines. We will restrict ourselves to an exploration of the last category, while realizing that the same fundamental concepts apply to them all.

ORIENTAL DRUGS AND THE HERBAL EMPEROR

Three legendary figures created early Chinese society. These three August Rulers were Fu Hsi, to whom is attributed the *I Ching*, the *Book of Changes*; Huang Ti, the Yellow Emperor, whom we have already met; and Shen Nung. Called the 'Heavenly Cultivator', he was father of both agriculture and herbal medicine, creator of the first Chinese pharmacopoeia, and mentor of Chinese physicians and folk healers until today. He is supposed to have written the *Shen Nung Pen Tshao Tching*, or *Pharmacopoeia of the Heavenly Cultivator*. This work contains 365 remedies as well as the basic teaching of Chinese herbal medicine. In actual fact *pen tshao* means a 'teaching based on an understanding of drugs', rather than a mere list.

Shen Nung, according to some apocryphal sources, lived about 3000 BC. Others say that he never existed. But it is probable that the legends of the man and most of his oral teachings were present in Chinese culture a thousand years before Christ. The book, his *Pen Tshao*, was known at least as far back as the second century BC, according to Joseph Needham.

The image of Shen Nung which springs to mind is of a

simple man, a sage, an innovator and a teacher. As one of the early books states:

The people of antiquity consumed plants and drank water. They gathered the fruits of the tree and ate the flesh of clams. They frequently suffered from illnesses and poisonings. Then Shen Nung taught the people for the first time how to sow the five kinds of grain and to observe whether the land was dry or moist, fertile or stony, on hills or the lowlands. He tasted all the herbs and examined the springs as to whether they were sweet or bitter. Thus he informed the people of what they ought to avoid and where they could go.[8]

His insight, combined with his experimental approach, was regarded as a heavenly gift, and throughout Chinese history pharmacopoeia have placed his name respectfully on their title page. For the Chinese physicians love this patriarch, a man who discovers drugs through wisdom, whose body and mind are a cradle of drug-testing put to the service of the people. He is relevant as an embodiment of the pharmacological insight which is the concern of this book.

Why was the first pharmacologist also the first ploughman? Although agriculture and pharmacology are strange bed-fellows, a look at the Pen Tshao brings home the connection. It is a guide for the maintenance of health by means of drugs, in the same way that an agriculturist teaches how to make plants flourish, how to irrigate, feed, and protect crops. They both have the same approach: to bring out the best in living things. These two sciences are unquestionably linked in the Chinese mind.

In the West the attitudes to the health of crops and the health of people are completely different. The Westerner cannot see a connection between agriculture and pharmacology. Shen Nung would say that today our crops were getting the better deal. The Western farmer will work hard using new strains of plants, intercropping, leaving fallow, thinning and treating; all of these are intended to prevent his crops from becoming diseased. There is little of the curative approach in farming. After all, who wants a diseased apple, even if most of it is still healthy? On the other hand, the Western doctor takes few steps to ensure disease resistance in his charges, and the pharmacologist has designed drugs which are curative, not preventive.

The medicines in the first *Pen Tshao* reflect the organic attitude to health. Medicines are gleaned widely from the natural world. Of the 365 remedies listed therein, 237 are botanical, 65 animal, 43 mineral and the rest unidentified.

The remedies are classified in a most interesting manner. They are placed in three grades according to their toxicity, in an order which the Westerner would find topsy-turvy. The most important group are the 'kingly', 'superior' drugs. They are characterized by being absolutely harmless, by being used for a great variety of health purposes by the sick and the healthy, and by their ability to increase vitality. These are plants such as:

Panax ginseng (jen-shen) (ginseng)
Adenophora verticillate (sha-shen)
Schizandra chinensis (wu wei tzu)
Glycyrrhiza glabra (kan tsao) (liquorice)
Ophiopogon japonicus (mai-men-tung)
Eucommia ulmoides (tu-chung)
Pachyma cocos (fu ling)
Zingiber officinale (shen-chiang) (ginger)
Ziziphus jujuba (hung-tsao) (jujube)

In the second grade are the 'ministerial' herbs. These common drugs are more powerful, are used against some diseases and are slightly toxic. For example:

Sophora angustifolia (k'u-shen)
Scrophularia oldhami (hsuan-shen) (a figwort)
Polygonum bistorta (tzu-shen) (bistort)
Angelica sinensis (tang-kuei) (type of angelica)
Fritillaria thumbergii (pei-mu)

Thirdly come the inferior 'assistant' herbs, whose toxic dose is close to the therapeutic dose. They are used to cure specific diseases. They are the last resort when all other methods have failed. For example:

Aconitum carmichaelii (aconite)
Platycodon grandiflorum (chi-keng)
Adonis amurensis (pin-liang-hua) (pheasant's-eye)
Veratrum nigrum (hellebore)
Strychnos nux vomica (vomit-nut tree)

There is also a subsidiary 'servant' class of drugs. They have the ability to conduct other medicines to the place where they are intended to act in the body.

This classification is, of course, the complete reverse of the Western list of priorities, which regards the powerful curative drugs as the mainstay of medicine and the mild drugs as accessories of little significance. Almost all Western medicines would be assigned to the assistant category by the Chinese pharmacologists because of their fundamental harmfulness. The classification of drugs is a reflection of the emphasis of each medical system. Chinese medicine values subtle drugs which can be used to 'tune' the body and ensure maximum vitality and disease resistance. Western drugs are designed to cure diseases once they occur, and the toxicity is tolerated as part of the deal. Chinese medicines largely follow the principle of *noli nocere* (harmlessness). Few poisonous plants are used, and if they are, the toxins are removed by processing. Western medicines are usually synthetic, but where plants are used it is usually the toxic plants in which the toxins are themselves the medicines.

In the two millennia since the first *Pen Tshao*, the principles of the Chinese use of drugs have changed very little. They have only become somewhat more complex and more erudite, and many more remedies have been discovered. For a descriptive look at these remedies in our times, we can turn to an interesting study carried out in the Soviet Far East. At the Institute of the Physiology and Pharmacology of Adaptation, Vladivostok, Professor Israel I. Brekhman, who was the head at the time, together with his wife, M. A. Grinevich, and colleagues, explored Chinese medicines in a unique fashion. They accumulated 158 remedies from China and South-east Asia, especially Vietnam.

They recorded the medicinal properties, the species, the manner in which the drugs were used and other details, and fed all this information into a computer. They were able to obtain all kinds of interconnections.[9] Three-quarters of the remedies contained from four to eleven separate plants. By comparison, three-quarters of Western medicines contain but a single constituent. The Chinese, apparently, tended to use the roots and tubers of plants rather than the leaves. Brekhman found that most of the plants were made up as concoctions, i.e. by boiling with water. The active components were established and found to belong to classes which were mild and safe. There were few of the alkaloids which are the strong plant chemicals used in Western medicine (e.g. morphine, reserpine, nicotine, papaverine). Brekhman also found much overlapping within recipes. Several different plants with the same kind of medicinal action were often compounded together in a single remedy. The doses were also surprisingly large. It was not unusual to find prescriptions recommending up to 100 gm (4 oz) of a plant mixture.

What were the remedies used for? Astonishingly, over half the remedies were *not intended to treat any specific disease*, but were used to affect the whole body in an *adjustive* manner. These were used to restore energy and function in the various internal processes of the body. In the West they might be lumped together under the crude designation 'tonic' or 'restorative' remedies. Others had a local action on specific diseased parts, or were for the treatment of serious diseases or relief of various symptoms. Every remedy, for whatever purpose, contained at least one of these tonic plants. The next most frequent were plants increasing the flow of urine or sweat, next were those protecting the body against harmful substances, then anti-cough remedies and sedative plants.

THE TECHNIQUES OF CHINESE DRUG THERAPY

The therapeutic concepts associated with the use of medicaments range from simple peasant herb brews effective against specific diseases, such as Vitex negundo against bronchitis, to highly complex concoctions based on the ultra-sophisticated reasoning of skilled professionals. These manipulate the internal energies like a man playing an organ. They may drain the 'fire' or the 'cold', augment the 'humidity' or dissolve mucus, work on the spleen while protecting the heart, or clear poisons while increasing vitality, all the time taking into account external factors as disparate as the phase of the moon and the facial features of the patient.

A typical example of a system in Chinese medicine which would assist in the detection and subsequent use of plants is the five flavours. Drugs were classified as bitter, sour, salty, sharp or sweet, the Chinese equivalent of our chemical groupings. The flavours correspond, as we have seen, to the relevant primal element, so that sour-tasting medicines affect the liver and have a solidifying 'woody' characteristic, while a bitter taste affects the heart and has a strengthening character. A sweet taste has a mild 'earthy' character and affects spleen–pancreas function. Sharp tastes affect the lungs and are 'metally' and dispersive, while salty tastes are delicate and 'watery' and affect the kidneys and urinary system.[2]

The healer has a point of reference in designing remedies. Medication must always maintain inner vitality. The inner resources of the patient in fighting the disease must be cosseted, protected and encouraged, while at the same time attempts are made to restore as much of normal function as possible. Treatment must reinforce the patient, not weaken him. For example, 'tung-tan sie-chan' concoction for 'moist heat' disease, resulting from blockages in the liver and gall-bladder, contains plants with strong bitter and cold qualities. But these must be balanced by liquorice to maintain the vitality of the stomach functions during the treatment. Atractylis ovata and liquorice harmonize and increase energy. Sweating and internal purification of the poisons of disease is accomplished without any harmful side-effects. Therefore the mixture is nicely balanced and is said to 'walk on two legs'. Sometimes concoctions are designed so that poisons are inhibited within the mixture. Aconite is powerful and toxic but its action is mollified by mixing with honey.[4]

The treatment must always be designed for the patient, as well as his disease. For example, a thin woman will be given Rehmannia sinensis as an accessory to other relevant treatments to disperse her 'fire', while a fat woman will be given Arum species to dissolve excessive secretions. As the patient progresses through stages of the disease, the treatment must be continually altered.

The Yin and Yang balance, the degrees of activity or of sluggishness of the functions of the patient, must always be maintained by remedies. For example the 'six remedies', 'lu-wei', contains:

Rehmannia glutinose (25g of root)
Cornus officinalis (12.5g of fruit)

Dioscorea batatas (12.5g of root)
Paeonia suffruticosa (9.4g of root)
Alisma plantago aquatica (9.4g of tuber)
Pachyma cocos (9.4g of tuber)

Plants are linked in pairs. Rehmannia stimulates the kidney energy and Alisma disperses or clears the powerful 'fire', the waste products, which result. Cornus and Paeonia do the same to the liver, Dioscorea stimulates the spleen and Pachyma disperses the consequent humidity. The dispersives allow a more powerful medicinal action by preventing harmful metabolites from accumulating, somewhat like increasing the flow through a stretch of river by opening the sluice gate. The symptoms guide the physician to choose his mix of remedies. Often he will determine the chief remedy, the master, fix its dosage, and let the other accessory remedies fall into place around the leader. Then servant plants are added to conduct the main components to the site of the disease. Thus, in the six remedies, Rehmannia is the master if the blood is poor and Yin energy weak, Cornus if there is giddiness and a tendency to fainting, Pachyma if urination is abnormal, Alisma, the water plantain, if there is too little urine, Paeonia if the heart is weak, Dioscorea is the kingpin if the stomach is weak and the skin is dry.

   A patient, let us say, arrives at a Chinese doctor loaded with the symptoms of severe dysentery which we know so well: chills and fever, pain in the stomach, diarrhoea with stools containing blood, and a fast and strong pulse. The doctor, after a suitable analysis of the organ systems involved, may decide that the vital energy of the patient is quite strong. His constitution is not yet undermined. Therefore he will give him medicines to clear the 'fire', promote urination and remove poisons, such as Pueraria (hair-grass) root, Sauscuraeae lappa, Coptis chinensis, Scutellaria baicalensis (skullcap), Pellodendrin chinseuse and Pulsatilla chinensis (meadow anemone). On the other hand, if the patient has been suffering for some time from mild dysentery, his constitution is weak, his inner energy has been drained. He is likely to show loss of appetite, lassitude, hollow and weak pulse and poor circulation. The priority is to recharge his inner batteries, following which the doctor assesses that the disease will subside by itself. Thus

Table 2: Chinese and Modern Medicines

	Chinese medicines	Modern medicines
Discovery	Trial and error over long periods. Deduction. Intuition-introspection	Trial and error over short periods. Deduction from pharmacological principles
The typical laboratory	The human body in daily life	The rat body attached to instruments
The range	Animal, vegetable, mineral	Vegetable and mineral but now largely synthetic
Typical principles	Co-ordinating Yin/Yang. Adjusting five elements. Increasing vitality. Removing poisons	Killing infecting agents. Receptor competition. Reducing symptoms
Values	Harmless subtle drugs best, powerful curative drugs worst	Curative drugs best, mild drugs worst
Examples of most important	Ginseng, Rehmannia, liquorice, Dioscorea	Cortisone, penicillin, morphine, barbiturates, digoxin
Examples of least important	Adonis, Veratrum	Tonic wines, old time cough remedies, herb teas, laxatives
Use of foods and spices as medicines	Yes	No
Recipes	Multiple drugs in water	Single chemicals in pure form
Doses	Large (1.0–100.0 g)	Small (0.0001–5.0 g)
Given	By mouth and skin	By mouth, injection and skin
Processing	Minimal, sometimes poisons removed	Maximal. Entire plant discarded apart from active principle
Typical drug successes	Increasing resistance to disease, managing chronic diseases, e.g. hepatitis, diseases of old age, removing debility	Total control of infectious diseases, e.g. pneumonia; control of some serious diseases, e.g. diabetes
Typical failures	Diseases in advanced stages. Epidemics. Accidents	Chronic diseases, cardiovascular diseases, mild but persistent disease, especially of old age

Aconitum carmichaeli (aconite), ginger, liquorice, Codonopsis pilosulae, Atractylodis alba and Coptis chinensis are given; these plants have a tonic power for basic health, as well as ability to clear heat and inflammation. The principle here is to 'establish vital energy so as to eliminate the harmful factor', while in the former case the treatment is the opposite: expelling the harmful factor in order to establish vital energy. In both cases one can assume that the 'harmful factor' is the bacteria which have invaded the digestive tract, plus the poisons generated by them. Indeed, modern research in China has shown that some plants, such as Coptis chinensis, are effective antibiotics, and has confirmed that the former recipe is more antibiotic, while the latter is more capable of raising the body's own defensive mechanisms!

Many of the Oriental medicaments are familiar to us: types of sage, mint, liquorice, aconite, opium, rhubarb. Some are spices: ginger, fennel, cinnamon; and some foods: glutinous rice, bean curd, honey and sesame. But many are utterly strange. In the vast search for effective medicines, everything animal, vegetable or mineral has been explored. Chinese medicine has become famous for its universality; 'Anything, indeed, that is thoroughly disgusting in the three kingdoms of nature is considered good enough for medical use,' writes one cynical Edwardian doctor.[10] Of course, this is true of all traditional medical systems. In the ancient Egyptian pharmacopoeia we read of the use of putrid meat and the moisture from pigs' ears, and in the Ebers papyrus an extraordinary remedy to keep babies quiet which consisted of the minute droppings of flies! 'Sewage pharmacy' appeared unreservedly in the pharmacopoeia of Europe 300 years ago. Traditional medicine finds no reason to forbid anything in nature on purely emotional grounds. This is particularly true in China, where man is seen as an integral part of a flux of organic materials in the biosphere.

We are now in a position to sum up our knowledge of Chinese traditional and Western modern drug therapy, as in Table 2.

THE BAREFOOT DOCTORS' MEDICINE CHEST

In 1578 a monumental pharmacopoeia appeared, the *Pen Tshao*

Kang-mu, compiled by Li Shih-chen. He selected material
from about 500 medical works written before that time,
gathering and categorizing the best medicaments and adding
new ones from his personal explorations. The book described
1892 different drugs and some 10,000 prescriptions. It has been
revised recently by the Nanking Pharmacological Institute,[11]
which categorized 2000 substances by Chinese and Latin
name, usage, history, preparation, constituents and other
details.

This pharmacopoeia is used today. But the brigade stations
are stacked with herbal and Western remedies. Doctors trained
in both systems work side by side in the commune and
country hospitals. A barefoot doctor will usually offer a
patient a choice of traditional or Western treatment. Sometimes one or the other is recommended because of the nature
of the disease. Traditional methods are often preferable in
cases of pre-disease states, mild infections, tiredness, migraines, and many kinds of chronic diseases, liver diseases,
anaemia, hepatitis, impotence and so on. Western medicines
are usually preferred in acute diseases, injuries, serious infections such as pneumonia, cholera and infections of the digestive tract, parasites, etc. Barefoot doctors are partly trained in
treatment with herbs, acupuncture, moxibustion, massage
and exercise therapy, as well as in the use of a medical bag full
of Western drugs.

This is the situation presented to Liang Li-Ying at the
beginning of the chapter. It often leads to extraordinary
confusions as attempts are made to fit Western drugs into the
pre-existing theoretical framework. The antibiotic strep-
tomycin, for example, is considered to cool the lungs, with the
side-effect of dispersing the ch'i. How similar it is to
nineteenth-century Europe, when the same chemicals were
also described in the language of the old humoralist school.
Treatments are also mixed. For example, high blood pressure
is diagnosed in the Western manner, but then differentiated
into liver-Yang-dominated and kidney-Yin-dominated types.
Both are treated by acupuncture, complex herbal and mineral
prescriptions, or by Western reserpine and phenobarbital.
Ironically reserpine is a chemical isolated in the West from the
plant Raowulfia serpentina which was originally used as a
tranquillizer in China and India. It has completed the circle.

Traditional remedies are still highly regional. The Tibetans use Himalayan herbs. The Mongolians, who brought yoghurt to the West, have a rich understanding of curious plant medicines; the Koreans are skilled in constitutional medicine, that is, matching simple 'diet and decoction' regimes to the individual. There are also multitudes of regional and familial folk remedies. Gradually, all these remedies are being gathered and added to the huge compilation of traditional remedies in the major medicine centres, and a new phenomenon is appearing: research.

Chinese research on traditional and Western medicines is influenced by the pragmatic social climate. Much effort is devoted to the standardization and manufacture of herbal preparations in suitable forms. This has led to large industrial concerns making enormous quantities of patent medicines, and factories manufacturing some 700 different types of synthetic medicines. There has been a distaste for basic research and knowledge for its own sake, especially under the Gang of Four. But laboratory research into traditional remedies has been steadily gathering momentum in recent years, and is generally concerned with the competitive testing of Oriental and Western remedies, reminiscent of the games of K'ang Hsi.

These comparative hospital experiments tend to baffle and infuriate Westerners. The Chinese scorn the Western method of the clinical trial. They find the double-blind procedure outrageous. Giving a patient a useless pill is, they feel, contrary to the natural relationship between healer and patient which is an important component of the whole healing process. They find the deception unethical and unrealistic.

Nevertheless, research is beginning. For example, experiments on the six-component remedy have been carried out on animals with impaired kidney function. The remedy was shown to greatly increase the kidney's capacity and to progressively lower the blood pressure over a long period. Chinese scientists believe that it relaxes the blood vessels supplying the kidney and works on the performance of the filtration 'plumbing' in the kidney itself. If this is true, it should be of great interest to those involved in the treatment of cardiovascular diseases in the West.

THE HARMONY REMEDIES

Certain drugs promote vitality and disease resistance. They manipulate body energy not so much to cure disease as to promote health, both in the sick and in the healthy. The physicians use them to charge up the various organ systems, balancing one against another. These are among the kingly remedies of Shen Nung, the most valuable and respected plants in the Oriental materia medica. They are subtle and difficult to understand for the Westerner, who has never met anything like them. They have been given the title 'tonic' medicines by outside observers. Now the word 'tonic' comes from the Greek *tonos*, tension. It implies something which is bracing, invigorating, mildly stimulating. But that by no means describes the essential feature of these medicines, their integrative harmonizing effect on body energies. There are no comparable drugs in the West and few principles in Western pharmacology which could be used as a frame of reference. Certainly the tonic remedies of the West – such compounds as sugar phosphates, glucose, B-vitamins and minute quantities of the deadly poison strychnine – are so different and limited in scope that it would be a primary confusion to put them both under the same hat. Therefore I would like to rename these kingly remedies *harmony remedies*. The justification will emerge later when we examine in detail the manner in which they are used.[12]

The remedies in Oriental medicine were sometimes called *great remedies*, powerful curative prescriptions, *small remedies* which remove mild disease superficially, *deferred remedies* which uproot chronic diseases, *emergency remedies* which control symptoms immediately, and the *tonic*, now renamed *harmony remedies*, which are used to increase inner vitality and energy, increase disease resistance and tune up the body. It is only these harmony remedies which are a huge question-mark to the Western specialist. The others he knows, at least in principle. Our challenge is not only to understand the harmony remedies but to bring them gently home into the life of Western man.

A list of the main harmony drugs is given in Table 3. The first few names are well known to anyone from the Orient and have also been coughed up by Brekhman's computer as the

Table 3: Chinese Harmony Remedies

Name	Description and part used
Glycyrrhiza glabra	liquorice (root)
Rehmannia chinensis	relative of figwort (root)
Panax ginseng	ginseng (root)
Poria cocos	fungus growing on pine tree roots
Zingiber officinalis	ginger (root)
Ziziphus jujuba	jujube, Chinese date
Paeonia suffruticosa	variety of paeony (root)
Dioscorea batatas	yam (underground stem)
Beuplurum chinensis	umbelliferous herb (root)
Eucommia ulmoides	bark of tree
Schizandra chinensis	herb (fruit and seeds)
Lycium chinensis	boxthorn (fruit)
Achyranthes bidentata	amarantaceous herb (root)
Salvia multiorrhiza	sage relative (root)
Panax pseudoginseng	ginseng relative (root, leaves)
Panax japonicus	ginseng relative (root, leaves)
Aralia cordata	ginseng relative (root, leaves)
Acanthopanax spinosum	spikenard (root, leaves)
Aralia racemosa	spikenard (root, leaves)
Angelica sinensis	type of angelica (root)
Nelumbo nucifera	the lotus (seeds)
Nephelium longana	dragon-eye (fruit)
Polygonum multiflorum	many-flowered Solomon's seal (all parts)
Smilax chinensis	China root (root)
Sika deer	antlers of young deer
Aweto	caterpillar infested with fungus
Tortoise	ground shell

most widely used tonic remedies. They pepper the pages of the ancient medical texts and pharmacopoeiae, and are widely used today. Almost every mixture has one. The same tonic plants are usually part of the Korean, Japanese, Laotian, Mongolian and Tibetan materia medica, although the further one travels from the Chinese mainland, the more individualistic become the medicines. They are mostly plants, but some animal products are used, such as young deer antlers, tortoise-shell, the trunk of the seahorse, the bladder of the sturgeon and the gecko lizard. There is also aweto, a Tibetan medicine which is a caterpillar infected with a relative of ergot. In the next chapter we home in on these harmony medicines and see what is inside them, how they are used and what science has to say about them. We will focus on one of them, which Shen Nung said was the greatest of all medicines: ginseng.

Ginseng and related Chinese harmony remedies are the agents which, in the eyes of traditional medicine, build up vitality and disease resistance. These are the drugs which at present the West has neither knowledge of nor faith in. Yet they are the kingly drugs of Shen Nung, the most important in the ancient pharmacopoeiae, the most harmless and yet effective. They are also the kind of medicaments which the West really needs at this time – the best of the possible remedies to come out of the fusion between old and young medicine in China.

These are the subtle 'hair-breaking' medicinal plants, whose very subtlety makes them most difficult to test using Western methods. Yet if we could demonstrate their effectiveness, the results could be dramatic. They could come as knights in armour to the aid of overloaded allopathic medicine.

The importance of ginseng is not only that it is already on sale in the West and therefore comes in the vanguard, but that it has also been the subject of scientific study. Besides, it is at the very top of the list of kingly remedies. An effective adapter or conductor is needed to transmit the experience of Oriental medicine more smoothly and speedily to the West. Ginseng is an ideal candidate for the job. It is the ideal bridge between East and West.

PART 2
Exposition

4

Ginseng

'SMALL ROOT GOES, GOES, GOES'

At the turn of the century, a middle-aged Muscovite, named Mikhail Prishwyn, packed his bags and left the city for good. He went to find himself amid the wildness of the Ussuri Mountains. There he met Lubin, the healer. This is what he writes:

One day I looked at the face of the old man as he was carefully choosing a herb. I dared to ask him: 'Lubin, you understand everything so well; tell me, am I sick or healthy?' Lubin answered:

'All people are healthy and sick at the same time.'

'So what is my medicine,' I persisted. 'Pantui?' He laughed long and said:

'Pantui is only given to restore lust to the impotent.'

'So maybe ginseng would help me,' I asked. Here Lubin stopped laughing and gave me a long gaze. He was silent. But on the next day he said, in his bizarre language,

'Your root of life will grow, grow, grow. Mine I will show you tomorrow.'

I knew Lubin did not say anything for the sake of it and I waited for the opportunity of seeing not simply a powder, but the genuine root, indigenous to the Taighur. In the small hours of the night the dog started barking and rushed to the depths of the valley. Lubin followed and I was right behind with the gun in my hands. When they came back, Lubin said,

'No need for gun; our people.'

Soon six Chinese arrived, handsome Manchurians armed from head to toe. Lubin repeated: 'Our people.' He said to them the same thing about me, this time in Chinese. The Manchurians bowed to me, faces glowing, then one after another, these tall people lowered their heads and went into Lubin's small dwelling. They sat in a circle and put something on the floor. All of them, as one, suddenly fixed their concentration on it.

'Lubin,' I whispered. 'May I look too?' Lubin repeated in Chinese: 'Our people,' and all the Manchurians looked at me with respect, moved a bit and invited me to sit with them and look at the 'thing'. That is when I saw, for the first time, Zen Shen, the root of life, which is so precious that six strong well-armed men were appointed to bring it. They had made a little box from cedar bark. In it on a bed of black soil there was a small yellow root, which looked exactly like our parsley root. I sat with the Chinese and we were all staring, when to my great amazement I noticed that the root had a human form: here was a separation between the feet, there were hands and there, a neck, and on it the head and even a little plait. The fibres of the hands and feet were like long fingers.

But my heart was struck by more than the similarity between the shape of the root and the human body, since, after all, there are so many shapes that can be found in the tangled forms of roots. I was more overwhelmed by these seven people wrapped in contemplation of the root of life. These seven seemed to be the last of millions who had returned to the earth during past ages. Millions upon millions who, like the remaining seven, believed completely in the root of life. Many of them had probably stared at it with trembling awe, just like these Manchurians who were drinking it with their eyes. I could hardly bear the power of their faith. The lives of all these millions of people seemed to me to be in relation to the enduring faith like the waves are to the sea. The waves began rushing towards me, the living, as to a beach, begging me to grasp the power of the root. Not with my flesh, because that will soon go, but with the wisdom of the stars and the constellations and maybe something beyond that.

After a long contemplation the Manchurians all began to talk at once, and to argue about tiny tiny details within the root. Perhaps they were arguing about a certain fibre which seemed to be more fitting to the masculine root giving it more decoration, while it was unseemly on the female root and therefore perhaps it should be carefully removed. There were an endless number of queries and problems of that nature that Lubin would settle with a smiling face. Everybody would accept his decision for he was the top authority in these matters.

Lubin told me that a poor ginseng gatherer had found this root but was murdered for it, and the treasure went to a certain tradesman who came an immense distance from China and paid a lot of money for the root. He also hired these six men to bring the root back to China for him but paid them too little money. They knew that the root was priceless and they could sell it for even more money to someone else; and so it goes, on and on.

'And so,' I asked, 'what will be the end of this matter?'

Lubin said, in broken Russian:

'No is end. Small root goes, goes, goes, and has much cure. Little people who found it sleeps, sleeps. Rich people then go, go, go.'

The Manchurians left this precious 'go, go' root with Lubin and went to sleep on the cold stone, from where they rose and left before sunrise.[1]

There can hardly be a plant that is held in so much awe by so many people. It is loved, worshipped and cherished in all the countries of the Far East. 'This demure herb of the woodlands of temperate Asia has held the esteem of the Chinese as the single most omnipotent medicinal herb for almost seven thousand years,' writes Professor William Embolden.[2] Wars have been fought over possession of forests where ginseng grows. One Tartar emperor built a palisade around a whole province in order to protect his ginseng against poachers who at times braved the death penalty in order to collect it. In 1709 the emperor sent 10,000 Tartar soldiers to search for ginseng, ordering that each soldier should give him two catties of the best and sell the rest for its weight in silver. Fabulous prices were paid for wild ginseng in imperial times; in fact ginseng has commanded higher prices than any other plant in the history of the world. An old root of the required quality would fetch much more than its weight in gold, and up to 250 times its weight in silver. There are reports of an emperor paying the equivalent of $30,000 for a single root. Even today a Chinese pharmacist in New York has offered $10,000 for a top quality wild root, and there is a huge specimen at the USSR permanent agriculture exhibition in Moscow valued at $25,000. No wonder there is a sarcastic epithet from Manchuria: 'Eat ginseng and ruin yourself.'

There is a rich mythology concerning man's first meeting with the root. Most of the legends tell of a benevolent nature deity within the plant. The ginseng root was not found by man. Man, we are told, was found by the root.

One story relates that the whole village of Shantang, in Shensi province, was disturbed nightly by a strange howling. Unable to tolerate the noise, the villagers gathered together and marched to investigate the source of the sound. They found a large bush and decided to dig it up. Underneath they found a massive man-shaped root which had been screaming for attention. The root was therefore named the 'spirit of the earth'.

Other legends relate that the root was discovered by messages transmitted in dreams. The legends are of the same genre
as those used to retell the discovery of important medicinal or
sacramental plants in other tribes, for example the discovery of
the coca bush by Andeans or of Amanita by Siberian tribes.
The legends are in accord with the notion that ginseng may
have been discovered by the intuitions of shamanism.

The enthusiasm for the root shown by emperors and peas-
ants alike is indubitable.[3] The Chinese, especially older men,
buy the most expensive pieces of root that they can afford. The
root is sold in balsa-wood boxes, sometimes lined with lead to
'preserve the radiations emitting from the root'. Inside, the
root itself is carefully wrapped in silk or tissue paper. It will be
taken home and nugget-sized pieces will be boiled in a little
silver kettle designed specifically for the purpose. Or the root
may be kept in brandy for years, the family eking out the
precious liquid by taking it in little sips, and offering a little to
the most honoured guests. Travellers to China, from Marco
Polo onwards, have invariably commented on its great value
as a medicine. 'This, with the Chinese, is the medicine *par
excellence,'* writes Dr Stuart at the beginning of this century:

the last resort when all other drugs fail . . . it is mostly reserved for
the Emperor and his household and conferred by Imperial favour
upon high and useful officials whenever they have a serious breakdown that does not yield to ordinary treatment . . . the Chinese
describe cases in which the sick have been practically in *articulo mortis*
when upon administration of ginseng they are sufficiently restored
to carry on items of business.[4]

Sir Edwin Arnold, author of the *Light of Asia*, sums up the
situation:

According to the Chinese, Asiatic ginseng . . . will best renovate and
invigorate failing forces. It fills the heart with hilarity while its
occasional use will, it is said, add a decade to human life. Have all
these millions of Orientals, all these many generations of men who
boiled ginseng in silver kettles and praised heaven for its many
benefits, been totally deceived? Was the world ever quite mistaken
when half of it believed in something never puffed, never advertised,
and not yet fallen to the fate of a trust, combine or corner?

There is a plethora of names of ginseng, reflecting its varied
reputation and the legends describing its dramatic entrance

into Oriental consciousness. Ginseng or, in Chinese, *jen-shen,*
means roughly 'man-root'. However, the Chinese characters
represent ideas rather than sounds. *Jen,* it turns out, has
multiple concepts connected with it, including the spirit of
man or the shape and dimensions of man. *Shen* or seng means
root, but also a 'crystallization of the essence of the earth'.
Thus a more accurate version of jen-shen means the 'crystallization of the essence of the earth in the form of a man'. This
powerful image also has a legend somewhere at the back of it.
It is related that ginseng is found where a bolt of lightning
strikes a clear spring, for the fusion of fire energy, water
cohesiveness and earth solidity produces this crystallized
essence.

Ginseng is also called 'spirit vessel' because of the kindly
nature spirit that was associated with it, and 'life root' and
'seminal essence of the earth' because of the belief that the root
was a condensation within the earth of energies vital to man. It
was called 'like the constellation of Orion' because Orion is
both man-shaped and the constellation which was thought to
have astral influence over ginseng. It was called 'yellow shen'
because of its colour, 'blood shen' because of its affinity with
human juices, and 'man gag' because it needed such lengthy
chewing. 'Magical herb', 'wonder of the world' and 'Tartars'
root' are names evincing its fame, while the more prosaic 'the
regenerative elixir which banishes wrinkles from the face', and
the similar Tibetan name, 'medicinal plant giving long life', relate
to its supposed medicinal power. The Koreans call it 'Pough-
wang', meaning Korean phoenix, because the leaves die every
winter to regrow again in the spring. There are many other
names in the countries of Asia, from Japan to Afghanistan.

THE PLANT

The botanical name of ginseng also reflects its reputation. It
was first named Panax schinseng Nees by a German botanist,
Nees van Esenbeck. In 1842 it was renamed Panax ginseng
C. A. Meyer by Carl Anton Meyer. Panax comes from the Greek
pan-axos meaning all-healing. It is from the same word as
panacea, which means cure-all. We find this name in Ezekiel
(27:17), where it is said that 'they traded wheat of Minnith, and
Pan-nag, and honey, and oil and balm'.

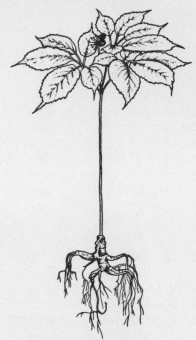

Figure 2 Panax Ginseng.

The plant belongs to the Araliacea family, in company with the humble ivy and the spikenard. Ginseng has a fleshy root which is thick and yellow. The root often bends sideways as it grows; it usually has one or two fat branches and from them sprout long wispy rootlets. At the top of the root there is a 'neck' which is in fact a short rhizome, or underground stem. Some roots do look man-shaped, even at a casual glance. It tastes slightly bitter with an undertone of aromatic sweetness.

The foliage, in contrast to the root, is rather plain. It has a straight stalk which reaches up to a metre in height, topped by an array of serrated leaves in groups of five. The pale green flowers only appear when the plant is three or four years old. The plant bears bright red edible berries which are its only means of reproduction. Birds like them and spread the seeds in their droppings. As the plant gets older, further stems appear, and a very old plant can grow a central stalk supporting up to five separate stems. At this stage the Chinese call the plant 'the hundred feet'. The plant is a deciduous perennial, that is to say

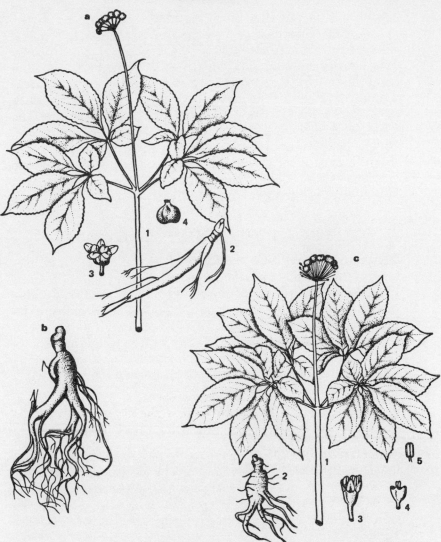

Figure 2a   Panax ginseng: 1. Habit sketch of aerial portion of a fruiting branch. 2. The underground portion of plant showing fleshy taproot, branches and adventitious roots attached to the *Lu-t'ou*. 3. A flower. 4. A fruit.

Figure 2b   A *Pa-huo* Tassel Ginseng from a sixteen–year–old root.

Figure 2c   Panax pseudo-ginseng: 1. The habit sketch of aerial portion of plant in fruit. 2. Underground portion showing short stem and fusiform fleshy primary root. 3. A flower. 4. An anther. 5. A flower with petals and stamen removed.

the leafy material dies every autumn and regrows in the spring. One curious aspect of the yearly regrowth is that it occurs from a bud situated at the peak of the root. The rhizome lengthens every year, and in order to keep the bud at ground level the root shrinks into the earth by an exactly equivalent amount. This annual shrinkage produces wrinkles on the neck of the root which have always been used to assess its age. The Chinese believe that the plant can be very old indeed. A Russian expert on ginseng, Grushvitzky, claimed he had found a root which was 400 years old.[5] A Royal Botanic Gardens expert doubted these fantastic figures, but conceded that he could find no evidence to the contrary.

THE ROOT THAT HIDES FROM MAN

Between the thirty-fifth and forty-fifth parallels, in the mountainous forests of the northern temperate zone of the Far East, lies ginseng country. Wild ginseng grows deep within deciduous forest on rich moist loam, hidden and protected. Its preference for shaded and inaccessible places has given rise to the name which is our subtitle. It was often found in association with a certain broad-leafed tree which provided maximum shade. This has led to the well-known Korean song:

The branches which grow from my stalks are three in number and the leaves are five by five; the back part of the leaves is turned to the sky. Whoever would find me must look for the Kia tree.

As Dr Yu of the Harvard Arboretum has pointed out, there is in fact no such tree as the Kia tree. The Korean characters for *kia* and *tuan* are very close. *Tuan* is the linden or basswood tree. Its Asiatic version is called botanically Tilia tuan. This confusion should have been detected long ago, for *kia* is Korean for false!

It is widely held that ginseng glows in the dark. Ginseng hunters used to go out at night armed with bows and arrows and shoot at the plant from a distance. The next day at first light they would go out and find the plant where the arrow stood. This has led to all kinds of legends with a distinctly ghostly flavour. A modern one is that ginseng emits some kind of phosphorescent radiation. This is unlikely; a more probable but mundane explanation for the light is that it is

produced by glow-worms, which, like humans, are attracted
to the plant.

Wild ginseng was never very common. Ginseng collectors
in China were called *va-pang-suis* and their profession was
extremely dangerous. They were preyed upon by vicious
bandits called the White Swans, who killed many of them to
get the root. The only redeeming feature of these bandits was
that they believed that no prospector should be robbed twice.
They would present a red-bordered flag to the unfortunate
victim to signify to other bandits that he had already been
cleaned out. These ginseng collectors still maintain much of
the old tradition, together with its fears and faiths. They
preserve the special rituals and the ancient jargon. They refrain
from meat and sexual intercourse for some time before the
search, and rely heavily on their dreams to guide them and
give them signs or warnings.

Nowadays wild ginseng has all but vanished as a result of
overcropping, deforestation and the ineluctable march of civil-
ization. The tuan tree has no precious neighbour. However, a
few roots can be found in the high mountains of north-east
China, in the wild areas of Heilungkiang, Kirin, Liaoning, in
the northern Hopei provinces and on the southern border of
Manchuria. Some of these roots are 'escaped' ginseng which
has somehow returned to nature from cultivation beds. There
are still ginseng prospectors in China.

In Korea, wild ginseng used to be found growing in
Pyongyanbuk-do province. Now the plant is well on its way
to total extinction in its wild state. There are perhaps a
hundred wild roots still growing. These supply the twenty to
eighty professional ginseng collectors or *shimmani* still searching, and a thousand amateurs. Although this scarcity would
seem to make collecting a fruitless enterprise, the ginseng
collectors know that because of the high prices paid for wild
ginseng they only need to find one root in their entire lives. It is
said that twenty men have already detected roots and keep a
careful but secret eye on them, waiting until they are mature
enough to be sold. The others scrape the deep valleys and
peaks of mountains such as Sorak, Odae, Chiri and Kaya in the
remaining forests and National Park land of South Korea. It is
this collecting which, as the head of the wild ginseng society
put it, is 'set to snuff out the wild root like a wind approaching

a candle flame'. There is no legal protection of the root at present and the government surely ought to take that step as soon as possible; whether it would make any difference is debatable.

The wild root is remarkably different from the cultivated root. It is long, thin and flexible, while the cultivated is short, fat and fleshy. The wild root can be bent double without breaking, which has led to the piquant description of its elasticity in one Chinese classic: 'like an angel's bosom'. It grows very slowly over long periods. The wild root is usually much older than the cultivated form and local sources hold strongly to the view that such roots are often two or three hundred years old. The roots are traditionally of child, dragon, phoenix, yin-yang, turtle and human types; the latter is, naturally, the best. The wild root has a strong aroma and a very strong taste which is easily distinguishable from culti-vated ginseng. With prices so high, it can be assumed that some attempts are made to transplant cultivated ginseng back to the forests. When professional collectors pull up a wild root they always plant seeds in the same place. The resulting ginseng is almost as good as the wild root and virtually as expensive. But when cultivated ginseng is put back to the forest it does not turn into the wild plant. Something has happened to it in 600 years of cultivation. It has suffered some kind of genetic drift away from its original form. This means, of course, that the few wild roots remaining are the last genetic resource of the original celestial root.

The last area still sufficiently populated with wild ginseng to support a small army of collectors is the Ussuri region of the Soviet Far East. There are still large tracts of wild land in the Taighur. Collectors, both amateur and professional, are strong and dedicated people. They would not be worthy of their name if they did not return year by year whether they found ginseng or not. Several writers, including Mikhail Prishwyn, and V. K. Arseniev, the author of *Dersu the Trapper*, write of the drama and the mystery of the search. They go after the root of life, and it is more than just a medicine they are looking for.

MASS PRODUCTION

The fields are seas of straw, the lines of rough thatched shades like waves. Lush green foliage flourishes under the cool thatch. The soil is a fine rich loam, prepared with a care and labour unequalled by the most exacting of farmers. The cultivation is long and difficult, and it has daunted expert botanists from Western Europe, for no one has successfully grown Asiatic ginseng there.

The Koreans have cultivated ginseng since 1300, traditionally at Songto, near the capital, and at Yong-san and Kamsan. Nowadays ginseng growing covers every nook and cranny of the Korean peninsula, producing thousands of tons of the root. The best comes from upland places such as Pocheon. But there is a surprising uniformity in the manner of cultivation, and in the roots that result. The tiniest little ginseng bed, a couple of lines of straw thatch next to a row of Chinese cabbages, produces similar ginseng to the giant farms covering acres on the choicest hillsides.

The fields are prepared on gentle slopes facing north or north-east. At one time the earth used to be carted in huge loads from the forest floor for use in the farms. The Koreans now prepare beds of crushed granite soil, adding clear sand and leaf mould. A mulch of rotted leaves, wood and sometimes other organic fertilizers such as chicken droppings or bone are added. No chemical fertilizers are permitted.

Traditionally, ginseng was always planted on soil which had never previously known a similar crop. It was imagined that ginseng took the essence of the earth for its healing power and devitalized the soil completely in the process. Fields used to remain fallow for ten to fifteen years, with supplements of organic material regularly ploughed in. Nowadays, mass cultivation cannot wait so long. The usual practice is to plant pulses which provide nitrogenous fertilizer, and then to leave the land fallow for two years, ploughing about twelve times during this period. This short-cut has allowed more ginseng to be grown, but the costs, it has turned out, have been high. 'Soil sickness' is rife among today's ginseng crops, causing rotting of the roots. In 1965, 80 per cent of Kumsan ginseng was affected by root rot and most discarded. Something like a quarter of the roots now grown in Korea are affected by rot in some way. This is due to various organisms that live in the soil, particularly fungi. Some experiments with biological control are in progress at the College of Agriculture in Seoul, but little useful information has emerged, except the finding that certain special fertilizers such as clam shell can reduce the disease agents in the soil.[6]

Ginseng is planted from seed taken only from four-year-old plants. The seeds usually require eighteen months to two years to sprout – another strange phenomenon to add to the list of the plant's peculiarities. Korean farmers have developed methods of hastening germination by keeping the seeds cool and dark in moist moss or sand. The opened seeds are sown in little trenches inside sheds made of rice-stalk matting. Sand is sprayed on top. Once in three days the seedlings are watered and the bed inspected to prevent crowding, decay and the attacks of worms and insects. The plants are always kept in the deepest shade.

In the second year after germination a soil of fine loam, sand and chicken droppings is added to prevent the seedlings from toppling. The seedlings are transplanted in the following spring. The plants remain in this bed one year and are replanted again; according to some reports, they are transplanted once more the next year. The beds for the maturing plants are covered with straw shades, simulating the forest environment. The roots are pulled up after six or seven years, carefully so that all the fine rootlets remain intact.

The elaborate care of the plant does not stop there. The roots used once to be carefully washed by hand and the earth removed with fine brushes. The roots were scraped and then taken to the steaming-house where they were steamed in earthenware vessels over boilers fuelled with pinewood, after which they were dried in the sun. Then they were subjected to several days of curing, hung by bamboo poles over charcoal fires in a special building. They were then taken out and dried in the sun. 'During this process the roots become very toughly hard, and their colour changes from carroty white to nearly cherrywood red. They break hard but crisply, exhibiting a shiny glassy fracture.'[7] This is the famous red ginseng, believed to be more powerful than the white which is sun-dried without curing.

The processing of ginseng is now a modern industrial procedure carried out in huge factories, with white-coated Korean girls standing by the conveyor belts. The same basic methods are used. The roots are washed by hand and machine. Then they are steamed in huge pressure vessels. They are dried in ovens as well as in the sun and then checked, sorted and graded. The root still comes out partly translucent. Upland ginseng is used to make red ginseng, and lowland ginseng, from Daejeon and its environs, is used for white ginseng. If it is processed as red ginseng this lowland ginseng tends to develop holes within the root. Ginseng is then sold as roots, or pulverized, tabletted, encapsulated, made into teas or extracts.

It is worth remembering that the ginseng root is the antithesis of the little white pill. Only within modern medicine is a drug so standardized that in every dose we find exactly identical amounts of exactly identical substances. With plant remedies there is always a great variety of forms to choose from, providing the advantage of diversity and the disadvantage of uncertainty. There are many different grades and types of ginseng on the market. The roots are noticeably different due to the manner of curing, of steaming, of gathering and of growing. Furthermore, each ecology nurtures a different kind of plant with different properties, due to differences in the soil, the weather and associated conditions. Such is the case with many plants with which man has a close relationship. There are hundreds of types of tobacco produced in different ways to give varieties of flavour which suit different people. We have a section on the varieties of the root in the appendix.

The whole industry in Korea astonished me. The Koreans seem to have adapted the traditionally complex art of growing ginseng with considerable skill and ingenuity to the modern world. It is no mean feat to export $70 million-worth of a plant which is so hard to cultivate and tricky to process. Yet there is a nagging doubt in my mind. The cultivated root is certainly much poorer in quality than the wild root. The short-cuts necessary for mass production may have reduced the medicinal potency of the plant even further. The worrying thing is that no one really knows by how much. There are no studies of the wild versus the cultivated root, of the forest-cultivated versus the field-cultivated, or of the factory-processed versus the hand-processed. For example, the Chinese stressed that ginseng was not to be boiled in metal vessels, yet ginseng is extracted in factories in enormous metal vats. Until these kinds of studies are carried out I will always be concerned that the root may be drifting into medicinal inferiority with each new development.

Extensive cultivation of ginseng occurs in China, especially in Kirin and Liaoning, where the imperial ginseng used to grow wild. The Chinese methods are similar to those of the Koreans. The Chinese do not export such quantities of pure ginseng. Most of it is grown for home use. However, they use considerable amounts in tonic wines, extracts and traditional medicines which they export all over the world, especially to Chinese communities abroad.[8] The Chinese have many elaborate ways of curing ginseng. They produce, besides red and white, some sugared ginseng roots which are pricked with needles and then soaked for twelve hours in sugar syrup before drying in the sun. The piercing, soaking and drying are repeated. Sometimes the branched rootlets are removed, sometimes they are tied to the tap root to give a whip-like tail; sometimes the pricking or stabbing with a bamboo knife is artfully executed so that the root takes on the shape of a man on drying.

During the 1930s, Soviet scientists had been carrying out extended tests with their wild ginseng. Then in 1945 the Soviets occupied North Korea. They found the Korean excitement over ginseng infectious. Their interest renewed, they collected many wild roots to be sent back to Russia for study. What they found is the story of the next chapter. As Richard Lucas writes, from contemporary diplomatic records and from his own experience at that time:

Evidence of continuing Soviet interest was revealed when a report announced that the Russians had confiscated an entire crop of ginseng from North Korea during the Korean conflict. Shortly after, team after team of Russian scientists were sent into neighbouring countries to study established ginseng plantations on the spot. As a result, the Russians now have tremendous plantations of ginseng in their own country, where the root is widely used for medicinal and tonic purposes. It is also exported in large quantities to Africa, India and elsewhere.[9]

The first Russian plantations, the hidden plots of Siberian trappers or of emigré Chinese, were situated in the Ussuri region. Now there are huge state farms, one of the biggest being known, not surprisingly, as Zenshen. The farms lie in the Ussuri, in Siberia, Byelorussia and south of Khabarovsk. Russian cultivation methods are today more technological than in other countries. For example, they found that by soaking the seeds briefly in a plant hormone called gibberellic acid they were able to cut down germination times dramatically.[10] They also carefully control the condition, humidity, aeration and illumination of the soil. The Russians, interestingly, have found that their methods allow them to grow Asiatic ginseng in European Russia and countries of Southeast Europe such as Bulgaria. Large-scale experiments are carried out in the forests of Northern Caucasus, especially the Tiberdin reserve. Recently, the growing of ginseng has been taken completely out of the natural environment. At Moscow State University ginseng is grown indoors, in glass vessels in a nutrient medium. The old Lubin would have found zenshen radically changed. Scientists have hauled ginseng out of the layers upon layers of its history, just as the last of the wild roots are now being pulled out of their dark recesses amid the rotten leaves of the forest floor. Ginseng will never be the same again.

GINSENG IN EUROPE

The West always knew of the Asiatic ginseng. Marco Polo and all the great travellers to China spoke of it. It may have been brought from the East on the silk route, together with other spices. Ibn Cordoba, one of the great seafaring Arabs, is credited with bringing ginseng back from China in the middle of the ninth century AD. Arab doctors after that time knew of the healing properties of ginseng, but this knowledge was apparently lost with the decline of Arab culture. Ginseng began to turn up in the West again at the end of the seventeenth century, when the rapacious East India Company and the equivalent Compagnie des Indies imported it. It was touted as a panacea at that time by apothecaries and quacks, but we know little of it for it is submerged under a flood of elixirs and miracle cures of doubtful origin and even more doubtful effectiveness.

A new chapter began in the reign of the Chinese Emperor K'ang-hsi, the man who put medicine in the arena. He favoured Jesuits because of their scholarship and sent one missionary, Père Jartoux, into the interior to make maps. The good father was struck by the power of ginseng. He wrote back to the Royal Society of London in 1711 about the plant the Tartars call 'orhota' or Chief of Plants. He related how he became very tired after a long period on horseback. His guide gave him a little bit of ginseng to chew and within an hour he could carry on with renewed energy, quite oblivious of his previous fatigue.[11] Ginseng thus became known in European medical circles. When a delegation from the King of Siam arrived in the court of Louis XIV, they gave the Sun King a royal gift of a first-class 'Gintz-aen' root. Ginseng became appreciated in France, especially by the aristocracy. It was imported into Holland and used by the most famous Dutch doctors in cases of exhaustion and debility. It became available in select pharmacies all over Europe, and entered some eclectic materia medica such as Geoffroy's, published in 1840. Ginseng was represented sporadically in European pharmacopoeiae during the nineteenth century, but the early part of this century saw it vanish from sight.

This was partly because of a purge of Galenicals (vegetable drugs). Besides this, when American ginseng reached Europe in the mid-nineteenth century, it began to replace the more expensive Asiatic ginseng in the apothecaries. The confusion of the true ginseng with the much less effective American ginseng led to much of its disrepute. Ginseng has only begun to resurface in recent years through a resurgence of popular interest in herbal remedies.

BOONE'S CARGO

Daniel Boone may seem an unlikely companion to the Tartars, but he too was a ginseng collector. He personally gathered large amounts of ginseng in America and purchased more from white settlers. In 1787 he started up the Ohio in a boat containing nearly fifteen tons of ginseng. The boat overturned and he lost it all. Undismayed, he returned and collected another boat load by the next year. He made more money from ginseng than any other commodity.

The ginseng he collected is American ginseng, Panax quinquefolium, a cousin of the Asiatic species. American ginseng is also found in the Himalayas. It has an unusual history, which comes as no surprise, since ginseng seems to gather extraordi-

nary tales around it like a botanical Ulysses. The Jesuit priest in
China, Père Jartoux, reported on his ginseng experience not
only to the Royal Society, but also in a Jesuit bulletin. He
mentioned that ginseng might be found in Canada, where the
forests and mountains resembled those in the ginseng regions
of China. Père Lafiteau, a Jesuit missionary in Canada, read the
bulletin and began a search for the root. He eventually found it
'by accident when I was not thinking of it, near a house I was
having built. . . . I pulled it up and with joy took it to an Indian
I had engaged to help me hunt for it. She recognized it at once
as one of those the Indians used'.[12]

Lafiteau's discovery brought the Chinese to Canada to
explore the purchase of ginseng. A ginseng rush began. Settlers and Indians scoured the hardwood forests for ginseng to
be shipped to Canton. The price in Quebec rose from two
francs a pound to eighty and it was sold for at least a ten-fold
profit in Canton. The Compagnie des Indies took over the
trade and shipped ginseng via France, at the same time sending
back repeated requests for more. This drove everybody into
the woods. The Indians were so busy looking for the root that

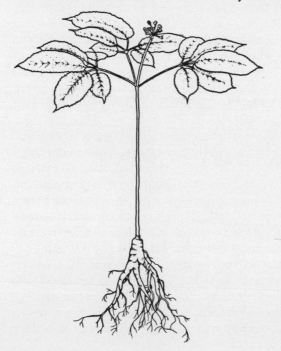

Figure 3
Panax quinquefolium
Ginseng.

the French had to gather in their harvests themselves. However, the ginseng was collected with more avidity than foresight. It was gathered out of season, regardless of age and without replanting. The root became rare. In addition, it was dried in ovens, and this made it unacceptable to the Chinese. The bottom fell out of the market, and the traders looked to the white American settlers in New England, New York and westwards for authentic supplies.

The hunt for ginseng in America was on. Whole villages were emptied of their inhabitants who went to the woods armed with mattock and sack in search of 'seng'.[13] Greater and greater quantities were shipped to China, at a huge profit to both the traders and the 'seng' diggers. The amount of ginseng exported increased steadily, reaching 622,761 pounds of dried roots in 1862. Many farmers survived drought and depression at the time by ginseng hunting. Fur trappers, including Daniel Boone, found 'seng' as profitable as furs and would return from the mountains with both. In fact, the American ginseng trade is still handled largely by the fur companies.

At the end of the nineteenth century wild ginseng became scarce, despite government attempts to regulate digging. Some enterprising farmers attempted cultivation, and a few made a great success of it. However, ginseng is attractive to other species besides humans and glow-worms. All kinds of insects, fungi and worms made cultivation a laborious and protracted struggle. In fact, virtually the entire American crop was wiped out in 1910 and an economic depression finished off the few farmers that survived.

A fascinating account of American ginseng gathering and growing at the turn of the century is written by a farmer and doctor, A. R. Harding.[14] His advice to farmers was to grow it much as the Koreans did. The seed was germinated under a sawdust or leaf mulch for eighteen months and the little plants carefully tended, cosseted and replanted until ready. Many growers found shady hardwood forests the best place to start their ginseng plantations. The high shade and good ventilation would produce heavy crops on sandy loam, but the gardens needed to be well spaced to avoid infections. As in China, the main problem with the forest-garden method was theft. The farmers had to keep a watchful eye on the plants for seven years, although one cannot imagine our Wisconsin worthies going so far as the Chinese farmers, who used to yowl eerily, pretending to be unearthly forest creatures, in order to frighten poachers.

The wild ginseng used to be found in most of the eastern states of the USA north of Missouri and Georgia. Nowadays, heavy collecting has reduced the areas where it can be found to the Allegheny mountains. It still grows well in the Catskills, where collecting has never been professionally thorough; but rather an amateur pastime for tourists and retired people. The American species is not in as much danger as its Eastern counterpart. The cultivated root is more like the wild root, and there is not so much demand for the wild root except by sensitive critical ginseng cognoscenti. Nevertheless, it is becoming rarer. Its export was banned in 1978. Most wild ginseng used to be exported, making up the annual export of a quarter of a million pounds of cultivated and wild root which went to Hong Kong every year, netting about $20 million.

There are currently large and small farms growing ginseng in limited areas of Tennessee, North Central Wisconsin and Kentucky. A letter from one Wisconsin ginseng farmer stated:

One third of the ginseng exported to China is grown within 15 miles of our farm. The land is perfect because the soil is rotted granite and rolly [sic]. The Chinese come here with sharp tongues but ready money to buy it up even before it is out of the ground. They say it is not as good as Korean, but that doesn't seem to stop them . . . also many of the big farmers sell the seeds to them. . . . The area people have for decades used it themselves and the present market is from $18–30 a lb but it is very hard to grow, very prone to diseases, and is sprayed and watched carefully. It costs about $13–15,000 an acre to plant, takes four years of backbreaking work and is a true gamble.

Strangely, neither the growers nor the dealers are really sure about their own commodity. They are influenced by the negative reports on ginseng which have appeared in America in the last fifty years. But dealers and growers nevertheless have a hunch that it may work so they keep on nibbling.

The Chinese import American ginseng because their own is expensive and in short supply, although they acknowledge the American as inferior to the Asiatic species. As long as demand outstrips supply, American ginseng will find a ready market in the Far East, although it is like shipping poor quality coals to Newcastle.

OTHER RELATIVES

Besides the cousin in America, Panax ginseng C. A. Meyer has some brothers in Asia, in particular Panax pseudoginseng var. notoginseng. This species has narrower, more serrated leaves, with seven leaflets rather than five and a shorter, fatter, more carroty root. This species yields the san-ch'i (Three Seven) ginseng, so named because of the number of its leaflets. It occurs wild in China in the mountains of Yunnan, Hopei and Kwangsi, and is now cultivated there. Almost 90 per cent of the cultivated commercial product comes today from Yunnan. The roots are pulled slightly earlier than ginseng and dried in the sun. They are then placed in a sack with wax and tumbled until they are coated and the skin is a shiny brown. The medicinal properties of san-ch'i are rather different from true ginseng but it is held in great esteem and is expensive.

We also find Panax pseudoginseng var. japonicus widely used as a medicine, especially in Japan where it grows wild. Panax bipinnafitidum is one of a range of species which can be found in the Himalayas in Nepal, Sikkim, Assam, North-east Frontier, Burma, Thailand and China. They are much more common than the true ginseng. I have seen specimens in Nepal and Professor Tanaka of Japan recounts a marvellous story of how he pitched his tent on a carpet of Himalayan ginseng in Bhutan. Like the relatives of a film star, the Himalayan species have gained respect by association with the Asiatic ginseng, and they are used as medicines in their respective localities; however, they have never been regarded as particularly out-standing. The ginseng family is summarized in Table 3.

Their classification is confusing. Some authorities feel that various Himalayan species should be subspecies of Panax pseudoginseng;[15] others feel they should be separate species; and yet others feel that many of the differences between them are due to the different sites at which they are grown and not to anything intrinsic in the plant. The question cannot be resol-ved until different plants are grown together under the same conditions, and since this difficult task has not yet been accomplished it seems that the confusion will reign on for some time yet. The classification put forward by Professor

Table 4: Varieties of Ginseng

Region	Species	Comments
China	Panax ginseng (jen seng) C. A. Meyer	Extensively cultivated, and exported to West. Many grades and commercial preparations. Wild root found occasionally in high mountain forests of Manchuria.
	Panax pseudoginseng var. notoginseng (jen seng san-ch'i) Panax pseudoginseng subsp. japonicus (chu-chieh seng)	Grows wild and cultivated in Yunnan and Kwangsi provinces.
	Panax pseudoginseng subsp. himalaicus Panax bipinnafitidum	Grows wild in W. China, Tibet.
Korea	Panax ginseng	Massive cultivation and export for 1000 years. A few wild roots currently found per year.
Japan	Panax ginseng	Cultivated roots originally from Korea, now well established, exported to China but of low quality.
	Panax pseudoginseng subsp. japonicus previously Panax repens	Indigenous species, exported to China.
Russia	Panax ginseng (Zen shen)	Cultivated roots originally from North Korea, for research and domestic consumption only. Occasionally found wild in Soviet Far East, Ussuri region.

Table 4: Varieties of Ginseng

Region	Species	Comments
America	Panax quinquefolium (American ginseng, five-fingers root)	Still grows wild, especially in Catskills; however, almost vanished in other areas through collection. Cultivated and exported to China.
Nepal, E. Himalayas, Burma, Thailand	Panax pseudoginseng subsp. himalaicus Panax quinquefolium Panax assamicus Panax bipinnafitidum	Found infrequently in East Himalayan forests. Rarely used in local medicine.

Hara seems, provisionally, to be most sensible and is the one used here.[16]

A number of types of root are substituted for ginseng by the unscrupulous. This used to happen quite frequently in China and Korea. Adenophora verticillata (sha shen) is sometimes sold as ginseng, as is Campanunoea pilosule, otherwise known as bastard ginseng (tang shen). These roots have some medicinal value, though nothing like that of ginseng. They are easily spotted, but some subtle meddling used to go on in China in which these roots were pricked and poked and tied with threads to make them man-shaped and elegant.

MAN-ROOT AND MANDRAGORA

Ginseng is often confused with the mandrake. The similarities between them are most odd. The mandrake is a man-shaped root, and this has led to its use in the West as an aphrodisiac, just like ginseng, following the Doctrine of Signatures (see page 42). Like ginseng, it is meant to house an earth spirit. This spirit strongly resists attempts to uproot it. A Chinese traveller in the Near East in the thirteenth century BC brought back reports of mandrake root which is man-shaped, 'just like our ginseng'.[2] The other similarity is the story first reported by that wordy Roman gentleman Josephus, that the mandrake glowed at night; this also seems to be due to its attraction to glow-worms.

In actual fact the mandrake, Atropa mandragorum or Mandragora officinarum, is completely unrelated to ginseng, both botanically and medicinally. Anyone drinking a brew of it believing it to be similar to ginseng will be in for a nasty surprise, for it has quite the reverse effect. The name of the mandrake comes from the Sanskrit *mandros agora*, sleep substance. It can also be made into a poison, as recommended by Lucrezia Borgia. Nothing could be further from ginseng.

THE USES OF GINSENG: SHEN NUNG AND THE *ENCYCLOPAEDIA BRITANNICA*

To hear the claims made for ginseng is to be thrust into one of two positions: either a romantic awe at this God-given root which is a most amazing panacea, or a total cynicism concerning a root which symbolizes man's capacity to make a fool of himself.

In China, ginseng is used to prevent tiredness, headaches, exhaustion, amnesia and the debilitating effects of old age. It is used supportively in the treatment of a large number of diseases of the heart, kidneys, nervous and circulatory systems. It is well known as a remedy to stay the decline in potency in older man and to assist women smoothly over the menopause. It is used by the sick to speed their return to health, by the convalescents to gain strength and by the healthy to remain so. In general, it is regarded as a restorative and prophylactic.

It is invariably chosen as the medicine for patients who suffer from any kind of general weakness, particularly 'those with signs of anaemia, lack of appetite, shortness of breath, accompanied by perspiration, nervous agitation, forgetfulness, continuous thirst, lack of strength and no sexual desire'.[8]

In Russia ginseng was always a folk medicine, used by healers such as Lubin, and in an unsophisticated way by those rural folk who could obtain it. Since the Russian ginseng jamboree in North Korea, doctors and medical personnel have used it widely and it has all the necessary authorization from the health ministries. The doctors are pragmatic about ginseng. They do not have the backing of an esoteric healing system in which ginseng has a recognized place. Rather, they have merged scientific and folk medicine into a homely and common-sense synthesis. The doctors consider ginseng to have tonic, stimulant, diuretic and gerontological (helpful in old age) properties. It is widely prescribed to adjust the blood sugar and metabolism in diabetes and other internal metabolic diseases. It is used to treat anaemia, insomnia, neurasthenia, gastritis, tiredness, depression, impotence, and any kind of weakness.

An Eastern materia medica sums up the claims: 'It nourishes and strengthens the body, stops vomiting, clears the judgement, removes hypochondrias and all other nervous affections. In a word, it gives a vigorous tone to the body even in old age.'[17] If even half these claims are proved, then ginseng will surely earn its reputation as a panacea and will be rightly called a 'wonder of the world'.

But this is not all. Ginseng is also reputed to have a short-term action. Chinese and Vietnamese troops would carry a root where possible to prevent their succumbing to stress and shock if they were wounded on the battlefield. Diplomats take it to stay awake in all-night marathons, and Henry Kissinger took it to cope with his stresses. Those in risky occupations take it to be more alert to danger and resistant to its consequence. This in fact was the use recorded by Père Jartoux in his famous letter to the Royal Society. Ginseng is used in China to restore the flagging energies of the dying, to give them time to receive their families, dispose of their properties and prepare to meet their ancestors. Rich men used to keep some excellent root aside for this purpose. It is said that when these people died, a special fungus used to grow inside the lid of the coffin which was somehow connected with their previous ingestion of superbly powerful ginseng. People would dig up the coffins and scrape off the fungus which was then sold as an extremely precious medicine called 'the mushroom of the dead'.

Ginseng was also credited with being an aphrodisiac. The Chinese stated that it gave them virility, especially later in life when they most needed it. Observers of Chinese aristocrats paint a picture of a robed man in the bedchamber, chewing a ginseng root and sipping rice wine. The emperors certainly used to take best quality ginseng as a condiment for breakfast, and then direct much of their energy towards the pleasure-house. It is today combined with deer antlers or sea horse tails as a patent virility remedy.

But others have equally strong opinions. We have already read the dismissals of pharmacopoeia and encyclopaedia in Chapter 1. A Smithsonian Institute report at the turn of the century stated that, 'Ginseng has no value as far as Western medicine can judge . . . its effects being purely psychologi- cal . . . but we have only scratched the surface of Chinese medical knowledge.' It is a lot more polite than are some modern medical men. 'Utter rubbish' is common. 'As far as we are concerned, it is completely useless as a medicine,' said a representative of a health ministry.

To make things worse, ginseng is an item of commerce and nothing can possibly sell so well as a panacea. Advertisers of ginseng products, aware of this fact, go right overboard. Their literature trumpets a veritable crescendo of claims. 'Why does the emperor drink ginseng? To cure his neurosis, headache, fatigue, senility, poor appetite, high blood pressure, low blood pressure, diabetes, sterility, cancer, arthritis, anaemia, rheumatism, allergy, bad skin, gout. . . .' Never has anything more absurd been said about a medicine since the American quacks touted their nostrums on soapboxes. A joke is only a hairsbreadth from absurdity, and sure enough one Belgian advertiser has unwittingly produced a few belly-laughs with the statement that ginseng should be taken if 'connubial intercourse is followed by deficient salivation causing dryness of mouse' [sic]. I have a little ginseng root pipe which states that the merits of the pipe involve the 'circulation of the blood, all healthy effect exhibition, nicotine removal, smoking saving and a long life'!

What a mess. What is beneath this pyramid of claim and counter-claim? Where is the kernel of truth? It is necessary to go back to the beginning again and carefully examine the traditional Chinese use of ginseng. This is stated eloquently and succinctly by the *Pharmacopoeia* of Shen Nung: 'It tastes sweetish and its property is slightly cooling. It grows in the gorges of the mountains. It is used for repairing the five viscera, harmonizing energies, strengthening the soul, allay- ing fear, removing toxic substances, brightening the eyes, opening the heart, and improving thought. Continuous use will invigorate the body and prolong life.'

This is ginseng in a nutshell. The 'repair of the five viscera' is the key, although expressed in Chinese terms. As we have seen, the five viscera are the basic working systems within the human frame, each with its own portion of the five elements and degree of the Yin/Yang polarity. Now ginseng was not only the chief of the kingly harmony remedies, but also the most Yang of them all. Its function on the body process was to *pu* (restore) the Yang. In other words, to promote a flow of energy, increase heat, and burn up stored and toxic substances. Ginseng had Yang fire. It promoted the expression of potential body energy which had become blocked, diseased or lethargic.

Ginseng's heat could be directed selectively at certain organ systems, homing in on them by combining ginseng in prescriptions with an appropriate 'servant' to carry it to the particular function in need. Thus the *Pen-tshao kang mu*, the classic Chinese pharmacopoeia based on Shen Nung's earlier work, stated that ginseng combined with Cimicifuga heracleifolia strengthens the lungs, with Poria cocos strengthens the kidneys, with Ophiopogon japonicus helps the heart and the pulse, with ginger, Zingiber officinale, increases strength, with liquorice, Glycyrrhiza uralensis, and Astralagus membranaceous removes or drains the fire from Yin organs (e.g. 'spleen', digestion and metabolism), and increases resistance and vital energy. It can be used with certain balancing factors to distribute and therefore increase ginseng's power, e.g. tangerine peel, or the jujube. It must never be used with hellebores, e.g. Veratrum nigrum, which cancel its effect. Ginseng is used more in combination than alone, and this sometimes makes for difficulties in distinguishing its special effect.[19]

These are all restorative, not curative, uses of ginseng. It is important to understand that ginseng is never used alone as a curative medicine. However, it is found in complex mixtures for the treatment of a variety of diseases. In these cases it is used supportively to provide strength to diseased organs and energy for the process of self-healing. Chieh-pin Chang described no less than 500 remedies containing ginseng for every kind of disease in a book written 1000 years ago. There are restrictions as to the stage of the disease at which ginseng may be given. The right time is usually when the disease is in retreat. If it is applied too early its strong Yang energy may possibly fuel the disease rather than the resistance.

At the same time, Shen Nung makes no bones about the fact that ginseng by itself is a strong revitalizing agent. He categorically states that ginseng is used to make the mind and the body work better and more efficiently. This use of ginseng against weakness, fatigue, stress, lassitude, debility, anaemia, reduced potency and so on is a regular theme that is aired again and again. It is surely the kind of use one would expect of it if the Chinese 'tonic' plants work at all, and if ginseng is, as claimed, the most potent of them all. Furthermore, there is no doubt that the Chinese make heavy use of ginseng in this way.

A Korean expert on plant medicines recently surveyed nearly 500 Oriental prescriptions. He found that 28 per cent of them contain ginseng, a proportion far higher than any other single plant medicine. More to the point, he found that no less than 57 per cent of those remedies in the mild 'kingly' class contained ginseng, 30 per cent of those in the middle 'princely' class and only 5 per cent of remedies in the more toxic 'assistant' class.[20]

Here are some examples of Chinese harmony remedies:

Four Gentlemen Soup: For someone with a weak stomach and poor appetite. A kingly 'tonic' remedy, especially for renewing strength after illness. Boil up:

      30g Ginseng
      60g Atractylis microcephala root
      3g Poria cocos
      1.5g Glycyrrhiza uralensis (liquorice)
      3   slices fresh ginger
      1   fruit of Ziziphus jujuba (jujube)

in 500 ml of water until reduced to half, and give some to patient before meals.

After Childbirth Pills: For a mother who bleeds excessively:

      Ginseng
      Cannabis sativa seeds
      Poncirus trifoliata skin

Roasted in bran and ground to a powder to be mixed with honey to make pills. On the other hand, if the mother is weak and feverish without bleeding, a soup made of ginseng, Angelica sinensis, glutinous rice and pig's kidney is recommended.

For generalized Yin depletion
> Astralagus membranaceous
> Ginseng: *equal amounts*

Ground into a powder, taken with Chinese radish soaked in honey.

White Tiger potion: For outer heat and inner coldness, dry palate, cold hands and feet, and body weakness:
> Anamarrhena asphodeloides: *6 parts*
> Powdered gypsum: *16 parts*
> Glycyrrhiza glabra (liquorice): *2 parts*
> Ground rice: *6 parts*
> Ginseng extract: *3 parts*

The same harmony plants seem to crop up again and again almost indiscriminately in both these vitality concoctions and in mixtures for the treatment of diseases.[19] In curative medicine each mixture contains non-specific remedies which prepare the ground, and specific substances which then root out the specific disease. Thus the tonic remedies are fundamental tools of the physician, and the specific remedies are the special tools. In the same way a mechanic has one reliable set of tools – spanners, a screwdriver, a hammer – to enable him to set to work on a car, and special tools – a hub extractor, a soldering iron, a valve grinder – for specific repairs. Ginseng is one of the most important and most frequently used of the general remedies, and therefore it has gained a little of the reputation that should by rights belong only to all the remedies of which it is a part. This is one of the origins of its designation as a panacea. Certainly no proper Chinese doctor will state that it is a panacea, a cure-all. It is instead, he will say, a basic health instrument.

It is the West, utterly misreading the principles of Chinese medicine, which has given ginseng the description of a panacea. The very concept of a panacea is a dream of the Western medical system, devoted to curative medicine. There is no place for it in the Oriental practitioner's language. His dream would be of 'all-health'. In actual fact, the Greeks did regard the word more as 'all-health' than as 'all-healing'; Panacea was a goddess, the daughter of Aesculapius, and they knew her not as the goddess of complete healing but of complete health.

If you try to slip into the Chinese way of looking at health, like a crab sidling into water, the wide range of uses made of ginseng begins to seem quite understandable. Imagine your body, without organs or tissues. It is more like a giant amoeba in which the processes of digestion, assimilation, reproduction, combustion, reaction, communication and consciousness are deep currents visible only by their eddies on the surface; the pulses, colours and textures which the doctor perceives on the outside of the body. The currents can whirl against each other, leading to a crashing maelstrom which wastes energy (excess Yang), or to a silent dead backwater which becomes stagnant and poisoned (excess Yin). The harmony medicines widen the channels. The currents flow smoothly and fast, each integrated with the next. The stream has more momentum – it is stronger and not so easily blocked.

If we now re-examine the list of claims made for ginseng, it can be seen that they are not quite so broad as one first thought. They have something in common. They invariably relate to conditions where the body has reduced vitality, situations where the restoration of Yang energy would be likely to be useful. The more extravagant claims are certainly misunderstandings of ginseng's subtle action.

THE CHEROKEES' 'LITTLE MAN': GINSENG'S RELATIVES IN USE

Two classic confusions have contributed to the current demise of ginseng. The first is that the cultivated root has the same properties as the wild root, which it does not. The second is that the root of American ginseng is the same as the root of the true Asiatic ginseng. This mix-up should never have happened. When negative reports were published on ginseng, especially one from the Smithsonian Institute, everyone accepted that there was only one ginseng and that it grew in the Far East and the United States. Studies were limited to the American species but the conclusions were applied to ginseng as a whole. It was a mistake that a first-year student should not have made, and only arose because of the lack of convenient dried specimens of the Asiatic ginseng in the West. Without this mistake, the history of ginseng in the West might have been utterly different.

Even a cursory study of the uses made of the American species shows that it is likely to be different from its Asiatic brother. For example, it was respected as a stomachic by the Iroquois, in whose territory it was found by Père Lafiteau, and the Ojuiba made a similar use of it. The Menonini and the Cherokees both called the American ginseng 'the little man' in their different languages, and used it as a tonic and against cramps and menstrual problems. The Creeks drank an infusion of the root for shortness of breath, croup and fevers, while other tribes used it as a supportive aid for the wounded. Ginseng, as all Indian medicines, tended to be associated with magic, incantation and ritual, compared to which the Chinese use of it is coldly rational and sophisticated.

The American Indians claim far less for their ginseng than the Chinese, and the use made of it is sporadic. It is neither their most important plant nor one held in the highest esteem. Similarly in China, Panax quinquefolium does grow but is used as a low-grade ginseng. The *Barefoot Doctor's Manual* describes it as a tonic, producing more saliva and increasing appetite. It is clearly not the chief of medicines.

The Indian remedies became part of frontier medicine, transmitted by quacks and travelling herbalists. Ginseng was entered in the early US dispensaries and could be found in the *US Pharmacopoeia* until 1882. The herbals of this period describe uses for the American ginseng which confirm its distance from the Asiatic species. Dr Williams's herbal of 1827 stated that ginseng eased 'inward hurts and ulcers' and recommended ginseng combined with calamus, angelica and white root (Asclepias tuberosa) for windy colic. Jonathan Carver held that ginseng was a great strengthener of the stomach. Barton, an early botanical physician, felt that the Indians did not 'so highly esteem the ginseng as their Tartar brethren in Asia', and felt that ginseng was by no means a powerful stimulant. The same comment is repeated in other records of those times.[21]

A. R. Harding, the dedicated physician and ginseng cultivator, had some interesting things to say about Panax quinquefolium, and he is a good guide to the use of ginseng in rural America at the turn of the century. He gives a recipe for a ginseng tea which he says 'is a most pleasant aromatic drink, with a good effect on the stomach, brain and nervous system.' The writer prefers it 'to all the whisky and patent medicines made. To all those who are damaged or made nervous by drinking coffee or tea, quit the coffee or tea and take ginseng tea as directed.'[14]

He believes it to act through removal of poisons in digestion: 'If I should advise or prescribe a treatment for the old "seng digger" who is troubled with dyspepsia or foul stomach, I would tell him to take some of your own medicine and don't be selling all to the Chinamen.' Harding perpetuated the error that ginseng is the same all over the world, that American ginseng is a mild aromatic tonic, and that the Chinese belief that the Asiatic ginseng is anything more than that is superstition. Harding confesses himself puzzled by the Chinese claims. He is aware of the strength of their belief in ginseng and cannot bring himself to dismiss it entirely. Particularly because, he says with astonishing crudity, 'they are said to be a people who neither "kiss nor cuss", and their physical sensibilities are so dull that a Chinaman can lie down on his back across his wheelbarrow with feet and head hanging to the ground, his mouth wide open and full of flies, and sleep blissfully for hours under the hottest July sun. There is nothing about them, therefore, to suggest that they possess the lively imagination to make them have faith in a remedy with purely imaginary virtues. Nevertheless . . . a plant not found by any medical scientist to possess any curative powers is used almost universally, to cure every type of ailment and has been used so for generations.'

Although I am reluctant to leave the tale of the use of Panax quinquefolium on a note of such ignorant prejudice, it does serve as a reminder of the persistence of the bamboo curtain into our day and age. European opinion of Chinese medicine is almost as prejudiced today, despite its more sophisticated mode of expression. It still says that the pub on the corner has the best beer in the world.

Other plants in ginseng's extended family are also used for different purposes, though, as we have already observed, they do not command the same respect as Panax ginseng. The best of the relatives is the Chinese Panax pseudoginseng var. notoginseng, *san-ch'i* ginseng. It is a weak tonic and is used more to stop bleeding, disperse blood which has leaked out of the vessels (e.g. in bruises), and reduce swelling and pain. It is prescribed for accidents, bruises, boils and bleeding, swelling, internal haemorrhage and irregular menstruation. Other species, Panax pseudoginseng subsp. japonicus and Panax major, are also used to disperse extravasated blood. The Himalayan ginseng species are used generally as mild aromatic tonics. Local Himalayan tribes and the Ayurvedic doctors of India use these varieties in cases of poor appetite, indigestion and nervous complaints.

A somewhat more distant group of ginseng relatives is used in both Chinese and Russian medicine, particularly today. The *Barefoot Doctor's Manual* states that Tetrapanax papyritera has 'cooling properties, clears fever, promotes diuresis, stimulates milk production', and is useful in cystitis and poor lactation. Acanthopanax gracilistylus 'dispels wind and moisture, strengthens sinews and bones, especially of the back and the knees'.[19] It is used particularly in rheumatoid conditions. The Russians use Echinopanax elatum, 'samnicha', in a similar manner to the true ginseng. It is frequently prescribed as a tincture of the root against debility, asthenia, depression and low blood pressure. They are also interested in the toning, strengthening effects of connected plants such as Acanthopanax spinosum, Aralia chinensis, Aralia cordata and Aralia racemosa. The last is the spikenard which is indigenous to both East and West. It was used as a medicine in America by the Indians and early settlers, and became accepted into the *National Formulary* in 1916. Carver made 'a most palatable and reviving cordial' from spikenard berries. The Indians used it in cases of blood poisoning, to cure earache and relieve asthma, for wounds and as a mild stimulant. Its uses are clearly not unlike that of Panax quinquefolium in America. All these ginseng relatives, including the American ginseng, have properties which are not grossly dissimilar. But the true ginseng stands head and shoulders above them.

SIGNPOSTS

In summary, we can see that ginseng is perhaps the most important of Chinese remedies. Exotic and extraordinary powers are claimed for it, but closer examination shows these to be overenthusiastic. A careful probe of the way the Chinese healers regard and use ginseng enables us to streamline the claims. Ginseng then appears as a non-specific vitalizing and harmonizing substance. It 'repairs Yang', and tunes and energizes body functions. It is not curative. Its use in sickness is intended to set the stage advantageously for the confrontation with the disease, and for this purpose it is combined in a large proportion of all compound remedies. It is said to have effects against fatigue, impotence and debility in old age. There is a mosaic of grades of ginseng. There are also a number of relatives with connected but inferior properties.

The claims made for it, even after some pruning, are remarkable. Yet can this be evidence that there is something very special in the ginseng root? The answer is no. We are attempting to prove the effectiveness of ginseng and the harmony remedies, using the language and the methods of the West. Science is very clear about enthusiasm: it is completely inadmissible as evidence. Nowhere is this more true than in investigations into drugs, where elaborate precautions are taken against subjectivity.

Unfortunately, the pursuit of objectivity leads to some very sticky situations, particularly because the importance of the *will* in the healing process is not recognized. The degree of enthusiasm for the ginseng root becomes a challenge to the principle of objectivity itself. Since the passion for a drug is not taken as evidence by science, it implies that the enthusiasm is baseless; those who are enthusiastic are regarded as quite probably deluded. This may be possible in a clinical trial with fifty people but is it possible when half the globe is involved? Can any expert say that one billion people are suffering from the placebo effect? Of course not. Delusions of that kind can affect some of the people some of the time but not all of the people all of the time.

Nevertheless, we will pursue our quest along scientific lines and discover whether or not these medicines can be objectively demonstrated to work. For the present, the myths can be used as signposts in the search for the real importance of this 'root of being'.

5
Analysis of a
'Celestial Medicine'

BREKHMAN AND THE RUSSIAN SOLDIERS –
A SPRINT INTO NEW TERRITORY

One cold morning in the spring of 1948 one hundred young Soviet soldiers set out to run a special three-kilometre race. A young candidate of science of the USSR Academy of Sciences waited anxiously at the finishing line as the soldiers tore across the countryside of Eastern Siberia on the outskirts of Vladivostok. Each soldier had been given a spoonful of a bitter-tasting liquid several hours previously. While half of them had drunk liquid containing nothing but flavourings, the other half had consumed a special ingredient disguised by the flavours. None of the soldiers knew which they had drunk. The race ended. The scientist pocketed his stop-watch and went off to calculate the figures. There was more than a twinkle in his eye as he wrote them down. The soldiers taking the ingredient ran the course in fourteen minutes thirty-three seconds, while those taking just the flavourings took on average fifty-three seconds longer. The difference was of major significance: if the soldiers were carrying batons in a relay race, the group taking this drug would arrive *forty-five minutes* before the others.[1]

This new substance was none other than an extract of ginseng. The man was I. I. Brekhman, of the Institute of Biologically Active Substances in Vladivostok, who later became a professor and head of the Institute. He can rightly be called the Grand Old Man of research into the Oriental harmony remedies.

He had asked himself those same questions which lie at the back of all of our minds. Were these plants drugs or placebos? If they were drugs, how could they be tested? If they acted in the restorative fashion claimed by the Chinese, they were new to science; what methods could be used to test an action that could not even be defined in scientific terms? The answer is obvious when you think about it. What does an engineer do when he wants to test the strength of a structure? He applies massive force to parts of it to see if it can survive a brief but intense stress. He makes the necessary assumption that such a treatment is equivalent to prolonged mild stress. Similarly, to test the vitality of a man you examine his capacity in an extreme situation. With these thoughts in mind, Brekhman chose stamina as an indicator of vitality. He tested ginseng on fit young men at the limit of their capacity. In actual fact the ancient Chinese also used to test ginseng in this manner, by sending men on a march of several miles. This was not, however, to prove that the root was effective, which they felt was utterly obvious, but to differentiate ginseng from its substitutes.

Brekhman's experiment was a breakthrough, the first time that ginseng had been properly tested on man, and the first time an objective effect on the human body had been demonstrated. For Professor Brekhman the experiment mapped his course for many years to come. For Russian science it provided an intriguing puzzle which began to occupy institutes, laboratories and scientific adventurers. For the Russian people it meant a supply of ginseng through their doctor with the stamp of official approval. Its echoes are still reverberating around the world today. One of them is the change in attitudes in Russia and elsewhere to Chinese medicinal plants and herbal medicine. Another is this book.

One swallow doesn't make a summer. It takes a mosaic of evidence derived from different kinds of studies before a drug's effectiveness can be regarded as proved. One of the problems with the three-kilometre run was that it was too physical to be a realistic measure of vitality. Vitality is the capacity of the whole being, not just the heart and legs.

So a new series of tests was begun. Wireless operators and telegraphists were employed initially, for they need to carry out fast physical actions for as long as possible, and they also need mental concentration and co-ordination. An early test went something like this. Radio operators were required to transmit a special text for five minutes – two minutes longer than the normal limit. All the subjects were healthy young professionals. They carried out the test eighteen times. They transmitted the text before and after they were given ginseng extract or a similar-tasting placebo. After taking the placebo the men transmitted the text faster but made on average 30 per cent more mistakes. After taking the ginseng they also transmitted faster, but made only 17 per cent more mistakes. These results were nothing to shout about but, like fruits dangling just out of reach, were sufficient to spur on more elaborate and careful studies with higher dosages. This time Brekhman's team used telegraph operators who had to encode a special text. Again, those given ginseng only slightly increased their speed of operation, but there was a major reduction in the number of mistakes. Those given the placebo made 28 per cent more mistakes than in the first test, while those given ginseng made 10 per cent *fewer* mistakes than in the first test. The same kind of study has been carried out with similar results with proofreaders and other groups of professionals.[2]

The Russians then found that giving ginseng to their young men over a long period could intensify the stamina effect. It gave results which were more consistent, and more significant. Ginseng seemed to be cumulative. This was expected, for the Chinese have always insisted that a one-off dosage of ginseng is of little benefit and these mild harmony medicines must be taken continuously for some time in order to build up an effect.

These results triggered off research outside Russia. For example, Professor Sandberg of Uppsala University, Sweden, travelled to Russia and China where he became highly intrigued by Oriental remedies. He has repeated these performance tests with thirty-three very willing young Swedish students. The trial was double-blind, that is, neither the student nor the experimenter knew whether a particular student had been given a ginseng plus vitamin capsule, or an inert placebo. He used two tests. First the students had to trace a complex spiral maze with a pen without touching intervening shapes, to test their psycho-motor function. Then they were presented with twenty lines of randomly grouped letters, and had to cross out certain letters according to three different rules applied simultaneously. This was weighted towards testing intellectual function. The students taking ginseng made approximately half the number of mistakes as the others on the first test, and two-thirds on the second.[3] The Swedish Health Ministry was sufficiently convinced to allow the manufacturers to claim that their product was an anti-fatigue preparation. The same experiment had been used by Swedish researchers to demonstrate the effectiveness of caffeine, which also improves performance in those tests.[3]

But there is something rather cursory about all this work. Today it is normal to test performance over the whole range of human activity, in the same way that an IQ test, if it is to measure anything at all meaningful, cannot be limited to, say, the matching of shapes. One would use a battery of tests, including coding with words and tests of psycho-motor skills, then different kinds of questionnaires on states of mind, mental activity, mood and so on. There are the tests of perception such as visual sensitivity, auditory and visual discrimination, and tests of ability to react to stimuli such as the testing of reaction time. Then there are all the various electronic assessments of brain function.

Sporadic reports have appeared in recent years in which human psycho-motor performance has been tested in these more elaborate ways after ginseng administration. Some of these studies were in old people's homes and for various reasons, particularly because of the complex range of other medicines usually taken by such a group, the data gained are not of great value in our attempt to understand ginseng. Also, these studies have not been particularly rigorous. For example a new study has just been announced by Professor Doerling of Hamburg, together with Dr Anton Kirchdorfer, representing a European firm. They gave strong doses of ginseng extract to sixty people and placebo to another sixty. The visual and auditory reaction times were tested by asking the individual to press a button or make some other response as soon as he saw a sight or heard a sound. The time between the stimulus and response was measured. Ginseng extract was claimed to increase the reaction times in 80 per cent of that group compared to about 17 per cent in the placebo group. They also carried out the so-called flicker-fusion test. The subject is shown a flashing light which gradually flickers faster and faster. There comes a point when the subject perceives all the flashes merging into a continuous light. This point is an excellent index of visual and mental sensitivity. When this test was used, the number of subjects showing improvements in the ginseng group was approximately double that in the placebo group. Unfortunately, there is little detailed information available on this trial, and it would be much better to state the amount of change rather than the proportion of people experiencing it, for the change might be too small to be of interest. These results therefore lack conviction at present.[4]

I have completed a study in collaboration with Dr Cosmo Hallström of a psycho-pharmacology research unit in a London hospital. We measured the performance of nurses who were undergoing one of their regular periods of night duty. After three nights of this, most of the nurses feel tired and overwrought from a combination of hard work and disrupted sleep patterns. They were given ginseng under double-blind conditions. The results were analysed using a standard computer programme. The nurses taking ginseng felt somewhat more capable, alert and tranquil during their work, they were better at a test of speed and co-ordination, they didn't seem to sleep as well during the day, but were nevertheless less lethargic afterwards. The results, like virtually all these studies on ginseng, were not large, but they suggest some kind of improvement in stamina and competence in people who are pushed to their limit.

But what does this mean? Is ginseng some kind of new mild and long-term stimulant? If that is so, surely the Chinese have been almost as deluded about its health-giving properties as if it were ineffective? In order to begin to answer these questions we must turn for help . . . to the mouse.

TIRED MICE

Before any new drug can be popped into the ever-open mouths of Western patients, a host of mice have drunk it, eaten it and had it injected into them, in doses varying from the minute to the mortal. Mice are, in the eyes of science, dispensable, and can therefore be experimented on as people can not. Moreover, animals do not, one presumes, believe in panaceas. There is no question of subjective bias. Studies are therefore more reliable than with man, although there is the obvious disadvantage that mice are not, after all, men, and drugs do not necessarily do the same things in *Mus* as they do in *Homo*.

Brekhman began to observe the effect of ginseng on mice after he had satisfied himself through studies on people that there was something in the root beyond fable. This sequence is the reverse of that usually expected in drug-testing, where animals are employed before a substance is judged safe enough for people. But these Oriental remedies have been taken for so long by so many people that Brekhman and all others involved in this work have little doubt that they are absolutely safe (see Appendix, p. 295). It is their effectiveness which is in question. Brekhman first developed a test to assess stamina in mice. Mice were put into water, where they swam until they were completely exhausted. They were taken out and allowed to rest, and then repeated the swim. The second swim of the tired mice is usually much shorter, perhaps a third of the first swim. In Brekhman's initial study 120 mice went through the trial. He found that, by injection of a small quantity of ginseng extract, the duration of the second swim could be almost doubled.[5] He repeated the test under various conditions and with different dosages to find the best conditions, and then he tried it out with mice in a long-term study. Mice swam once every five days for two months. After the first two sessions, half the mice were given ginseng extract every other day for thirty days. At the end of two months the average of the animals given ginseng was regularly double that of the others.[6]

This work solidified the evidence. Here at last was a secure test of ginseng's anti-fatigue properties. The mice were put through an efficiency test which is more severe than is possible in an experiment on man, and the effect of ginseng was correspondingly greater, as it should be. Such a positive result puts nails in the coffin of the proposition that ginseng acts purely psychologically, just as the success of veterinary acupuncture informs us that acupuncture works on the body independently of the attitude of the mind. But the real importance of the mice test is that it is a laboratory tool for further studies. Now, for example, a ginseng preparation can be tested to see how strong it is, it can be standardized by firms and, more tantalizingly, the root can be broken down into its constituent parts. Then, by testing each in turn, the actual chemical substance which is increasing the stamina of the mice can be identified.

The test has often been repeated in different parts of the world. For example, some new trials were instituted in a research laboratory in London with minute doses of ginseng, in order to answer the criticism that early studies had used unrealistically large doses. Ginseng was then given to different groups of mice for two, three, or four weeks. After two weeks there were small increases in swimming time, but after four weeks the mice were able to swim an extra 50 per cent longer than those without ginseng.[7] In other words, the amount of ginseng which corresponds to that taken by man was quite sufficient to produce large increases in the stamina of these mice at their absolute mousely limit.

The problem with the mouse swimming test is that it is somewhat laborious and unpleasant. It has been replaced in the Soviet Union by a test in which mice climb a moving rope. If these tests are to be used to test the strength of different ginseng samples, each sample must be given to mice and many hours spent, stop-watch in hand, watching mice swim or climb furiously.[8] Since there are differences in the abilities of individual mice, just as there are when humans race each other, large numbers of mice must be used to arrive at a consensus.

While it is tedious to the scientist, it is utterly harrowing to the mice. Many find mice studies cruel and unnecessary, others find them tolerable and inevitable. This is not the time for me to take sides in this bitter argument. These studies are all standard techniques no more or less uncomfortable to the mice than research going on in virtually every hospital and laboratory in the world. As long as the goal is the attempt to explain ginseng in Western terms, one is dependent on whatever unpleasant tests science can offer. I would only suggest that a more harmonious method should be used for the routine testing of harmony drugs. Ginseng affects the growth of cells; that could be used as a basis for testing.

On the other hand, these tests are not scientifically crude, although it may seem that way. The swimming test or a similar running test is generally accepted as a test of stamina with which to measure the effect of stimulants. It has been used most recently as a definitive test of the stimulant effect of caffeine by German psycho-pharmacologists.[9]

In fact, only a few months ago scientists announced the discovery of a new animal model of depression. 'Our procedure provides an animal model of at least some aspects of depressed mood which is readily amenable to experimental manipulation.' So what is this new model that is exciting psycho-pharmacology? None other than a swimming test with rats![10] It is most ironic that those who 'rediscovered' the possibilities of this test write, 'The method described here might be capable of discovering new types of anti-depressant agents hitherto undetectable using classical screening tests.' I would heartily agree, but would respectfully suggest that the authors acknowledge those who have said it all before, and that they might like to try out their method on a few old roots.

Russian studies usually have a certain methodological naïveté and lack the finesse of top-quality work; for example, the double-blind method may be used, but the results are not submitted to the deepest statistical analysis. When Russian scientists tackle a problem, however, they grasp it in their teeth, like the proverbial Russian bear, and worry it to death. What these studies lack in quality they make up for in quantity. Anyway, our criticism does not give us a reason *a priori* to ignore their results, only to seek confirmation of them. Much of the research on the harmony remedies which started in Russia has been confirmed and extended elsewhere.

A more serious problem is that Russian work is written in a turgid and heavy style which makes it difficult for Westerners to read. This, together with the need for translation, has often been used as a convenient excuse by Western scientists for ignoring Russian work, especially in the field of experimental medicine. Brekhman, being Russian, has only told his story properly to half the world. So has another pioneer.

CHOPPING BEHAVIOUR

Petkov is intelligent and eminent. Yet nobody in the West seems to understand him. Is it because his ideas are gibberish? Is it because his experiments are unrepeatable and worthless? Or is it the listeners who are befuddled, not the speaker?

Professor Wesselin Petkov is head of the Faculty of Pharmacology in the Institute of Specialized and Advanced Medical Training, Sofia, Bulgaria. A man of great experience, he has published scores of scientific publications and has an imaginative cast of mind. He would be a greater disturbance to mainstream pharmacology if he were listened to. An investigation of ginseng is only one of his projects. In an examination of the way the seasons influence the effect of drugs, research clearly inspired by Chinese medicine, he discovered that the digoxin heart stimulants upon which millions of people now rely have different strengths in winter and summer. This is revolutionary work, and should have had more impact.

He has been studying ginseng for about twenty-five years, starting with batches of fresh roots flown from China and replanted with remarkable success in Bulgaria. He has come to some exciting conclusions which are quoted but misunderstood by those investigating ginseng, and ignored by others.

Taking the logical step from the mouse-swimming studies, to find what kind of stimulatory effect ginseng could have on the brain he carried out behavioural studies. The effect of drugs on behaviour is a subject in its own right, termed behavioural pharmacology. Mind-acting drugs, including stimulants, sedatives, tranquillizers, anti-psychotics, narcotics and hallucinogens, are all elaborately tested by examining their effect on the behaviour of animals in the laboratory and of man. This type of research had its origins at the beginning of this century in the work of a Soviet physiologist named Ivan Pavlov.

Pavlov was the first to consider a brain as a kind of processing unit into which one could place stimuli and out of which would come a corresponding response. In his classic experiment, he gave dogs food in association with a completely neutral stimulus such as a ringing bell. The dogs soon learnt to link the bell with the food, and eventually responded by salivation to the neutral stimulus by itself. The same can be achieved with punishment as the 'conditioning' stimulus. This type of training is called classical conditioning.

Petkov began his experiments on ginseng by examining its effect on the speed of Pavlovian conditioning of rats. He placed a rat in a transparent cage with a wire snaking along the floor. When an electric current was switched on, the rat could escape by jumping up to a wooden bar. A bell was rung in association with the shock, and eventually the rat became conditioned to jump whenever the bell rang. An extract of white ginseng roots was given daily to some of the rats two hours before the trial. The rats receiving ginseng learnt the conditioned reaction more quickly than the others. By the end of the second day of testing the ginseng-treated rats gave from 80 per cent to 100 per cent (average 90 per cent) correct responses to the bell, whereas the others gave from 40 per cent to 90 per cent (average 70 per cent). Petkov noted that the rats given ginseng climbed down more hastily from their wooden perch when the signal ended.

Then Petkov introduced a complication. He sometimes presented the rats with a harmless buzzer which was not followed by a shock. At first they jumped, through habit, and he measured how long it took the rats to learn that they need not jump up when they heard the buzzer. The buzzer here is a negative conditioned stimulus – it encourages restraint. The ginseng-treated animals learnt more quickly. After the fourth day of training 85 per cent of the rats in this group ignored the buzzer, whereas only 50 per cent learnt not to react to it in the group without ginseng.[11, 12] This is an important finding, for it indicates that the animals are more adaptable, not simply more stimulated. They are better at switching off as well as switching on.

To cap these, Petkov has also carried out Pavlovian-type behavioural studies on humans.[13, 14] Volunteers were given a ginseng preparation disguised by flavourings, or the flavourings alone. Their responses to cues were tested. For example, they learned to say words in response to certain sets of stimuli. The stimuli were then changed, and the rate of adaptation to new response rules measured. Petkov also measured their general state of arousal, and found it to be increased. His subjects apparently learnt more easily and performed better in these tests when they had taken standard doses of ginseng.

There is nothing wrong with the quality of Petkov's behavioural studies. They were competently executed and repeated in various ways as any such trials should be. Professor Petkov's not inconsiderable reputation in the USSR rests on his work, and it has been confirmed by other Soviet and Japanese scientists, including Brekhman.[15] He has used it with Chinese red roots, Korean white roots and fresh Bulgarian roots, with substantially the same results, and his doses are not excessive.

BALANCED AROUSAL

What do these studies mean? Petkov uses Pavlovian thinking. Pavlov saw the brain as a thought-less, will-less black box. Its natural state is, like a sleepy telephone exchange, inhibited and quiescent. When it receives a stimulus, e.g. an electric shock, through the sense organs, the signal passes to the information-processing area of the brain, the cerebral cortex. Here it excites the pain centre, which sends a message down the lines to the body to take action. Other areas of the brain – the food centre, sex centre and so on – are woken up and shut down as stimuli come and go. Thus, if excitation could be imagined as light, one would see a spot of light travelling over the brain, waking up different areas as an individual receives various stimuli during daily life.[16]

How does the brain switch attention from one stimulus to another, e.g. from bell to buzzer? Either because the stimulus is replaced by a stronger one, or because the animal learns to suppress it. Pavlov called the suppression 'active inhibition'. The healthy ability to depress one centre and light up another, to excite and inhibit, constitutes the adaptability of the individual in Pavlovian terms.

Ginseng helps the animals to respond more quickly. Petkov imagined that it primed the brain, causing more rapid excitation. At the same time, since animals realize more quickly that the buzzer is innocuous, the process of inhibition or damping down is also speeded up. This explains the fact that the animals do not stay so long on their perch after the shock or bell has stopped. They are more adaptable. Therefore, ginseng affects the function of the cortex 'through simultaneous reinforcement of the process of excitation and inhibition'.

This conclusion shook Petkov. He saw ginseng as a new type of stimulant, which did not simply excite brain areas like other stimulants, but increased the control of these brain areas to produce more excitation or inhibition as required. While other stimulants tended to produce jittery over-responsiveness, ginseng, he felt, was *the first truly balanced stimulant*. There is no denying that Petkov's conclusion is of critical importance to our understanding of ginseng, though he was hindered by the Pavlovian framework within which he sought for explanations.

He marshalled other kinds of observations in support. He noticed, for example, that the rats reacted more quickly. In order to demonstrate that their aroused brain was also more adaptable, he swapped the stimuli some way through the test, so that the buzzer became associated with the shock and the bell with no-shock. The rats had to unlearn everything and relearn the opposite set of responses. Again, he found the mental agility of his rats considerably improved with ginseng.

Petkov also carried out some studies on the bio-electrical activity of the brain, in an attempt to confirm directly that ginseng increased the level of mental activity and attention. This involved analysis of brainwaves measured by the machine known as the EEG, the electroencephalograph. The first crude measurements of the EEG of cats given extracts of ginseng showed minor and complex changes which, despite valiant efforts on Petkov's part, are almost impossible to explain properly. However, when he stimulated the brain with sound or light, he gained some very clear answers. The ginseng-treated animals appeared to release a greater burst of energy from the auditory region of the brain when a sound was made, and from the visual region on presentation of a light. To make this more obvious, Petkov turned down the volume. He eventually reached a point where the stimulus was so low that only the ginseng-treated cats gave clear wiggles on the record in response to the stimulus. Again he felt sure of his interpretation: that ginseng had produced a greater level of excitation or sensitivity of the brain.[12, 17]

Pavlov's research has been eclipsed by more complex and subtle views of the brain. Physiologists now realize that excitation does not go directly from the sense organs to the cerebral cortex; it first passes through a primitive region called the reticular formation which controls brain sensitivity and activation,[18] and determines the level of wakefulness. If I burn my finger there is, besides an immediate reaction, a message sent down to the reticular formation which tells it to charge up the rest of the brain. Thus patterns of excitation in the cortex 'recruit the reticular formation systems and receive from them their charge of energy'.[18] At the same time, messages are sent down through the reticular formation to bring the body in line with the arousal state of the higher attending and perceiving brain. The reticular formation joins and regulates the arousal states of mind and body.

For a modern view of what Petkov's results mean, let us take his papers to a behavioural pharmacologist working at London University. 'Have you read Petkov's papers?' we ask. 'Yes,' he says, 'I have glanced through them.' 'What do his results mean to you?' 'Nothing. Absolute rubbish,' he says contemptuously. 'Why?' 'Because his conclusions are extravagant, childish and incoherent and don't follow from his experiments.' Then we go away. We edit the paper and take out all the ossified prose and excessive rationalizations. Now we take the papers back, and ask the same question. He no longer discusses the papers and now takes the experiments at their face value. 'Ah yes, interesting basic classic conditioning studies.' 'What do they show?' 'They show that this odd substance, ginseng – what the hell is it, do you know? – this drug, if we can call it that, seems to increase the learning ability of the animals. Now lots of drugs can affect learning, as you know. Some do it simply by increasing the general state of arousal and alertness. This seems to be the case here. The animals are more alert and aroused, since their reactions are quicker and the evoked potentials are stronger. There seems to be an improvement in higher neural mechanisms of learning, because the animals are more adaptive. They can switch a stimulus more quickly from positive to negative and learn to ignore the buzzer more easily. This may be due to improvements in the cholinergic system' (now he is talking about brain chemistry, the strong point of Western brain analysis), 'in the reticular formation and the hippocampus. It is not clear whether the animals are simply more sensitive and discriminate more easily between the buzzer and the bell when they take this ginseng, or whether they are actually more psychologically adaptable. This is a bit of a puzzle, although the results of his switching trials do suggest adaptability. The suppression of the conditioned stimulus when the buzzer sounded is nothing special, and can be explained as part of a sharpness of responses due to overall increase in attention. Amphetamine can do many of the things that Petkov reports for ginseng. On the other hand, amphetamine acts on the catecholamine neurones. Ah! There is a strange fact. No known drug can achieve all-round increases in both speed and performance in all types of complex learning tasks. This is a surprise. It cannot really be classified with any stimulant that I know of. Dear me . . .' and here we leave him to his puzzlement. All will be explained in good time.[19]

The fact is that Petkov's own cortex had become as excited as that of his rats when he completed his behavioural studies. He was aware of the implications of a drug which could at the same time produce both excitation and inhibition. There are already drugs which stimulate (e.g. amphetamines) or sedate (e.g. barbiturates). These drugs can often do the opposite under specific conditions (amphetamine becomes a sedative in children). But there would be an astonishing possibility of improving the function and power of the mind with a drug that was capable of facilitating both *simultaneously*. Petkov believed that he had found such a drug in ginseng.

This would imply a new kind of remedy, that stimulated without excitation, insomnia or discord. A remedy that might help man cope in some as yet unknown fashion with the loads he places upon himself. 'After various kinds of experiments on men, it was established that daily doses of ginseng preparations during 15–45 days increase physical endurance and mental capacity for work, as well as industrial activity. The increase in work efficiency was noted not only during the treatment itself but also for a stated period of time (a month and a half) after the treatment was over.'[5]

This extraordinary claim, if true, could cause a confrontation with a whole segment of modern pharmacology. This cannot be done only on the basis of the lonely Petkov, crying in the dark. He is too easy to ignore. He belongs to the Soviet school of psychology which is suspect, isolated and strongly Pavlovian. He is understood only by those who, like the neo-Pavlovians, understand the mind as a cascade of reflexes. He need not be believed unless he is understood, and his tendency to obscurity and tortuous explanation need not be forgiven unless his basic research findings are believed. Therefore he is caught in a mesh which ensures his obscurity, and he writes in Bulgarian which seals it up. But his work is a foundation stone, next to Brekhman's, upon which we must build an impregnable castle, solid with evidence. Then the gauntlet can be flung down.

LEARNING AND FORGETTING

Another stone can be neatly laid alongside Petkov's. It comes from the East. Japanese and Korean scientists acknowledge Petkov with a brief Oriental bow and then take his work several stages further on. Anxious not to fall into Petkov's trap of conceptual exile, they use Western-style textbook methods of behavioural research.

The Japanese have a singular advantage which shoots them straight into the modern world of controlled drug-testing: they possess the major active principles (essential ingredients) of ginseng in pure form. We describe what they are in the next chapter. Japanese chemists have isolated them, and they work next door to the pharmacologists, who have flocked round these pure substances, truly the essence of the root, like bees round nectar. The practice of playing science with an unknown brown soup came to an end. With it fell one of the major criticisms that have helped to keep the wraps on research into ginseng. As long as scientists were playing with the crude material, other experts could ignore the work since, as Alex Comfort once said: 'We cannot be interested in the ginseng root while it is still a lot of gubbins.' This attitude always was unjustified, for it implies that nothing on this planet that was not produced by a chemist is worth taking an interest in. But now it is irrelevant.

Professor Takagi, an urbane and affable man, and his team at the department of Chemical Pharmacology of the University of Tokyo, Japan, took the crystals and began at the beginning. Imagine, they thought, that someone had given them unknown material. Substance X. What properties does it have? The obvious approach was to put it through a battery of tests covering most of the different types of pharmacological activity known to man. Some of the studies were on the effect of ginseng on the mind, and it is these which are relevant to us here. Where Petkov used classical conditioning, the Japanese team asked the questions of the Western behavioural pharmacologist. They used operant conditioning, learning trials in which the animal is trained to carry out a task, like training a cat to use a cat tray, in contrast to Pavlovian conditioning in which the animals respond by means of reflexes, such as salivation or fear reactions.

In ignoring most of the previous work, Takagi began his studies with more industry than insight. He published several papers describing projects in which he gave such high doses of ginseng constituents to his animals that the results are of no use to anyone. Having learnt their lesson, the Japanese began testing the components of ginseng using normal doses. Now the results came in thick and fast. The animals seemed more keen to explore and investigate their environment – a sign of general vitality and interest in the world about them. Among other things, the team measured the extent to which animals went through holes in their cage to an unknown region outside, and how much they ran up nets at the side of their cage. Ginseng components could increase these exploratory activities. The difference was especially noticeable when the animals were already tired from previous exercise.[20]

Korean scientists at the College of Medicine of Seoul National University watched the behaviour of their experimental animals even more carefully and were able to split it up into separate behavioural aspects. Here the scientist is a watcher, almost a voyeur, not a Pavlovian taskmaster. First, the Koreans confirmed that ginseng components given to rodents could facilitate the learning of simple responses, increase activity and reduce the need for sleep.[21] They re-examined the activity of mice with the more objective light-beam apparatus, in which the number of times an animal crosses a beam of light is measured automatically. Activity increased by up to 50 per cent with the smallest doses.[22] The largest doses had the opposite effect. Let it be said that there was a certain amount of less than brilliant scientific work from both Japan and Korea in this field. Yet while it would be wise to be cautious about the extent of the changes in some of the tests, there is now no longer any reason to doubt the basic findings, which have been repeated again and again in the most prestigious research centres of the Far East. The effects of ginseng seem much broader than we first thought, certainly broader than any known stimulant drugs, as Petkov noted.

This makes us aware, however, that there is still an important piece missing from the story: the piece of evidence that might link Petkov's concepts of a drug causing both activation and inhibition in the brain, to those of the Far Eastern scientists who talk, in the modern behavioural argot, of performance, arousal and activity.

When the piece came it was unexpected. Japanese scientists found that some components of the ginseng root were seda- tive. They depressed mouse activity and ability to learn, while increasing sleeping time.[23] This was so contrary to the known general arousal produced by the whole root that it threw an international conference on ginseng in 1974 into a brief startled confusion. Peace was restored when it was shown that other constituents were stimulatory, improving learning and activ- ity just like the whole root,[24] though more powerfully.

The ebullient Dr Saito, in what is probably the best of these series of behavioural studies, examined the single most seda- tive and single most stimulatory components of ginseng. With the stimulatory substance he showed that rats explored their laboratory environment more. When they were put into a Y-maze, a Y-shaped path with cheese at one end, they got to the cheese in a shorter time and they made very few mistakes. More sophisticated tests were carried out. The cheese was switched to the other limb of the maze and the time it took the animals to learn the new location recorded. The stimulatory substance significantly increased the ability of the animals to adapt to their new situation and correctly unlearn and relearn. A conditioning trial demonstrated that the animals were better able to learn to avoid a shock, to learn association between the shock and a neutral stimulus, and to discriminate between two sounds similar to the sound connected with the shock. The test, known as a one-trial passive avoidance test, was carried out on two consecutive days. Without the stimulatory com- ponent, only about 25 per cent of the animals had learnt what to do after the first session, but when it was given before the learning session, 70 per cent of the animals learnt correctly. In all these studies, the sedative component showed the opposite effect.[25]

This offers one solution to the question posed by the lonely Petkov: how can a drug increase the processes of both activa- tion and inhibition at the same time? How can a drug both stimulate and sedate? Perhaps it does both because of its range of active constituents, each producing a different degree of arousal or sedation. Some idea of the music of the root has been obtained through the energetic research of the Japanese and Korean scientists. It has many different instruments, some rousing, some depressing, some strong, some weak, and some ineffective in this particular musical arrangement, but possibly coming into their own during another concert. Suddenly it becomes clear how there can be so many different grades and values of ginseng, how a root picked on one mountain may be worse than a root picked on another, how the cultivated root may be worse than the wild, the Japanese than the Korean, and the American less stimulatory than the Korean. The quality varies according to the exact mix of the components in each root. You do not eat a medicine when you eat a root, you eat an *aggregate* of medicines.

Actually the answer to this balanced arousal is more complex and more interesting, as we shall see in Chapter 7. The mystery of how the root works is not solved by calling it a mixture; it is enriched.

BRINGING OTHER KINGLY REMEDIES INTO THE LABORATORY

In Chinese medicine, each of the kingly remedies is thought to restore harmony in a different manner. One heats, one moistens, another solidifies, and another lightens, and the remedy is chosen according to the type of activity which is deficient or overdominant. However, it is difficult to find testing models to examine these various properties. Laboratory testing is crude and ungainly. The stamina test is mostly used to measure the effect on vitality of these medicines. Thus they are all lumped into the same class for the purpose of proving that they have at least some effect. This is like trying to recognize a food by determining if it fills the belly.

Using the usual basic principle that tonic drugs reveal their worth most clearly when a person undergoes a taxing experience, Russian scientists have tested a range of local harmony plants and found increases in physical and mental efficiency in single and especially in prolonged administration.[26] Healthy and sick volunteers were, for example, put through learning and responding trials of a type similar to those used by Petkov. Their performance rating particularly increased with the Oriental remedy Schizandra chinensis. Animal tests of stamina were also used, such as the swimming test with mice and the test in which mice are made to climb a continuously moving rope. Araliaceae plants, such as Echinopanax elatum and Acanthopanax sessiliflorum and their constituents, helped the mice to swim longer.[27]

The Japanese found the same with some of the more traditional non-araliaceous Oriental kingly plants such as rehmannia, cnidium and cassia bark. Dioscorea and ligusticum, which are not kingly remedies, did not increase mouse activity. The quality of all these trials is now so standardized that the results are not, in my opinion, disputable. Schizandra has been of particular interest. An unusual early Chinese report at the First Conference of Chinese Physiological Sciences in 1956 stated that ginseng and schizandra were both able to increase the learning ability of mice in the conditioned reflex test. As the authors, Ku and Chen, reported, they could get the animals to learn faster at low doses, but as they increased the dose there came a point at which learning deteriorated. In fact, some Russian scientists feel that ginseng and schizandra are equally powerful in improving the efficiency of cerebral activities. A few of the plants, particularly Aralia manshurica, seemed to be especially excitatory. Animals given this plant ran about rather more and wave changes appeared when they were tested by the electroencephalogram. At the same time, these more strongly stimulant plants enabled animals to wake up earlier when heavily sedated.

THE DEER AND THE SPIKY SHRUB

One day, or so the story goes, a young Russian doctor named Gorovoy noticed deer greedily eating the leaves of a thorny plant commonly found growing wild in the Russian Far East. He found that the plant was Eleutherococcus senticosis Maxim., so called because senticosis means prickly in Latin. It belonged to the Araliaceae. Kew Gardens was given some by Carl Maximowicz, the director of the St Petersburg botanical gardens after whom the plant is named. Eleutherococcus joined the other araliaceous medicinal plants on trial in the laboratory, and it outshone them all, rivalling or even surpassing ginseng itself. Brekhman found that it was a first-class tonic plant medicine, and he studied its effects on both animals and people. In mouse stamina trials, he found that an extract of the roots increased the duration of work by 25 per cent. A preparation of the leaves increased capacity by 44 per cent and of roots and leaves by 70 per cent. The increase in stamina was even greater in long-term administration.[28] Again, telegraphists and proofreaders were used as the human guinea-pigs. The effects of eleutherococcus extract were as good, if not better, than those of ginseng.[6]

The changes have been rung on the various available tests of stimulatory ability. For example, the Vladivostok group found changes in the EEG of rabbits indicative of arousal. They showed that eleutherococcus could reduce the effect of strong sedative compounds such as barbiturates, chloral hydrate or ether, and more quickly restore the sensitivity of the nerves of the narcotized animals. They have also demonstrated that rats trained to respond to a buzzer in Pavlovian conditioning trials were more sensitive to the stimulus, that is, they could discriminate more easily between two similar buzzings.[29]

Active principles have also been isolated from eleutherococcus, so active that one gram of each was sufficient to make 8000 mice swim an extra third longer than their usual limit. This was more than any of the ginseng constituents, the most stimulatory of which could only do the same to 6000 mice.[31] Brekhman in fact found eleutherococcus better in his trials than ginseng.

Although similar in pharmacological effect, Eleutherococcus has advantages over ginseng. In the presence of high levels of physical work for man and animals, the stimulant and tonic effects of ginseng were found to be of shorter duration and weaker in comparison to that of Eleutherococcus. . . . In hyperactive individuals Eleutherococcus also possesses some calmative effect.

Brekhman then carried out the obvious test. He gave eleutherococcus extract to some of a large group of athletes before a ten-kilometre race. Those taking the extract chopped an average of five minutes from the average time of 52.6 minutes set by the others who had taken a placebo. The athletes apparently improved their reaction times, their endurance and concentration as a result. This may stretch the reader's belief. If it is true, would this plant not smash world records in dozens for Soviet runners and lead to pocketfuls of gold medals in international sports events? We will look at this question again (pages 248 to 252).

In the USSR eleutherococcus is more popular and cheaper than ginseng, for whereas eleutherococcus is always available, ginseng is continually in short supply and is in Russia an expensive medicine for those able to afford it. Eleutherococcus can be gathered like bracken from the forest. There is a reserve stock which is spread over ten million hectares of forest land. The Soviet Union now makes enough eleutherococcus extract for twelve million of its citizens to take a course every month. It exports it to the West as 'Siberian ginseng', which is a complete misnomer but boosts sales. In both the United States and the Soviet Union one can buy bottles and cans of Siberian ginseng drink.

Strangely, it was empirical trial and error in the laboratory, combined with the intuition of a few scientists, which led to the discovery of its profound and important qualities, in AD 1962 not 1962 BC. There is no mention of it, as far as can be judged, in Shen Nung's pharmacopoeia or any of its descendants. Nor was eleutherococcus apparently known as a Russian folk medicine. It is an example of that rare species, a new national plant medicine discovered by modern research.

But it is a local Soviet discovery, and thus far has not benefited from international research. Neither Shibata, Petkov, Kim nor any of the other scientists investigating Oriental remedies with their special skills have taken any interest in it. There is no real reason why they should, for they have no experience of its use as a medicine and it is not grown in their locality. Therefore eleutherococcus has not yet had the collective stamp of approval from interested scientists around the world, and we await amplification of this Soviet discovery.

THE DEER

By a strange twist of fate, the deer turns out to be as much a medicine as the shrub it is eating. The deer is the source of an Oriental drug which has been a hot topic for centuries, debated acrimoniously for as long as the chemists challenged the Galenicists. The antlers of the young sika or spotted deer, taken before they become bony, have been used since the earliest times in the Orient. Together with the gecko lizard, tortoise-shell and certain other preparations, they comprise the group of kingly remedies which are of animal origin, and just as ginseng is the most precious and effective of the plant harmony remedies, so these antlers, named 'pantui', are the choice animal harmony remedy.

In China the pantui is prepared with plants in mixtures and patent medicines, or processed into pills in modern pharmaceutical factories. The traditional use of pantui is as a general tonic in debility, old age, impaired vision and hearing, rheumatism, uterine haemorrhage, spermatorrhoea, and other diseases.

In the USSR the proper pantui is obtained from the noble spotted deer (Cervus nippon) which sheds its antlers every autumn and grows a new set in the spring. The soft antlers are collected in July, dried and made up in an extract. The deer used to be found wild in the Ussuri region. Nowadays, like ginseng, they have been hunted so successfully that more or less the only place they can be found is in the protection of certain Soviet state farms. Here pantui is extracted and used almost entirely for medical research. The pantui that is consumed so widely throughout Russia is in fact from the maral deer (Cervus canadiensis asiaticus), a much more common relative. The antlers from these deer are bought by the State and processed, particularly in the Khabarovsk Pharmaceutical Factory. Here the horns are briefly boiled, dried, ground, extracted and refined to give a preparation called pantocrine.

There is nothing more likely to raise the hackles of the Western medical world than the prospect of taking pantui seriously. Pantui, along with rhinoceros horn and many other animal preparations, has been the butt of numerous jokes ever since pharmacologists felt that the isolation of active principles allowed them to leave the medieval world behind for ever. Mention of deer antlers is almost sufficient grounds for excommunication in certain quarters.

Nevertheless, the facts will eventually have to be faced, since they won't go away. The Russians have produced several volumes of medical studies on pantui, almost as much work as on ginseng.[31] They cover everything from clinical studies to laboratory trials to stock-raising. Research has been in progress for fifty years, mostly centred in the Institute of Biologically Active Substances, Vladivostok. Virtually no Western experts are familiar with these medical studies.

The Russian work is a coherent, though heavyweight,

research effort which has produced firm results. The experiments stand up to criticism *in toto,* though some individual cases may be of crude design. The whole thrust of the work leads ineluctably to the conclusion that there is some kind of new medicine in these antlers, again of a type hitherto unknown to the West. Despite the jokes, the onus is now on all of us in the West to prove the Russians wrong. Otherwise, it is our loss, not theirs.

Early studies in the thirties confined themselves to research on the blood supply. The real testing began only as recently as 1969. Dr Taneyeva at Vladivostok found that pantocrine increased stamina in the now classic diagnostic mouse-swimming test,[32] and simple psycho-motor performance tests with people produced faster correct responses and fewer mistakes. A more physical test of stamina is the bicycle ergonometer, a fixed bicycle with an attached workmeter, which is a standard instrument for measuring human physical work. In one experiment men cycled on the ergonometer, after which they were given pantocrine or a placebo and two hours later checked again. There was a slight increase in the total work achieved by the placebo group, and a very considerable increase in the pantocrine group.[33]

A three-kilometre race was run by fifty young men, repeating the very first race which brought Chinese medicines into the scientific spotlight. A single administration of pantocrine thirty minutes before the race produced an average time of 14 minutes 41 seconds, compared to 14 minutes and 48 seconds in the placebo group. Again the effect was cumulative if pantocrine was given for some time. The data is convincing enough, at least as a first step. Brekhman uses the swimming test together with sex hormone and blood pressure tests to standardize pantocrine preparations. The Soviet health ministry have introduced a State standard for single-forked antlers (USSR State Standard 3673–4) which is regularly checked for its pharmacological activity by Brekhman's three tests. Single-forked antlers are used for export, while two-forked antlers are for home use. They yield twice as much pantocrine per antler.

Recently Brekhman pioneered a new preparation called rantarin, an extract of the velvet-covered horns of the reindeer. The reindeer is extremely common. There are perhaps two million head of domesticated and 600,000 head of wild animals in the Soviet Union. At the same time it is a close relative of the spotted and maral deer. In a series of tests similar to the ones described above, Brekhman and his co-workers demonstrated that rantarin is on a par with the pantocrine from the maral deer.[35]

We have no choice but to agree with the Chinese and include pantui in the class of harmony remedies. Yet it has many enigmatic features. It will appear again in our discussion of the sexual implications of tonic medicines. We conclude for the moment that pantocrine has some kind of anti-fatigue properties which may or may not be on a par with other arousing harmony medicines. The noble spotted deer is a somewhat dark horse.

EXISTING WESTERN HARMONY DRUGS?

As we shall see later, certain drugs already known in the West are mild, effective and safe modulators of arousal. But the effect of even these agents in our own house has been severely underestimated. They are better than we think they are, but it needs a little encouragement to pull out and reconsider the discarded drugs. Perhaps the example of ginseng will force the re-examination of the drugs in the dark corners of the Western pharmacy to see if anything there may have unsuspected ginseng-like properties.

The Russians have found a compound called dibazol. In the West it is known as bendazole or 2-benzyl benzimidazole. It is a cast-off. When I looked for details of its sale by drug companies, I discovered only that it is marketed in France. There is no reference to it in the *US Pharmacopoeia* and the *Merck Index* knows of it but does not ascribe to it any medicinal properties. The Russians have found that it has certain mild effects on stamina and arousal. Many used to take this medicine in the Soviet Union as a kind of safe and mild poor man's ginseng. We will later return to it to see if this claim is justified.

We should also examine a strange compound called centrophenoxine or meclofenoxate. It has an origin which is crazily sensible. French scientists at the psycho-pharmacology laboratory of the Hôpital Ste-Anne, Paris, carried out some studies on the effect of plant growth hormones on the mind. There is no *a priori* reason why hormones which control leaf growth should change human mental performance (despite our descriptions of people as blossoming or flowering!). But some plant hormone derivatives did work. The best of them was the p-chlorophenoxy acetic acid (pcpa) ester of dimethyl-amino ethanol (DMAE), which was reported to improve the regulation of blood pressure and temperature, and to be a mild stimulant.[36] Strangely enough, the DMAE portion had already been discovered to have subtle stimulational effects on the brain. It is marketed as deanol, and a series of clinical trials over the years has suggested that it produces improvements in concentration, sleep patterns and clarity of mind.[37] But centrophenoxine, the combination of DMAE and pcpa, produces a longer-lasting and more profound arousal than DMAE alone, and is now used in some places to assist brain function in the elderly. There is much debate about its effectiveness.[38] Is it too a kind of poor man's ginseng, which is too subtle to be visualized in the instant-cure situation? We will return to it.

Let us briefly recap. The point of departure was a story of harmony medicines which have captured the hearts of the entire Orient for many thousands of years: plants which were the most important medicines available to physicians in the traditional healing system. The first steps were the demonstration that ginseng increased energy, stamina and the capacity to carry out demanding activities. Then it was discovered that learning was facilitated. We reached the first milestone where we reflected that evidently ginseng is not just a fable, but given the right approach, could be proved to work. It was also clear that ginseng had something to do with arousal, but unlike stimulants it increased performance, capacity and adaptability, not just stamina. We continued with the discovery that the root contains some components which are stimulatory and some sedative, which may account for its balanced arousal. We saw that ginseng was not an isolated curio, and that the tonic harmony remedies of the ancient pharmacopoeiae mostly contained the same kinds of constituents and performed similarly when subject to the provings of the laboratory. No contrary evidence has appeared from any quarter, and there is more research which we haven't mentioned.

If these newly arrived medicines wake us up so that our abilities are enhanced more accurately, safely and harmoniously, then they should sweep away the classical stimulants from the pharmacy shelves. The toxic and ineffective stimulants would seem 'humiliating memorials of the credulity of the physicians who prescribed them'. It would be a new age of more effective self-administration. The evidence for this, and the astonishing possibilities that this brings, will be discussed in Chapter 10.

But is the traditional concept of restoring Yang only something as meagre as a safe version of a cup of coffee? How is it that ginseng is used as a drug for a wide variety of health-maintenance purposes? The Chinese claim that the harmony remedies, particularly ginseng, reinforce vitality and disease-resistance. Stimulants of any type have nothing to do with vitality; in fact, they drain vitality rather than augment it. After all the preceding evidence, all the conclusions concerning its effects on arousal, we are still somewhere at the beginning. We still have to discover the real nature of these harmony remedies.

6
Taking It Apart

THE ROOT GIVES UP ITS SECRET SUBSTANCES

Like a child who plays with his food, it seems that man cannot help playing with his medicines. Perhaps he is aware at some level that medicines manipulate him and he wants to get his own back. So he delves deep inside them and tries to pull them to pieces in his desire to get to the root of them. In the case of ginseng, what is at the root of the root? What strange and curious substances have accumulated there as ginseng matures slowly over years and years in its rich humus forest bed? What powerful alchemy has produced a celestial medicine?

It is recorded that the first man to pull ginseng to pieces chemically was Garriques, who in 1854 found within American ginseng roots a type of chemical called a *saponin.*[1] A saponin, from the same root as 'soap', is a substance which produces a foam when dissolved in water. It does so because, like soap, its chemical structure is composed of an oily part and a part which dissolves easily in water and drags the oily part with it into reluctant solution. But while the water-soluble part in soap is alkali, in the saponins it is a sugar molecule. For this reason these saponins are sometimes also termed *glycosides,* from 'glucose'.

Are these substances the ones which produce ginseng's effects on the body? This is the real question and it is a difficult problem for the scientist. Any attempt to find out the nature of the effective (usually known as *active*) constituents in a plant is a bit like trying to reconstitute an ox tail from oxtail soup. Where do you begin? The simple analysis of the gross constituents of the ginseng root may show no great differences from those of a parsnip root. So where lies the difference? It is only possible to determine which components are active medicinally if the analyst has some method of testing what he has got. So the explorations within the root were held up until the discovery of a reliable method of testing the effect of ginseng in the laboratory, that is until Brekhman and his mouse-swimming test.

After that breakthrough things were different. Now a chemist fished with a purpose; for he knew what a fish looked like. The root could be split up into parts and each part tested to see if it increased mouse stamina. In this way the medicinal chemicals can be gradually located and identified. Professor Elyakov and his team at Moscow University raced ahead and by 1962 had isolated a group of constituents which affected Brekhman's mice. The stamina substances were saponins, Garriques would have been happy to know. When discoveries are made in science they often tend to cluster together, the ideas evolving synchronously. This happened in the discovery of the active constituents of ginseng in 1961–2, a great year for ginseng. Lin in Taiwan and Professor Shibata and a large group at the University of Tokyo, as well as the Russians, all reported saponins, while the same year Professor Hörhammer and other German plant chemists at the University of Munich announced the discovery of certain other non-saponin compounds.[2] Since that time hundreds of papers have appeared presenting the fine detail, but it was the humble yet sharp Professor Shibata who cracked the saponin code and identified them completely.

Plant saponins or glycosides are normally of two types, terpenoidal and steroidal. Terpenoids and steroids are quite closely related. Steroids are ubiquitous in the animal kingdom. Examples are cholesterol, cortisone, oestrogen and progesterone (the female sex hormones – constituents of the birth control pill), testosterone (the male sex hormone), vitamin D and many other compounds. An example of a steroidal glycoside is digitalis, the heart stimulant. Steroidal glycosides are usually quite toxic; indeed, some of them are used as arrow poisons. Triterpenoids are a kind of vegetal analogy of the steroids, found only in the plant kingdom. No one is quite sure what they are doing there. There are triterpenoid glycosides in very many plants; oft-quoted examples are liquorice, thyme, sugar-beet, senega and ivy. Being oily, triterpenes and steroids will form part of the oil of a plant, unless combined with sugar to make the soluble saponin. Since all living creatures have watery tissues, and all living processes are carried out in water, the saponins are able to get right into the tissues while the oils cannot.

Behind the august grey portals of the National Gallery in London, a discovery was made which is of peculiar importance to our story. Dr Mills, a chemist, worked there on new substances which may be useful for the treatment of paintings. In the resin of the dammar tree he found a triterpenoid compound called dammaranediol and determined its structure. Shibata, with delightful serendipity, discovered that the triterpenes of ginseng were almost identical to dammaranediol and thus he described them as dammarane-type. Now this does not give anyone the excuse to lick the paint from restored oil paintings in search of subtle medicines. For the triterpenes in the dammar tree are in the pure oily state, while in ginseng they are in the form of saponins.

Although some of the credit for the full identification of the saponins must go to Elyakov and his team,[3] it is Professor Shibata who has pursued the main ginseng medicinal constituents to the end with a relentless intelligence. He has identified them as *dammarane-type triterpenoidal glycosides*.

Shibata found fifteen separate glycosides of this type which he has named ginsenosides. He gave them the code R (Ra, Rb, Rc, Rd, etc.). All of them have been isolated and their structures are completely known.[4] They are given in Table 5. They fall into two groups of compounds, each group consisting of different sugars combined with the same core triterpene. The two core dammarane-type triterpenes are called *protopanaxadiol* and *protopanaxatriol* ('diol and 'triol for short).[4]

VARIATIONS ON A THEME

Variations in the quantities of the pharmacologically active constituents occur both in different parts of the plant, and in different roots grown under different conditions. For example, red ginseng contains slightly more Ra and Ro than white ginseng. Recently, Professor Tanaka announced that the rhizomes of the Japanese ginseng grown on the western mountain slopes of Japan contain utterly different saponins from those grown on the eastern slopes. It comes as no surprise that

Table 5: The Active Constituents of Ginseng

		Ginseng Saponin Content		
Root	Aglycone	Korean P. ginseng	American P. quinquefolium	Japanese P. japonicus
Ra	'Diol	▇		
Rb₁	'Diol	▇▇▇▇▇	▇▇▇▇▇▇▇▇	
Rb₂	'Diol	▇▇		
Rc	'Diol	▇▇▇▇	▇▇	
Rd	'Diol	▇▇	▇	
Ro	Oleanolic	▇	▇	
Re	'Triol	▇▇▇▇	▇▇▇▇	▇▇▇▇▇▇▇
Rf	'Triol	▇		▇
20-gluco-Rf	'Triol	▪		
Rg₁	'Triol	▇▇▇	▇	
Rg₂	'Triol	▪	▪	
Rh₁ & Rh₂	'Triol	▪		▪
Leaves				
F₁	'Triol	▇▇▇		
F₂	'Diol	▇▇		
F₃	'Triol	▇		
Chikusetsusaponins				
Ia	'Diol			▪
Ib	Oleanolic			▪
III	'Diol			▇▇▇▇
IV	Oleanolic			▇▇▇▇▇▇

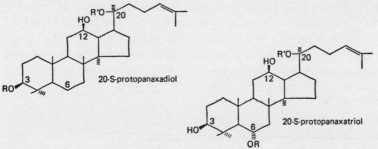

20-S-protopanaxadiol

20-S-protopanaxatriol

plants of the same species grown under slightly different conditions have widely divergent constituents. We expected as much in our look at all the varieties of ginseng and their values, but it is useful to have clear evidence of such differences. For in the race for standardization and productivity in agriculture it is all too easily forgotten that subtle changes of plant management can produce extraordinary variations in its constituents. This subtle alchemy of the growing plant has helped to put off the modern pharmaceutical world from explorations of plant medicines, for it makes standardization of a plant medicine difficult or impossible. Each plant should properly be described not only by its species but also by its ecology. This principle has been widely ignored.

If there are differences in the medicinal components of plants grown on the two sides of a mountain, how much more so in plants grown on two sides of the globe. The American ginseng is a different species, and the saponin spectrum reflects this[5] (see Table 5). Panax pseudoginseng var. notoginseng, the well-respected Chinese san-chi ginseng, has a mix of saponins somewhere in between the American and the true Panax ginseng, with a great quantity of Rg, more than any other type of root,[6] while the Japanese ginseng contains saponins so dramatically different from those of the true ginseng that they are given a series of new names, chikusetsusaponins, after the Japanese name of this plant.[7]

These analyses mesh in a most remarkable manner with the traditional claims made for these plants. If we draw up a list of saponins within the plants and grade them according to the relative quantities of the 'triol saponin which they contain, the list will have true ginseng on top, followed closely by san-chi, reflecting their traditional ranking. Some way behind we find the American ginseng, with its quantities of the non-dammarane triterpenoids, and a traditional reputation reduced in proportion. Finally, we have the Himalayan ginseng and the Japanese ginseng, which have such different constituents that one can challenge the botanists and suggest that they shouldn't belong to the Panax pseudoginseng family at all. They have a lower regard and a different traditional use compared to the other ginsengs.

In other words the traditional reputations of the ginseng family are roughly proportional to the degree of triol glycosides within them. If the roots of the various species were sold in an Oriental trading post, their prices would, unbeknown to the purchaser, reflect the 'triols within them. This takes on a special significance since the 'triols were the glycosides which the Japanese scientists found were more arousing, while the 'diols are the sedative components.

The connection can hardly be fortuitous. It is as if the millennia of Chinese experimentations in the laboratory of the body have come up with the same results as a few years' experimentation in the laboratory of the university. This finding tends to confirm the accuracy of the drug discoveries of the traditional physicians; it justifies the reputations enjoyed by the various ginseng species.

In the year 756 a famous Buddhist priest and physician, Kan-Jin, arrived in Japan from China. He brought with him many types of medicinal plants which were placed in the Royal Storehouse of Shosoin in Nara, Japan, where they have been for the last 1200 years. One of them was ginseng. Professor Shibata obtained some of this ancient ginseng which was still in relatively good condition. He extracted the saponins and found a range unlike any that he had seen before. They looked a bit like a cross between the japonicus and himalaicus subspecies.[8] It was an intriguing scoop; rarely can one go back so far in time to test drugs, and then find them so full of interesting compounds. It eclipses even the story of the man who was stung by a 300-year-old nettle while photographing Linnaeus's collection. At the very least, one now knows that if ginseng is properly cured it cannot go off on the kitchen shelf!

NEW HORIZONS

Medical people reading about these investigations will breathe a sigh of relief, thinking that now the real story is beginning. Romantics and those interested in natural remedies will heave a sigh of despair, thinking that now the real ginseng is coming to an end, reduced to pure white crystals of glycoside. Both are wrong. For one of the conclusions to emerge forcefully from current work is that although active principles are known and can be proved to be effective in certain laboratory tests, the whole root is still hiding many of its delights from us.

It would be foolish to be deluded by the sheer presence of the saponins into thinking that they encapsulate ginseng's activity. Quite a variety of components has been found in the root by pure chemical analysis, unrelated to any biological tests. (For those who are interested, the oil of the root contains certain steroids, particularly B-sitosterol, with smaller amounts of stigmasterol and campesterol,[9] as well as pure triterpenes, a sesquiterpene known as panacene, some poly-acetylene compounds such as B-elemene and panaxynol,[10] and several new similar compounds found by a large group of chemists and pharmacologists in Poland.[11] Besides these there are known to be actual fats, and a compound called kaempferol, also found in senna and other plants.[12] Small quantities of B vitamins were found, as well as folic acid,[13] sugars,[14] amino acids, certain peptides,[15] and some minerals, including manganese, copper, cobalt, vanadium, iron, zinc, and others.[16])

The saponins have always been regarded as the main active constituents of ginseng, because they mimic the action of the whole root in some tests on mice, as we have seen. Yet in Chapter 2 we described how a drug can only be pursued in the laboratory if there is a system with which to test it; for example, tranquillizers were only developed when scientists understood how to make animals anxious. As different test systems are developed, chemists can repeat the fishing process again and may discover a completely different range of active constituents of ginseng about which we know nothing today. Already, Japanese scientists who tested purified extracts of the root for substances affecting the blood pressure of laboratory animals eventually separated the constituents in various ways and came up with pure white crystals which lowered blood pressure. The crystals were analysed and found to be, not saponins, but a substance called choline which is already present in the body and involved in the control of blood pressure. Roots apparently contain 0.01–0.1 per cent of choline.[17] Meanwhile Korean scientists announced that the root contains an anti-oxidant, which they identified as 'maltol'.[18] There is more to the root than meets the test-tube.

Research on the active constituents, though still continuing, is now becoming far less theoretical. With the identity of the saponins absolutely known and the major species of ginseng

analysed, research is turning to commercial possibilities. New
methods of analysis have permitted the definition of minute
quantities of saponins almost small enough to detect ginseng
in a man's blood after he has taken some. Another line of
investigation is the culture of living ginseng plant material in
the laboratory. Tissue culture began in 1966 when Russian
scientists announced that they were growing ginseng material
from pieces of the plant minced up and placed on dishes
containing nutrients.[19] It became possible to start the culture of
living ginseng tissue from pieces of leaf, root, stem and petiole,
as well as from different species. Virtually all of the saponins
were made in their proper quantities by the ginseng tissues in
culture.[20] Such cultures have been kept going for several years
in America.[21] The cultures produced about 0.4 per cent of their
weight in extractable saponin, which is roughly ten times less
than the dried roots. But the success of these efforts so far
indicates that it will not be too long before the production of
the ginseng saponins becomes a purely industrial matter without any need for dirtying hands by growing the root.[22]

This would make ginseng constituents relatively cheap.
One would buy powdered ginseng tissue or extracts of it. But
it will inevitably reduce the variety and potency of the medicinal mix within the plant, which includes many, many compounds besides the saponins. It would be a further step in the
decline of the root, compounding the loss in quality resulting
from cultivation.

Tissue cultivation is also a step along the road to a not-too-
distant scientific horizon: the chemical synthesis of the ginseng
saponins, the production of saponins by chemical manipulations in the laboratory. In theory at least, one can expect one
day to make the saponins out of petrochemicals or, more
probably, from a more common plant. Already, Korean scientists have been able to break down some of the saponins into
smaller parts and build them up again,[23] but these are like a
small child's first faltering steps and this operation alone
takes months.

There will be undeniable advantages in the wide availability
of cheap saponins to all who may need them. There will also be
cases where one or other group of saponins will be needed,
specifically. The production of saponins can and will be
justified on these grounds. Yet there is a great danger in this:

that saponin pills will eventually supplant the ginseng root completely. The arguments for and against saponin pills are typical of the confrontation between ginseng and Western pharmacology, for they crystallize the Western quantitative-rational approach to drugs and the Eastern empirical-intuitional approach. We will return to this again later on. One thing is clear. Even if it is possible to duplicate the most advantageous cocktail of the various individual saponins by using synthetic materials, there are plenty of medicinal components left in the root. We don't know how important these are.

THE SUPPORTING CAST

The Chinese acknowledge ginseng to be their star performer. It is also right up front in the West, collecting all the myths, praise and money. It is the spokesman, attracting the curiosity of Asian scientists who have thrown themselves, fascinated, into the work of unravelling its mystery while simultaneously drawing the fire of Western experts. But behind ginseng is a supporting cast of other Oriental plants waiting in the wings – the harmony remedies, out of the limelight but of no less importance to the Oriental practitioner who calls upon them while designing his individual therapies. Their fortunes outside the Orient will rise or fall with those of ginseng. Do they support its case? Have they followed ginseng into the laboratory to be collected, extracted, injected, analysed and chromatographed? Or are they a mutinous crew who give contrary answers when asked penetrating questions?

Liquorice is one of the most famous plant medicines in the world. It is still taken everywhere in Europe and it is a key kingly plant remedy in China, though it is possible that the Chinese variety of Glycyrrhiza glabra or Glycyrrhiza uralensis is somewhat different medicinally from that grown in Spain or Pontefract and sold in the corner sweetshop. Its main constituent is glycyrrhizin, which is also a triterpenoid glycoside. There are additionally a series of related but minor glycosides, like chemical echoes within the root.[24] It is quite clear that the main glycoside is responsible for only some of the activities of liquorice.

Another important harmony remedy in our list is the

Bupleurum species, used in cases of debility, especially when due to liver disease. The indefatigable Japanese have isolated the major active principles from Bupleurum falcatum, which they call saikosaponins. They are triterpenoidal saponins again, of an oleanolic-acid type of sapogenin.[25] An exciting project has begun at the Research Institute of Oriental Medicine at Kinki University, Osaka, Japan, under the direction of Professor Shigeru Arichi, who has given purified saikosaponins to laboratory animals which have a kind of artificially induced hepatitis. The saikosaponins assisted in restoring the function of the liver and encouraging repair. Professor Arichi's team is now giving these saponins to human hepatitis patients in a clinical trial.

The analysis of the constituents of Oriental medicinal plants turns up similar saponins again and again. To cite more examples, Shibata's associates have found several triterpenoid saponins from Platycodon grandiflorum, an important Chinese medicinal plant (not strictly a mild harmony remedy), which they called platycodisides.[26] Another key Oriental remedy is yuan-chi, the root of Polygala tennifolia, used both as a sedative and to strengthen the nervous system. Here, too, triterpenoid glycosides spread themselves on the instruments.[27] An analogous American remedy called Polygala senega, senega or snakeroot, is one of the few plants in the modern Western pharmacopoeia. The Oriental species is used for the brain and the whole body, while the American relative is used for a more limited local purpose: as a cough medicine, just as the Asiatic species of ginseng is used for whole body treatment while its American brother is traditionally used for stomach troubles. Careful chemistry showed that, like the other root, the two species of snakeroot have linked groups of saponins with slight differences.[28]

Another kingly Chinese medicine, compounded into many of the tonic concoctions, is the Chinese date, the jujube, Ziziphus jujuba. Shibata has isolated some saponins which he called, naturally, jujubosides.[29] By carefully breaking up the saponins, he found that they have a basic dammarane-type triterpenoidal structure. Here he scored a hit, for he noticed that its breakdown products were similar to those found in one of the most important Indian traditional Ayurvedic plant drugs, known as brahmi or Bacopa moninera.[30] Not only can this medicine now be added to the widening triterpenoid list, but Shibata's discovery also indicates that the key plants of both Indian and Chinese medicine have dammarane-type saponins as their main active constituents.

As soon as a biological effect had been proved, eleutherococcus too was packed off to the Moscow chemists to search for the active principles. Using the mouse-swimming test as their hook they fished out the root . . . glycosides, *plus ça change*, although this time they were of a rather different nature.[31]

Pantui contains a high complex mixture of organic and inorganic substances. The Protein Chemistry Laboratory at Moscow State University, together with Elyakov and his team, has been given the task of unravelling its constituents. This research has shown that pantui also contains steroids and glycosides of unknown composition.[32]

Most of the Oriental harmony remedies so far examined have triterpenoidal glycosides within them. Ginseng and its relatives contain these novel kinds of substances which may be the key to their unique traditional uses as harmony medicines. And incredible as it may seem, medicinal plants everywhere in the world may owe their healing powers to these compounds, unsuspected by more than a handful of chemists such as Shibata and Elyakov. This includes plants which were once widely used but have been abandoned by a medicine that does not understand them. The tranquillizing valerian contains oleanolic triterpenoids not unlike those found in ginseng leaves. Sarsaparilla, the tonic drink of our grandfathers' day, is rich in saponins, some of them triterpenoid. Could it not be a mild version of the Oriental tonics with their similar constituents? Molasses has them, as do liquorice and senega.

As more plants are analysed, it will presumably become common to find these same active principles in widely different plants which nevertheless are used by traditional healers for similar purposes, just as the very rare dammarane-type terpenoidal glycosides were found in ginseng, jujube and brahmi. The opportunity of discovering more and more of these active principles is wide open to anyone who seeks to try his hand; for it is clear that the triterpenoidal glycosides so far discovered are just the tip of the iceberg. The Russians have continually turned up these terpenoidal glycosides when

studying plants taxonomically (by family) rather than eth-
nomedically (by reference to traditional medicine). In the
Araliaceae, for example, they have found triterpenoidal saponins in Aralia manshurica, Gypsophila pacifica and Clematis
manshurica. Within the Araliaceae there is often an overlap
where different species have some similar or identical active
constituents. Russian researchers have studied no less than
1730 Central Asian plant species from 104 families. Triterpenoid saponins were found in 627 species.[33]

Have we uncovered a vast untapped reservoir of mild
medicines? A sea of active principles whose very gentleness
has kept them hidden from the bullish investigations of pharmacologists with their laboratory models of diseased animals?
Will we now understand in scientific terms the action of a large
number of folk medicines which were always a mystery,
because those few who studied them did not know in which
chemical quarter to search for their active principles?

But was anything previously known concerning the medicinal value of these saponins? For of course it would be embarrassing to open a textbook to find that such saponins are
already well known, as, for example, narcotics. It turns out
that the dammarane triterpenoid saponins have never been
noticed to have any particular medical or biological property.[34] Even more astonishing, the science of pharmacology
has not found any specific medicinal activity in any of the
triterpenoid saponins as a whole, aside from their general
'soapiness'. Unlike the steroidal glycosides, the terpenoidal
glycosides are not used as medicines in the West. It is important to understand that this does not mean that they are
inactive. It means that so far no activity has been noticed in the
laboratory. Why is this? We have stressed that new drugs are
only discovered by first finding some model with which to
test them. Pharmacology has never had models to test for the
activity of these saponins.

Now we know that we are dealing with something completely new, we can expect discoveries. The ship can set sail for
uncharted territory without fear of reaching some apparently
new land which turns out to be a few miles along the shore
from the point of departure.

7
The Hormone Hypothesis

THE QUEST FOR A THEORY

It is absolutely essential that we develop a coherent medical model of the way ginseng and the harmony drugs work. It would be the valid passport into Western medicine. We need an underlying theory to guide us.

Such a theory must be scientifically expressed; it is true that in China ginseng is already 'understood' as a pharmacological agent, but this awareness is part and parcel of Chinese culture. There is nothing in our heritage to give it a framework. We cannot talk about it in the Chinese way as a warming medicine for Yang deficiency. That is borrowed language and means little to most of us.

How are we to know which are the central actions of the harmony remedies? Testing for arousal and performance was relatively easy, and it gave us a simple answer. Then with a jolt we realize that the answer is only as good as the question. If we now ask a broader question, we may get a broader answer. Do these harmony drugs have a more fundamental effect on the mind and body, of which stimulation is merely one consequence? If these harmony drugs reinforce some deep Yang energy within the body, would not stimulation automatically result if we looked for it? Have we not been testing our motor in a motor rally and, flushed with success at the winning of races, failed to look under the bonnet?

Suddenly we realize what is behind these tests. What really has been tested in the motor rally, in the mouse-swimming test, by the telegraphists crossing out letters and by the Russian athletes running races? One thing – stress. Stress is behind each of these tests. Fatigue is only a type of stress. Stress occurs when a man tries to concentrate on coding letters in the radio room, or when a mouse tries to learn how to escape an electric shock with a scientist peering in on its cage and the fluorescent lights glaring overhead. An organism at the limit of its capacities is in stress.

INSIDE THE *MILIEU INTÉRIEUR*

If these are the kind of situations which make the effect of the harmony drugs particularly clear, we must delve into the body to see how it copes at such times. We should ask what stress is. So let us digress a little in order to understand this critical concept.

Man is more adaptable than any other creature. The Sherpas are healthy living in the rarefied air of the Himalayas, the Bedouin likewise in the burning deserts of Arabia, and beyond them both is the man working on the sea bottom, using artifice to stretch his adaptability even further. Other animals are less adaptable. A seal can live in freezing seawater, its body at a cosy 37°C, but it would only last a moment in a sand desert. At the furthest extreme from man are single-celled creatures. If the environment changes, they die.

Yet man is composed of the same biological materials as these creatures. To what, then, does he owe his superadaptability? It turns out that the vital processes of man are as vulnerable as those of the most primitive of creatures. However, a considerable physiological industry is at work with the sole purpose of ensuring that within the body there is a sea of warmth, richness, calm and clemency. Man's physiology is continuously making adjustments to maintain a constant environment inside the body, whatever conditions occur outside. If the environment is cold, the muscles shiver to make heat and the blood vessels change their size to conserve it. If it is hot, another set of responses begins, including sweating and expansion of the blood vessels. Either way, the vital processes nestling deep in the core of the body remain at their optimum temperature, undisturbed.

The vital processes are bathed in a secure watery shell which acts as a buffer or shock absorber against the external environment. This stable internal world, called by the French physiologist Claude Bernard the 'milieu intérieur',[1] requires a considerable amount of energy and organization to maintain it. The dynamic balance was given the name 'homeostasis' by the famous psychologist Walter Cannon. Within the brain are measuring devices taking continual readings of the internal situation. These sample the *milieu intérieur* and instruct the machinery of the body to boost or drop the temperature, the sugar level, the salt level, the blood pressure and so on. They maintain this 'balance that results from the continual and delicate compensation by the most sensitive scales'.[1]

FIGHT OR FLIGHT

But this is only half the story. The greatest threat to life processes occurs when the body suffers some attack or challenge. Whether pursued by a hairy mammoth or a man with a gun, demands are placed on the body which are just as potentially disruptive to the internal environment as starvation or freezing weather. A stronger kind of reaction is necessary. It is the obverse of the gentle peace-time maintenance of equilibrium. Now the heart speeds and increases blood pressure so that blood can rush to the muscles, supplying oxygen and fuel and removing waste. Hearing and smell become more acute and the pupil of the eye widens, taking in more information. Breathing becomes faster, while the blood vessels near the skin contract to reduce loss of blood in case of injury. Sweating increases so as to cool down a system heated by strong muscular exertion. At the same time energy and blood are shifted away from functions such as digestion which are not relevant to coping with risks. The saliva dries, the stomach secretions are reduced, the bladder and bowels relax . . . *and the mind becomes alert and aroused.*

Cannon called this a readiness for 'fight or flight'.[2] The situation is one of *stress*. Stress rocks the boat; the captain must wake up and do something about it. Stress is the response of the body to demands made upon it:[3] chasing, fighting, competing, changing body rhythms or a hard day at the works. There are degrees of stress. A ski-jumper would experience a brief burst of intense stress, while his spectators resonate with an empathetic burst of mild stress.

The emotions are sometimes regarded as ancient mechanisms for marshalling all the forces of the body under the banner of the will.[4] This may be true, although it explains emotions no more than the creasing of the face musculature explains laughter. However, it is clear that all types of emotional excitement – whether fear, rage, love, hate or even hunger – are accomplished by the same series of fight-or-flight bodily activations. Strong emotion is therefore stressful, particularly grief.

DRUGS AGAINST STRESS?

A whole new vista opens up. If these harmony remedies have something to do with stress, it might explain much of what we have already observed. If we look back on all our evidence so far, one clue emerges: an essential difference between the harmony remedies and the stimulants is that stimulants seem to affect behaviour all the time, but the harmony remedies only seem to act when the person or animal is experiencing some kind of powerful challenge. For example, spontaneous activity is not affected by ginseng, nor is sleep, nor are the brain wave-patterns, but exploration, racing, and learning in the gruelling Pavlovian style are affected. Performance under stress invariably improves, as Brekhman's intuition told him.

If the foundations of research have been the solid evidence that ginseng and certain other harmonizers increase arousal and the quality of performance, the next step is to find out whether this effect is indeed connected with stress. One way would be to see if the ginseng arousal allowed laboratory animals to deal more effectively with specifically stressful challenges which do not require stamina. These studies have been carried out by a group of us in London. We decided to give mice ginseng for their entire lives, from just after birth until death. During this time we could watch their health and also test their ability to deal with stress. At certain intervals we would take a mouse out of its cage and place it in a novel situation: a flat round plate, known as an 'open field'. Mice like dark corners, as we all know, and when the mouse is placed on this white flat area, it feels exposed and vulnerable, and consequently experiences mild stress, a situation we reinforced by making noises. The mouse is divided: on the one hand it wants to explore this new situation and sniff out any potential threats or gastronomic possibilities; on the other hand it is frightened and wants to hide. The conflicting urges lead to a mixture of explorative activity (inquisitive running about) and the fear reaction (crouching).

Animals treated with ginseng crouched much more than the control animals and moved less. Its effect must therefore be quite distinct from mere stimulation, which would have produced more random sallies. It doesn't necessarily mean that ginseng increases the emotions concerned. The animals may or may not have felt more fearful. But they certainly acted more fully upon whatever degree of fear or anxiety they did experience.[5]

If the degree of stress was stepped up a bit by adding mild electric shocks to the white wilderness, the animals clearly responded more to the stress. It seemed that the animals actually experienced *less fear* after ginseng. Many of the control animals became severely frightened and defecated on the open field, while the animals treated with ginseng defecated less and showed less alarm.[6] They showed the same kind of improved reaction to stress during avoidance-learning trials. In place of the paralysing experience of fear in the stressed situation, there was an increase in purposeful action, including an understandable aggression against the experimenter.[7]

Indeed, if we look back over all the behavioural studies, the general principle emerges that the more stressful the experience, the stronger the ginseng effect. Petkov, for example, with his severe Pavlovian trials (which are known to be very stressful[8]) found a stronger effect of ginseng than Saito with his mild find-the-cheese tests.

We can conclude that the effects of ginseng on mental states are connected with the readiness produced by stress, the fight-or-flight arousal. They are not the result of pure excitation of the brain, as Petkov thought. In that case, does ginseng affect other components of the response of the body to stress?

THE KEY: THE BATTLE FOR SURVIVAL

The Russians had some inkling of this. Brekhman, and others, were aware that their early work gave a minimal and distorted picture of the root. They realized that stress was involved somehow. So over a period of twenty years they subjected tens of thousands of small animals to extremes of stress: some were placed in very hot or very cold environments or bombarded with lethal X-rays, others forced to carry out excessive physical work or prevented from taking any exercise at all. They were placed in artificially high or low pressure and accelerated in centrifuges. They were subject to chemical stresses, such as poisons, narcotics, toxic anti-cancer drugs, high doses of the heart drug digitalis and other substances, and biological stresses such as bacterial infections, malaria, surgery, the implantation of cancers, and artificially induced diabetes.

Many would say these tests were objectionable because of the suffering endured by the animals. In the UK these studies would never have been permitted by the Home Office. Yet they were methodologically adequate; and there was no doubt of the result. Ginseng and those harmony remedies tested by the Russians were able to increase the resistance of animals indiscriminately against all the stresses.[9,10] For example, rats who received something like 50,000 times as much radiation as a chest X-ray died after a short time. They survived twice as long if they had been given eleutherococcus or ginseng beforehand.[11] These studies have been repeated in the research centres which we have met before in this book. The Chinese chose to home in on the resistance to malaria parasites and typhoid vaccine as typical biological stresses, and artificially lowered atmospheric pressure and oxygen as physical stresses,[12] while the Koreans studied extremes of temperature and the effect of X-rays.[13] Both confirmed that ginseng improved the chances of survival in extremis. Other harmony remedies were effective in this way, including san-chi, pantocrine and, especially, eleutherococcus, as well as some Araliaceae plants, Schizandra chinensis berries, and possibly Beuplurum chinensis. The purely stimulant plants such as Aralia manshurica and chemicals such as amphetamine did not improve the animals' general resistance to stress. If anything, they made the animals more vulnerable.[14]

The Russian scientists now probed a bit deeper into the body. Instead of simply watching how the animals fared under severe stress, they looked at how their specific physiological processes coped with the imbalances. They artificially raised blood pressure and found that the medicines could reduce it. They lowered blood pressure and found the opposite. When they loaded the animals with sugar, they could eliminate it better. On the other hand, the medicines could raise low blood sugar. We will take a close look at these effects of the plants later. What is important here is that the medicines were shown to *assist the restoration of homeostasis or harmony*.

Now there are well-known pure drugs that can raise blood pressure, and there are others that lower it; there are some that lower blood sugar, some that help the body resist X-rays, and some that can assist in the removal of poisons. But each of these has a single defined effect on the body which always occurs, whether the body needs it or not. They also only work in one direction. A harmony drug can have all or any of these properties. It has no apparent effect in the absence of stress, but as soon as stress is applied it restores body processes to normal, *whatever the direction in which they have strayed*. In other words, the stress sets the drugs working, and the body's general resistance is increased. It is a current axiom of the science of drugs that there are no substances in existence which can raise the general resistance of the body beyond that normally expected. The harmony drugs have been overlooked.

The ability of these drugs to adjust or restore harmony in the *milieu intérieur* when, and only when, stress is applied led Brekhman to call them 'adaptogens': drugs which increase adaptation, or adjustment to changes in the environment. I call them harmony drugs because it is more in tune with both the Oriental and the present Western conceptions of them. It will now be clearer why I use this word.

HORMONES AND HARMONY

Let us try and take our quest one stage further. Where and how do these harmony drugs help the body bear extra loads? First we need to understand how the body copes with stress: what mechanisms does it use?

The brain records changes or threats to the stable inner environment, and flashes instructions to the physiology to make the necessary adjustments. Messages are sent from the brain by special housekeeping nerves called the autonomic nervous system. One part of this system is concerned with maintaining the equilibrium during continuous minor fluctuations, the other part with alarm. It prepares the inner environment for fight-or-flight. This part also induces the adrenal gland, lying just above the kidney, to secrete a chemical called adrenaline. This substance is now so well known that the word adrenaline is used as a synonym for arousal in everyday language. While the nerves provide instantaneous mobilization of body defences and preparedness, adrenaline begins to course through the bloodstream as well.

The electric-adrenaline answer that flashes through the body makes for readiness. But this is only the beginning of the story. When the soldiers are in the middle of a three-kilometre run, the adrenaline stimulus of the starting gun is only a dim memory. They are involved in a new kind of situation: the maintenance of their maximum capacity, rather than its initiation. Stamina is required to cope with the situation.

Slower, more pervasive changes are now taking place. A back-up system is being brought into operation to maintain the state of arousal. The adrenaline system is like the instant mobilization of the troops, while the long-term changes are like the supportive readiness of the home front. This readiness is organized by hormones, chemicals which issue from certain glands around the body and coordinate the various activities: for example growth hormone (involved in uniform and orderly body development) or testosterone and oestrogen (involved in the development and maintenance of sexual activity). Adrenaline too is a hormone, concerned with speedy arousal. The particular hormones which chiefly orchestrate the long-term preparedness of the body are called *glucocorticoids*. They are key hormones with which we shall be concerned in this book. Thyroid and growth hormone also play a minor role in the body's metabolic mobilization. The glucocorticoids are made in the outer layer of the adrenal gland, the tissue of which is separate from the adrenaline-secreting inner layer. This outer layer makes about thirty hormones, which have many functions throughout the body. Besides the glucocorticoids, it produces mineralocorticoids which are mostly involved with salt and water balance, and a minor quotient of sex hormones.[15] When the glucocorticoids of man are analysed, it turns out that one single hormone makes up about 95 per cent of their quantity: cortisol, or hydrocortisone.

The following figures (4 and 5) show the nerve and hormone systems, as well as the list of actions of the glucocorticoid stress hormones.

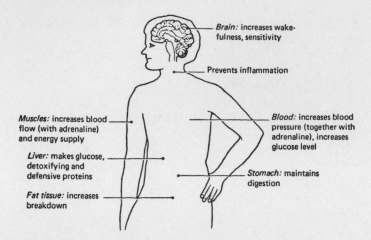

Brain: increases wake-
fulness, sensitivity

Prevents inflammation

Muscles: increases blood
flow (with adrenaline)
and energy supply

Liver: makes glucose,
detoxifying and
defensive proteins

Fat tissue: increases
breakdown

Blood: increases blood
pressure (together with
adrenaline), increases
glucose level

Stomach: maintains
digestion

Figure 4   The human body and the effects of the stress steroids.

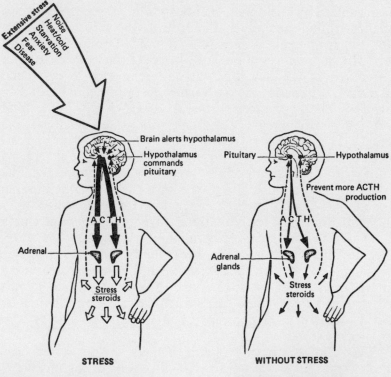

Extensive stress
Noise
Heat/cold
Starvation
Anxiety
Fear
Disease

Brain alerts hypothalamus

Hypothalamus
commands
pituitary

ACTH

Adrenal

Stress
steroids

STRESS

Pituitary

Hypothalamus

Prevent more ACTH
production

ACTH

Adrenal
glands

Stress
steroids

WITHOUT STRESS

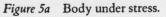

Figure 5a   Body under stress.

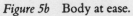

Figure 5b   Body at ease.

THE HYPOTHALAMIC PUPPET-MASTER

The adrenal glands are only the manufacturing plant. They make the hormones from the starting materials. They receive directions from a pea-shaped organ in the brain called the pituitary. These instructions are brought on a master hormone called adrenocorticotrophic hormone (ACTH for short), which means literally the 'adrenal-cortex-feeding' hormone. The pituitary controls most of the hormones of the body, measuring their amounts and making necessary adjustments.

But even the pituitary cannot decide which level of the hormones is appropriate for any circumstance in which the body finds itself. Real decisions are made by a further control-centre, at the top of the hormone hierarchy. This is a most remarkable unit of the brain called the hypothalamus. It receives information from the brain on events outside the body, assesses the conditions within the body and instructs the pituitary to make appropriate hormonal adjustments to the *milieu intérieur*. The hypothalamus is the core of the entire harmony maintenance system of the body. Embedded in the lower or 'visceral' brain, it is well placed to interact above as well as below, to send and receive signals from the conscious thinking part of the brain as well as to run the automatic responses of the body. Through its executive wing, the pituitary, it instructs hormone messengers to stimulate or suppress the metabolism, the appetite, heat production and salt elimination. When arousal is necessary, it instructs the pituitary to release ACTH and the glucocorticoids begin to surge through the body.

The remarkable fact about this organ is that it is not only the puppet-master which, out of sight, pulls the strings to control all the puppets which keep the body in order; it also has a powerful controlling influence on sexual activity and on growth and reproduction. Even more than that, it can stimulate the emotions. We might have suspected as much, knowing how emotional excitement puts the body on alert in the same way as any other kind of challenge. A Swiss scientist, Hess, made the early seminal discovery that electrical stimulation of the hypothalamus of a cat would result in instant and total rage, or fear or pleasure, depending on the point stimulated.

The hypothalamus is thus at the centre of body-housekeeping as well as body-defence. All body systems are related to each other in a flux, with the hypothalamus at the centre. The hypothalamus is at the interface between mind and body, coordinating the readiness of both, and it is measurer and master of the state of preparedness.

GINSENG AND THE STRESS HORMONES

When I first set out to construct some kind of picture from the multitude of studies on ginseng, I felt as if I were submerged under a great river in full flood. So many reports purported to show so many different effects on the body; ginseng seemed to affect blood pressure, blood formation, the nerves, the brain, blood sugar, muscle action, the liver, the kidney, and so on. It was beyond belief. Then I stepped back from science and suddenly realized that the river is exactly like the flow of energy in the whole being, and all the scientific material seemed then to be like efforts to cut this river into cubes of water. The scientific reports seemed so broad in scope because they were all manifestations of some deeper action.

Now, looking at the mechanisms of stress, it seemed absolutely clear to me: the liver, the sugar metabolism, the blood, the muscles, stamina, mental arousal . . . what are they all? They are tools of the mobilized body. By what means is this mobilization achieved? By the glucocorticoid stress hormones, which are involved in these long-term changes, and in the resistance to stress. A glance at Figure 5 will show how closely the physiological effects of the glucocorticoids match the range of reputed effects of ginseng. Maybe we should take a closer look at those curious glands, the adrenals, which disseminate the stress message throughout the body.

The adrenal glands are very much involved in the effect of the harmony drugs. In the first place, the increased resistance to stress induced by ginseng is substantially reduced when the adrenal glands are removed.[16] They are necessary for most of ginseng's effects. There is now a large body of evidence showing that when ginseng is given to relaxed animals there is more manufacturing activity in the adrenal glands. New cells are made,[17] likewise more steroid.[18] However, these changes are not so important and consistent as those seen when the animals are subjected to stress. Then ginseng has a dramatic impact on the adrenal glands. It is so clear and noticeable that, like the mouse-swimming test, the study has been taken up by researcher after researcher in order to show something unequivocal about ginseng.

In stress, ginseng helps the adrenal glands to mount an immediate hormonal response; more stress hormones are released and more manufactured. But when stress stops, the adrenal glands shut down more quickly. If stress is long and severe, the glands conserve their resources and do not release so much hormone.[19, 21] These effects, which have been demonstrated so far in ginseng, pantocrine, san-chi, eleutherococcus and their active principles, are not enormous. But what is important is that the adrenal glands are responding more sensitively and effectively to stress:

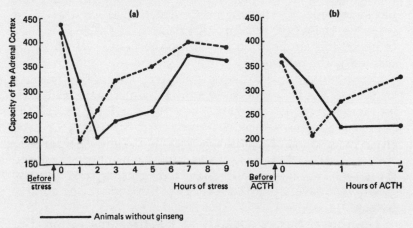

Figure 6   Animals are subjected to the stress of a hot environment (Fig. 6a) or injected with the stress master hormone ACTH (Fig. 6b). The capacity of the adrenal gland is measured at various times after the stress is applied. The animals which had been given ginseng had a stronger adrenal response and a faster recovery rate. (Redrawn from Kim, C. et al, *Lloydia*, Vol 33, pp 43–8, 1970.)

Ginseng, it seems, is making the hormone stress response more efficient; *tighter*. This is a seminal finding, one which underpins the hypothesis that will now be developed of how the harmony remedies actually work. It has two kinds of implications which we discuss at the end of this chapter. Firstly, the body will be more resistant, capable of mounting a more powerful protracted defence against stress. Secondly, this battle will do less harm to its battleground – the body. I believe this gives us a first real inkling of the value of the harmony remedies.

'GINSENG DOESN'T JUST GO TO YOUR HEAD, IT GETS EVERYWHERE'[22]

We are not out of the wood yet. The adrenal effect is an eye-opener and clarifies much. But the adrenals are merely the playthings of the higher centres of regulation. They dance to the tune of the pituitary gland, the melody being conveyed by the peptide hormone ACTH. The hypothalamus plays this pituitary pipe. If the harmony drugs sharpen the stress response, the whole system must be involved. The first place to check this supposition would be the next level up in the hierarchy, the pituitary.

We should be able to check if ginseng acts on the pituitary by seeing if it still works on animals which have had their pituitaries removed. It turns out that as long as ACTH is given, ginseng still works without any pituitary or even any stress at all. It produces just the same sharper and tighter adrenal response as if the pituitary had been there and the stress had been real.[21,23] Indeed, ginseng can actually modify the severity of the ACTH commands to the adrenal tissues.[24]

This throws the ball squarely back in the adrenal court. But there is some very recent conflicting evidence that the pituitary may be involved after all. A change in the quantity of a key chemical in the adrenal glands called cyclic AMP occurs during the first thirty minutes after ginseng administration, and is prevented by removal of the pituitary gland.[25] This finding would indicate that ginseng does cause a direct increase in ACTH master hormone after all, which directly contradicts the above.

Conflicts like this in science indicate the end of the old road.

They are also the gates to the unknown. I began to add some spice of conjecture to the soup of experiment.

Perhaps, I asked, the conflict would be resolved if we stepped up to the next level? Perhaps the pituitary too, like the adrenals, plays a passive role, and the hypothalamus, which controls the pituitary, is the root of it all. After all, nothing moves in the hormone defences unless it be commanded by the hypothalamus. Since the harmony remedies affect the *control* of the stress hormones, it would seem likely that they involve the hypothalamus. Also, the hypothalamus is the hormone door connecting mind and body; would this not be a fitting place for such remedies to work?

On the other hand, even if the hypothalamus were in some way central to the story, other parts of the stress system would also be involved. We need not exclude the adrenal glands or even the pituitary because of the evidence we have discussed. Nor should we entirely exclude the *targets* of these glands – namely, the tissues and organs which the steroids switch on. For I had demonstrated that ginseng affected isolated body cells which were grown in a glass dish without connection to glands, hormones or any other part of the body. I realized then that the stress-control system functioned as a whole. To attempt to dismember the system in order to find out *the* site of action of the harmony drugs was like trying to separate the dog from its bark.

AN HYPOTHESIS

I should like to propose that the harmony remedies amplify the effect of certain hormones. They act wherever these hormones act.

Ginseng, eleutherococcus and others are involved with stress steroids. When one takes ginseng, let us imagine that it spreads throughout the body priming or readying sites where the stress steroids normally attach. This would produce little effect when there is no stress. However, when stress occurs the steroids also flood the body and now find their path into the tissues facilitated. Thus smaller amounts are needed for an equivalent effect.

This does not mean that every place in the body is affected equally. The brain areas involved in the fundamental control of stress, particularly the hypothalamic puppet-master which is in charge, are, I believe, the special focus of these particular harmony drugs. The hypothalamus itself becomes more sensitive to stress hormone. The sensitized hypothalamus produces much more ACTH and stress steroid when stress occurs. But if stress is prolonged the sensitized hypothalamus becomes touchy; measuring the level of stress steroids in the body, it shuts down the stress hormone system more rapidly. This would explain how the stress steroids are conserved during stress or shut down more quickly when stress stops.

I feel that it is more than coincidence that the active principles of most of the harmony remedies are triterpenoids. It supports our picture, for triterpenoids are quite similar to steroids in chemical structure. It is quite conceivable that their paths meet within the tissues.

I believe that the range of active principles in the various drugs generally act in the same way, but they 'prefer' different sites: ginseng and eleutherococcus may prefer the hypothalamus, beuplurum may prefer the liver, and so on. Yet they overlap, attaching to other sites all over the body. There are precedents. Testosterone, for example, acts primarily on sexual tissues, but also to a lesser extent on other tissues around the body.

I began to search for evidence to back up these ideas. I found out that the ginseng active principles did indeed spread throughout the body after ingestion,[26] which indicates that they have at least the possibility of acting everywhere. However, no experiments have ever been carried out on the effect of these Oriental remedies on the hypothalamus. So I initiated some experiments at Chelsea College, which were executed by a bright Ph.D student in the pharmacology department called Deepak Shori, under the tutelage of Professor Ginsberg.

Laboratory rats had their adrenal glands and ovaries removed so that there was no chance of any internal production of the stress steroids. Then for eight days they were given either ginseng or placebos. Following this the animals were injected with pure corticosterone (the main stress steroid) which had been 'tagged' so that it was possible to detect it in the tissues (like ringing a bird to find it again). The corticosterone was found again, in the brain, but here was the surprise. In some areas of the lower 'visceral' brain (particularly the hippocampus) of those animals which had been given ginseng, severalfold greater amounts of the tagged corticosterone were found than in the brains of the other animals! Clearly ginseng treatment had produced a massive sensitization of those lower brain areas (in which the hypothalamus is located) to the steroid.[27] This supports the hypothesis in a general way, although we cannot exclude certain other possibilities at the moment, particularly that ginseng may be affecting the general metabolism of steroids.

Nevertheless, the result is an eye-opener. Nothing like it has ever been found before in this field of research. Certainly no such huge effect on the body is usually seen as a result of ginseng treatment. This work is, of course, a beginning, not an end. Much more research needs to be carried out before we can properly understand what is going on. But here at last is firm evidence of ginseng's connection with the stress steroids. Here too is a demonstration of a strong and clear effect of ginseng on the brain – not the cortex in its lofty box, but the lower brain that regulates and monitors internal harmony.

RETHINKING AROUSAL

We have a basic theory. Let us see if we can apply it to the questions voiced in Chapter 5. There we described how the first attempts at investigating the harmony remedies in the laboratory found noticeable improvements in endurance, alertness, concentration and the ability to carry out complex tasks. We came to the preliminary conclusion that the harmony remedies promoted performance and integration of mind and body, especially in the face of tiredness and stress. Then we mentioned that they were safer and more effective at increasing performance than classical stimulants. But how is this achieved, and how does it relate to our theory?

The reticular formation is the conductor of wakefulness. It kicks the entire brain into action when part of it perceives such a necessity. At the same time, it tells the hypothalamus of the situation and the hypothalamus sends the cascade of nerve-adrenaline instructions down to the body to mobilize itself. However, not all arousal comes from the higher brain perception of alarm, food and so on, as Pavlov would have it. Hunger can wake us up. So can fear. The stress of alarm can produce incredible activation. A normally slothful, sanguine person can be turned into a demon of energy when he is at risk or when faced with a deadline. Motivation, the will, and the passions can do the same from inside, whether or not there is stress from outside. Indeed the will, when harnessed, is one of the most powerful tools for arousal.

The primal powerhouses of the emotions are connected with centres of the lower brain, centres which we know are sensitive to the state of the body. Hormones can wake up the mind in this way. How many of us have experienced times when we want to sleep but some alarm or anxiety keeps the hormones shooting round the body, kicking our mind into reluctant wakefulness? Hormones are involved in sexual *arousal*, or the nest-feathering activities of expectant mothers close to birth. This hormone excitement is one of the avenues to wakefulness. The reticular formation is here tickled from below rather than kicked from above.

This has a special relevance to us, for we have proposed that the arousal produced by ginseng and certain other harmony remedies is connected with stress hormones. Their effect on competence, learning ability and stamina indicates that, unlike any other known stimulants, they influence the lower brain's powerhouses. I propose that the arousal of the harmony remedies is hormonal, not neuronal. It is close to, or identical with, the kind of arousal produced naturally in states of readiness by the action of hormones on the brain, that goes hand in hand with motivation or emotion, not the kind of jagged excitation produced by signal amplification in higher brain areas.

In order to be consistent with my theory, stamina and wakefulness must also be a consequence of the stress steroids. Is there any evidence that these hormones can actually stimulate? Support for this has come only recently from an unexpected quarter. During certain behavioural studies at the University of Utrecht, in Holland, Professor de Wied noticed that if he gave pure ACTH to animals he could produce distinct psychological improvements. It became apparent that ACTH and other hormones of the pituitary have a direct line into the brain to modify its behaviour. They act on the visceral brain, on areas concerned with vigilance, emotion, arousal and homeostasis.[28]

De Wied then discovered that the stress steroids also affect behaviour, but in an opposite manner to that of ACTH. Animals learn more easily as a result of ACTH injection, are more adaptable and sensitive when they are given glucocorticoids. Like ACTH, the corticoids were found to bind directly to the brain.[29] This was completely unexpected: hormones which were previously thought to flow out of the brain's black box to instruct the body in fact also circulate within the brain. Those hormones have been called psychohormones.

Doctors and psychiatrists have also noticed that their patients who were given ACTH or corticosteroid for medical reasons often developed a profound increase in vitality and energy. This was especially true of the aged and chronically sick, who sometimes experienced a 'miraculous' relief of severe physical complaints. But these hormones are not panaceas.[30] The effect is only temporary:

I had an American housewife with dermatomyositis who had been taught how to play the piano when she was little and had continued for the entertainment of the children, but didn't get very far. When she started on large doses of ACTH she was suddenly able to play the most difficult works of Beethoven and Chopin – and the children of the neighbours would gather in the garden to hear her play. . . . But she also became a little psychotic and so her dosage of ACTH had to be lowered, and with every 10 units of ACTH one sonata disappeared. It all ended up with the same old music poorly performed.[31]

Behind vigilance and alertness, behind stamina and performance, there are two fundamental driving forces: energy and will. It is these which ACTH primarily affects. This was made clear in experiments in which animals were trained to find food and subsequently the search was made difficult or impossible. The animals which had been given ACTH continued much more doggedly after the goal.

The corticosteroids complement ACTH. While ACTH improves motivation and performance, corticosteroids provide the focusing. They increase selectivity in the face of danger. ACTH and the corticosteroids join in a dual supercharge of the mind. 'ACTH analogues and steroids may therefore contribute to the integration of information from the *milieu extérieur* and *milieu intérieur* which is probably essential for recognizing stimulus-specific cues,' writes de Wied.[29] In other words, they are basic behavioural adaptations to changes in the environment. The more threatening the environment, the more they are needed.

The fascinating thing about these discoveries is that the kinds of improvements produced by hormones are precisely like those recorded for the harmony drugs: greater capacity, mental performance and memory, improved sensory awareness, faster learning, and quicker relearning in a new situation, as well as reduced errors. They were, as with harmony drugs, very far from the kind of pure excitation of the classical stimulants. ACTH, like the harmony drugs, is long-lasting, and does not have the side-effect of jitteriness. Similarly, ACTH was found to affect the vigilance system of the brain but not spontaneous random running about.[32]

It means that they must act through the same path. My view of the process is this: triterpenoidal saponins prime the pump in the hypothalamus, which in turn accelerates a flood of ACTH-type proteins around the brain and of ACTH itself around the body, producing hormone arousal, mental energy and will, vigilance, stamina and coordination. There is evidence that this occurs without connection with the adrenal glands.[33] The fact that the balanced arousal is so close to the kind of arousal produced by psychohormones tends to confirm the hormone theory of the way these remedies act.

We can see, in retrospect, how superficial was our early view. We suggested that the harmony remedies are so balanced in their effect on our functions only because they are natural products and contain a range of components which balance each other. The quality of ginseng's stimulation is then not a special consequence of its particular active principles, but only of their convenient mixture. This position is now untenable. The unique balanced character of the arousal produced by these compounds arises in virtue of their interaction with psychohormones, and is therefore written into the structure of the active principles themselves.

How then can we interpret the fact that Japanese researchers found some principles which were stimulatory and some sedative? I believe that an answer has been found by Dr Staba of Minneapolis. Using his sophisticated methods of chemical analysis, he has shown that when ginseng is eaten the 'triols (stimulatory active principles) reach a higher dose level in the tissues than the 'diols (sedative active principles). The sedative/stimulatory differences are only the result of the amounts of each saponin in the body,[34] as is known to happen with other drugs. The music of the root is 'pharmacokinetic' music.

We can also, with respect, overturn Petkov's view of ginseng's action. He imagined that it stimulated the higher brain which then woke up the body. I believe that the hormone arousal story tells us the opposite. The hypothalamus is sensitized first and then generates readiness in the cortex via the reticular network.

There is even a simple laboratory test for the difference between the two types of stimulation. If the harmony drugs act via ACTH-type substances which are proteins, they would require manufacture of proteins to work. Stimulants which cause excitation by locking into nerve cells should not. This study has actually been carried out. The psychophysical effects of eleutherococcus were found to be absolutely dependent on the manufacture of protein, while the effects of amphetamine were absolutely independent.[35]

The arousal produced by the harmony remedies is, in summary, directed discriminatory and motivational energy. It is an exaggeration of normal ability, not a caricature; an arousal that can help an organism adapt to its environment and get on better in the world.

HORMONES AND OTHER HARMONY REMEDIES

There is a gross imbalance in research. For historical and commercial reasons ginseng has stolen the show. Yet it is only one of a group. Now that we are getting to understand the root, we should see how far we can bring in the other harmony remedies.

We can be fairly sure that eleutherococcus, san-chi and pantocrine, as well as their active principles, act on the stress steroid system in the way we have described for ginseng. Chinese evidence would also implicate schizandra and its active principles. Some of the Araliaceae plants, particularly Raponticum carthamoides and Rhodiola rosea, have a considerable pedigree of Soviet laboratory work, mostly through their ability to increase resistance to diverse stresses.[9] They have also been found to preserve homeostasis in true harmony-remedy fashion. But they have not been directly tested on the adrenal glands. Most of the other harmony remedies have hardly been tested at all. We can only infer that they operate in a similar fashion within the body because they are arousing without being excitants, and they have similar glycoside active principles.

Not all Oriental harmony remedies need be arousing, and they do not necessarily work on the stress steroids. Our requirement in scientific terms is only that they are safe and mild medicines which maintain homeostasis in the face of stress. Liquorice is such a harmony remedy, and fortunately it has been considerably researched. We have seen that it contains a triterpenoidal saponin, glycyrrhizin. It also affects the steroids from the adrenal glands, not the glucocorticoid stress hormones, but the mineralocorticoids.[36] The mineralocorticoids have certain opposite effects to stress steroids. While stress steroids mobilize the body's defensive army, the mineralocorticoids balance it, particularly since they retain water and salt within the body. Thus liquorice does not cause arousal. There is some interest in liquorice in the West for the treatment of gastric ulcer, a use never imagined by Shen Nung, but born out of more modern necessities. However, doctors found that ingestion of liquorice for long periods had certain side-effects which could be abolished by removing the triterpenoid glycoside. These were alterations of salt levels in the body and of the blood pressure. However, these subtle actions are the very ones which put liquorice into the category of kingly remedies. The saponin is the valuable portion to Eastern physicians but the unwanted portion to their Western counterparts. It is effective for those who know how to use it and inconvenient to those who don't. One man's meat is another man's poison.

Now that the ice has broken, perhaps more of the vast cornucopia of these remarkable materials with their similar active principles will be explored. We should also explore existing Western drugs for this purpose. After all, we made the strong point that drugs for health would actually slip through the net of normal drug discovery according to Western methods. If the test methods described in the previous chapters are applied, one ought to be able to catch them.

This was how the Russians discovered the very first medicinal compound that had 'adaptogenic' properties. It was not ginseng at all, but dibazol, which was originally made and used as a compound to lower blood pressure until the late Professor Lazarev of Moscow put it through its paces. With Dr Rozin, he tested it on mice subjected to the usual wide range of noxious influences, including radiation and toxic drugs. It was active in increasing resistance and he named it the first adaptogen.[37] Subsequently it was tested for its effects on healthy people, and widely marketed. However, it has been superseded by eleutherococcus, which is much more effective.

Centrophenoxine is a safe compound which, as we saw in Chapter 5, is used to improve mental function. Is there any evidence that it can affect the stress system? There is evidence that it can improve homeostasis, particularly temperature control, blood pressure and blood sugar. French scientists have already suggested that it acts on the hypothalamus.[38] Then, to astonish us all, along comes Petkov who begs to inform us, in a scientific paper published in Italian, that he has been studying the effects of plant growth stimulators on animals for years before the French team thought of it. He confirms that centrophenoxine can stimulate learning and improve memory. Then he demonstrated that centrophenoxine could prevent depletion of the adrenal glands, and the effect was similar in quality to that of ginseng. He wrote that they are 'united by their common ability to regulate the . . . reactivity of the organism'.[39] He also noticed that centrophenoxine stimulated the activity of the thyroid gland, while stress reduced it. He therefore regards centrophenoxine as having an effect on those brain areas, the hypothalamus or pituitary, which control the stress responses and homeostasis. Petkov's conclusion is that centrophenoxine is a kind of poor synthetic ginseng. I would not go as far as that. It is generally less potent. But I would place it within the harmony drug category and hope that some more research can check that decision.

Ginseng was brought to the notice of the West because it stopped Père Jartoux from falling off his horse, but that should not set the tone of our interest in it. We are still after the crock of gold: health. Competence and activity are only part of it. Is there any connection between the stress hormones and disease? If there is, it would place in our grasp the elusive understanding of how these harmony remedies affect health.

It is important for our thesis that we fully understand the harmful effects of stress, so we will examine it in some detail.

THE DARK SIDE OF STRESS

Stress is a two-edged sword. On one hand, it is necessary. All creatures are moulded by the challenges of the world. Without calling on extra resources on occasion, man's adaptability would atrophy like an arm in a permanent sling. Mild stress is an aid to performance, presumably through the mechanisms of hormone excitement. It was certainly necessary to our ancestors for 'the alarm reaction of fight or flight made them ready in a flash to combat at peak efficiency, or to run away, depending on their evaluation of the odds. Moreover the physical exertion of a hunt served to burn up accumulated fuel and so release emotional tensions; the hunters could return to the camp with pleasantly tired bodies and feelings of satisfaction or triumph.'[40] Inner balance requires a modicum of stress. But there is a darker side to stress. Mobilization of resources can be costly and sacrificial as well as stimulating. Alarm systems begin to take more than they give, to cooperate in self-destruction, not in self-preservation. An executive sits at his desk – the blood vessels constricting, the pupils dilating, the digestion inhibited, adrenaline charging up the muscles and sugar supplies, the thyroid hormones and glucocorticoids shifting the metabolism, the whole body ridiculously ready for fight or flight. But nothing happens except tension, as this turmoil builds inside him and doesn't move further than the telephone.

Continuous overload is experienced by a remarkably large segment of the population. Most people in cities suffer from overstimulation, from noise, diverse threats and disturbances, crowding and a need for constant watchfulness. The mind can, of course, be a source of stress to the whole system even in the absence of unusual external threats. Complete relaxation is impossible to anxious people, since the mind is always working to maintain inner defences.

Studies have shown that each person has a certain constant and individual level of the stress hormones, a *hormone finger-print*, which is laid down very clearly. It is now felt that the personality of an individual is at least partly connected with his hormonal fingerprint. In one study, for example, people who were more emotionally expressive and more outgoing all made more glucocorticoid hormones. More guarded individuals had low levels of glucocorticoids.[41] Cases of anxiety and personality disintegration are always accompanied by excessive production of glucocorticoids and the relevant master-hormone, ACTH, as the body responds faithfully to the directions of the brain, in terrible abuse of fundamental defence mechanisms.

The effects of the environment are superimposed on the individual hormone fingerprint. A situation that opens the adrenal sluice-gate in one person may be without hormonal consequences in another. For example, research in the Vietnam war found that stress hormones always increased in anticipation rather than in action. Soldiers responded to a highly dangerous situation by a flurry of activity. They produced lots of adrenaline but there was little stress and little change in their stress hormone levels. It was the officers who demonstrated their load of responsibility with raised glucocorticoid levels.[42]

It is important to realize that people who can turn their stress load off at the end of a demanding task do not suffer from long-term detrimental stress. As Frankenhauser has pointed out, 'The speed at which baseline levels are regained may determine relative potency of harmful versus beneficial consequences.'[43] It is quite clear from hormone analyses that people do differ in the manner in which their system returns to normal after stress. Those whose hormone levels return quickly are generally less neurotic and more capable. They tend to be less uptight, more sanguine and better adjusted. In other words, you are best off if you can produce a high level of hormone on demand, and then drop it down quickly to a low level when the demand stops. On the other hand, research brought the chilling message that in stressful occupations, people become less capable of switching off their hormones; they are tired, worn, and in the end, ill.[44]

We can now make the obvious connection. If ginseng and

related harmony remedies make the stress hormone system more efficient, i.e. switch it on and return it to normal more quickly, is not this exactly what is needed to resist the harmful consequences of stress? Is this the basis of the belief that ginseng can improve health?

THE SOFT KILLER

What are the consequences of continuous mobilization of the resources of the body? Stress is only involved in something like half of all known disease! It is particularly relevant to the major killers of the modern world – heart attacks, strokes, high blood pressure, cancer and respiratory diseases. Although there is dispute about how much influence stress has on these diseases, there is no doubt that it is a contributory factor. It is *the* major cause of life-style illnesses such as gastric ulcer, colitis, asthma, certain kinds of skin conditions, migraine, impotence, irregular menstruation and menopausal disorders, insomnia and high blood pressure. These diseases occur on a colossal scale. Dr Pelletier in his excellent book on stress states that twenty to twenty-five million people are afflicted with high blood pressure in America, and thirty million with insomnia. He states, 'Stress-related psychological and physiological disorders have become the number one social and health problem in the last decade.'[45]

Stress undermines resistance and leads to various diseases which at first sight seem little to do with stress or the individual. It may be thought that stress is clearly irrelevant to infections. After all, one can inject microbes into an animal and it will fall ill. But if we ask why a certain person will fall ill with a certain disease at one time and not another, we unleash a barrage of uncertainties. It is impossible to escape the fact that psychological factors and life-experience are partly involved in susceptibility to most diseases. Only in the recent past have they been lumped under an umbrella of ignorance called 'environment'.

I remember the case of a friend of mine who spent some time in India in the very best of health despite a fairly casual attitude to the problem of contagious disease. At one point he entered a crisis in which he called into question his entire Western, university-trained personal identity, and immediately contracted viral hepatitis for his pains. Such experiences are a common part of our everyday life. There is a very great deal of scientific work which demonstrates that when the body experiences stress, susceptibility increases and the pathogenic organisms which are always around us take the opportunity provided and start to multiply. Episodes of infectious diseases such as urethritis or herpes virus are familiar to doctors as difficult diseases to remove because they recur at times of stress.

One series of studies illustrates the research on this subject. Mice were put through the stress of conditioned-avoidance trials. These are of the same type as those used to demonstrate an effect of ginseng on arousal and learning. After a long period of stressful training, the mice were found to be much more susceptible to virus diseases such as polio. Mice housed in crowded stressful conditions are much more likely to become infested with parasites.[45] A recent major article on the subject of disease resistance concluded, 'Even susceptibility to microbial infectious diseases is thought to be a function of environmental conditions culminating in physiological stress on the individual, rather than simply exposure to an external source of infection.'[47]

There is now considerable evidence that cancer is also a disease which can arise partly as a result of lowered resistance. In one study with mice which were susceptible to breast cancer, the number of mice incurring the disease jumped from 7 per cent to 90 per cent by crowding. The author concluded that 'the data suggest that moderate chronic or intermittent stress may predispose such mice to an increased risk of mammary carcinoma. . . .'[48] Cancers often appear after an emotional crisis later in life, and researchers feel that intense emotional stress can activate dormant cancerous centres in the tissues.

Why should this happen? Resistance to disease in man is controlled by the immune system, a complex system involving the spleen, the lymph, the thymus and the bone marrow which acts to kill invading microbes or to remove foreign material from the body. One branch of this system secretes defensive proteins called antibodies. Another employs white blood cells which are conditioned to react to certain types of foreign substance. For example, some may only respond to certain materials on the outside of the coating of a typhoid bacillus. Thus, when a typhoid bacillus enters the body's bloodstream, these cells multiply in the spleen and overwhelm the invader. The immune system is now known to be a defensive screen against those of the body's own cells which turn parasitic, i.e. against cancers. But the quality of the immune system is critical. If it declines, bacteria can slip through the net and start infections, and cancer cells can start a growth. The quality tends to deteriorate somewhat with age.

It is very interesting that hormones are known to be able to influence the immune system. A certain amount of thyroid hormone is necessary for the cells of the immune system to react, and growth hormone is also required. The glucocorticoids have *a powerful inhibitory effect* on parts of the immune response. This is why they are used to treat diseases like arthritis, skin diseases and allergies which occur when the immune system goes off the rails. With more glucocorticoids in the body, it becomes more difficult to mount a defensive reaction. Why should this be so if the glucocorticoids are part of the body's system of resistance to danger? The answer is that the immune response, when activated by an invader, produces fever, swelling, pain and redness, which is called inflammation. It is a necessary part of its defensive mechanism. Clearly it is inappropriate to have inflammation occurring while one is in a flight or fight situation. One repairs wounds after the battle, not in the middle of it.

The mineralocorticoids, the other steroids produced by the adrenal cortex, have the opposite effect, of promoting the immune system and encouraging inflammation. The contrasting effects of the two classes of steroids, first discovered by Hans Selye, provide a subtle balance by which the level of immune activity is controlled. There are, however, still many doubts as to how much effect each of the hormones has on the immune system, and on which part of the system.

Studies on the competence or quality of the immune defences show clearly that even mildly stressed animals had immune cells of reduced competence. This was seen as directly due to the excess corticosteroids circulating unremittingly around the tissues of an animal in stress. If the hypothalamus, the master-control of the inner equilibrium, is damaged, there follows a profound deterioration of the immune system.[46] The situation is complex, and other hormones are certainly involved which can under certain conditions of stress restore or even increase the immune competence.[49] Yet it is clear that the continuous distortion of the equilibrium can undermine the body's natural defences against sickness. Good health needs balanced hormones. Continuous stress subtly undermines the balance, and the result is disease.

THE HEALING LIGHT

At last we have emerged from a long tunnel of science into the healing light.

The harmony remedies tighten up the control of stress. The stress hormones are a two-edged sword. The harmony remedies sharpen the attacking edge and blunt the self-destructive edge.

They should make the body less vulnerable when faced with extreme stresses, and aid a *healthy person* in overcoming demands placed upon him. This raises the possibility of their use when man finds himself at risk, a special application which we deal with in Chapter 10. Our chief concern in this book, however, is not with moments of severe stress, but with the insidious effects of unremitting stress, effects which make us prone to disease and disability. The harmony remedies might help to protect us from these effects.

Is there any evidence that ginseng can make the stress response less damaging to its owner? Yes, there is some data indicating that the cells of the body and the immune system are not inhibited so much during stress.[50] In one Korean study, animals that had undergone the stress of surgery had severely depressed white cells of the immune system. This could be prevented by giving ginseng before the operation.[51] Japanese researchers studied patients who suffered from various cancers and had most of their immune system destroyed by strong anti-cancer drugs. They found that if they gave them ginseng's active principles, their immune cells returned faster and they survived longer than expected.[52] A Russian medical researcher found that eleutherococcus could similarly prevent the stress of surgery from weakening the defences of mice with cancer.[53] The Russian team found that the classical clinical signs of stress steroid overload (such as stomach ulcers) were much reduced.[10] Clearly, ginseng and eleutherococcus are protecting individuals from the dark side of stress, presumably by leading to a more efficient use of the adrenal tap.

Knowing as we do how long-term stress produces disease, we can only conclude that the harmony remedies can improve resistance to disease.

We have learnt that the ability to turn the stress reaction off distinguishes those people who are sanguine, healthy and vital from those who are more anxious, disease-prone and worn out. Therefore the harmony remedies can be taken to increase general health and vitality, rather than to achieve specific tactical attacks on disease.

This is a radical conclusion. Indeed, when I first wrote those words I was aghast: For the whole of life is a challenge. Through challenges man lives, learns and evolves. From a final challenge he dies. Am I really saying that drugs can aid him in this? In simple terms, they can. That conclusion arises ineluctably from the experiments and the argument described in this chapter. It is strange to us only because it is outside our normal expectations. Medicines for the healthy are, however, the backbone of traditional medicine. Now that we have seen the way the Chinese use such medicines, and have proof that the Chinese were right to use them in this way, our expectations and preconceptions about such medicines may change.

Drugs which locate their action in the middle of the flux of hormones would easily have the range of powers the Chinese claim for them. They would be effective during the course of multitudes of diseases, for diseases appear only halfway through a play in which disharmonies hold the stage for the first act. They would be precious, for restoration of inner homeostasis is a hard-won goal. Many, many medicines are known to change bits of the body machinery, but there are few indeed that can increase the smooth running of the whole. They would be difficult to discover, for they would appear to affect no part of the body, and to cure no disease unless examined with a highly sensitive eye on the control systems of the organism. They would be applicable to every kind of person and every kind of life-style, for we are all sometimes run-down, sometimes vulnerable and sometimes potentially ill, and our hormones are sometimes out of sorts through unavoidable stresses or abuses. Finally, we can see how difficult they would be to understand and to use, for the main-tenance of homeostasis is not like the throwing of a metabolic switch to alter one particular diseased facet of our complex physiology. It requires a shrewd insight into each person's optimum balance, requiring constant adjustments and restora-tions which are not isolated, but must be fitted into the life-style, food, climate and stresses experienced by the indi-vidual.

This leads us beyond pathology, into the restorative prac-tices which are as essential to the medicine of the East as they are irrelevant to that of the West. Their goal is more than improved resistance to disease. It is also *vitality*. Now vitality, like health, is a disincarnate word. An attempt will be made to add some flesh to it with the help of the concepts of Oriental medicine in Chapter 11. Vitality is one end-point of health practices, and a yardstick of their success. There are subtle interconnections between health, resistance and vitality; surely the efficient control of the *milieu intérieur* is in the middle of this web? The hormones of the adrenal and thyroid glands, as well as others, are responsible for regulating the flow of materials and energy through the tissues, such as those of the liver, kidneys, heart and muscles. Any means whereby these controlling agents can be made more sensitive or economic will result in a balance of energy that is neither a wasteful burning of fuel, nor a stagnating torpor. This may be one of the main preconditions for vitality. In this way, the harmony remedies could be used to assist in attaining the best balance. They would form part of a range of therapies to encourage vitality.

Naturally, these are mild medicines. They will not by themselves transform vulnerable mortals into resistant superheroes. But the fact that they work in the way we have shown is remarkable enough. We should find out their limits, and how they should be used to best effect.

PART 3
Implications

8

Towards a Pharmacology of Harmony

PREVENTION – PURE AND APPLIED

In the pitiless Siberian winter of 1972, 1000 workers at the Norilsk mining and metalwork complex received an unexpected fillip. Each took 2ml. of eleutherococcus extract every morning for two months. That winter their frequent influenza and catarrh dropped to one-third of that of a matched group of workers who did not take eleutherococcus. Half a million roubles were saved.[1] Next year it was the turn of 1200 heavy truck drivers at the Volzhsky car factory in Togliatti. They didn't know that their usual thermos full of tea, given to them as they drove out of the gates of the factory, contained eleutherococcus. The same result occurred: less influenza, fewer working days lost. The programme was stepped up. A large team of doctors gave eleutherococcus to no less than 60,000 car workers at the same plant, and their health improved compared to others at the same place.[2]

Schizandra, the classic Oriental harmony remedy, has also been tested, reducing the sickness of 700 workers at a factory in Chirchiksk, and 328 schoolchildren during an influenza outbreak.[3]

This kind of testing had been going on for some time. Twenty years ago a similar trial was carried out in which 800 subjects took dibazol for some time during an epidemic of influenza.[4] It was repeated in France[5] and it led to another trial which was so vast that it is difficult to comprehend it. During an outbreak of the A2 form of influenza in 1969, some quarter of a million people in the city of Chelyabinsk took dibazol for nine days.[6] The incidence of colds and influenza was roughly two-thirds that of a sister city. Surely this should go into the *Guinness Book of Records* as the largest trial of a medicine ever carried out. Yet who has heard of it in the West?

These studies bewilder. If these medicines can help to protect us from common chest diseases, are they not of extraordinary importance, especially to the wheezy millions of the northern climes? As the Russians insist, the savings in terms of productivity alone would be vast. In terms of medical care the savings would be vaster, and in relation to the quality of life, incalculable. And yet . . . one cannot quite believe these fantastic studies. Is there something crazy about them, some Soviet daydreaming which generates health only on paper?

Given the great difficulty of actually proving that a medicine which is reputed to improve health has accomplished its object, I believe these Russian trials have succeeded. Without exception, they showed the same trend, towards improved resistance which continued for some time after the medication ceased. The trials certainly suffered from methodological faults, a consequence of the usual Russian predilection for scientific broadswords rather than rapiers. A comparison of disease in one city against disease in another is begging for criticism. But even if some of the improvements in health were psychological in origin, it is impossible to explain away *all* the trials by a placebo effect. This confirms that the remedies can increase resistance of some people to common diseases. Mass prophylaxis with these medicines is possible.

The special feature of these trials is that drugs are given to healthy people. We understand treatments, such as vaccinations, that protect us from specific infections. But the twentieth century is a time when suddenly and strangely it has become an anathema to take medicines to increase general health. It makes doctors nervous. 'Healthy people only need drugs to get high,' states one. 'They should take fewer drugs, not more.' Another asks, 'Why should healthy people take any medicines?' This question could never have been asked in any other medical system in the history of this planet, except possibly by the hard-line empiricists of ancient Greece. And what of the answer? Another question: 'Is anyone completely healthy?'

MEDICINES FOR THE HEALTHY

Now I would agree that a completely healthy person should

not need any medicines at all. Such people will reach a ripe old age and die of no disease in particular in their armchairs. They have probably had few diseases in their life and taken fewer medicines. There is no need for them to take prophylactic medicines. However, they are the exception rather than the rule. Most of us go through at least periods of poorer health, and in health I include overall well-being. Many of us live our entire lives in a grey area between health and disease, only requiring an extra little push to plunge into some degenerative condition later in life. Our goal is fulfilment of our potential, and this includes our potential to be old and to be healthy in old age. Few of us can achieve this goal unassisted.

Shouldn't we try to achieve it? If the Chinese set their sights on such a goal 5000 years ago, why cannot we do the same in the sophisticated world of today?

Restorative and preventive drugs are necessary when we do not achieve maximal health from our life-style. It is part of the husbandry of health. As highly skilled doctors of all traditions attest, our bodies are *impregnated* by the way we live. Actions and habits, seasons and foods, stresses and restorations are never absolutely neutral. Husbandry of health is a lifelong project, as is destruction of health. Morbidity-oriented health care is unable to provide health husbandry, although it will provide a curative safety-net. The only way in which our goal can be achieved is by therapies for the healthy, for example, the use of harmless, preventive, 'kingly' drugs which should exist side by side with the curative drugs.

The harmony drugs reduce the damage caused by stress, presumably through an action on the brain-body hormone system. As a result, they should prevent disease. They act on the person, not the disease. There is no evidence that the harmony remedies inhibit or affect the growth of infective organisms. If anything, ginseng has been found to assist the growth of bacteria.[7] Some studies have been published indicating that ginseng and eleutherococcus may inhibit viruses in tissues,[8] but it is notoriously difficult to prove that this is a specific effect of the drug. It may be an artificial situation created by the test itself. It is important to realize that a person genuinely at the peak of his health will not be affected by these remedies. His resistance is maximal. If such a person is going to drink typhoid-containing water, he takes his chance; there is no point in his chewing a piece of ginseng root first. On the other hand, the drugs should help the tired, stressed and unhealthy, those weakened by chronic disease, and those who are vulnerable and likely to get much more than their fair share of sickness.

Why am I applying the same prophylactic terms to the use of the harmony drugs by stressed people as the use by the chronically ill? Can one compare a person who is tired from long-distance lorry-driving with another who has just come through a serious operation? Yes, one can: each has the potential to go higher or lower on the scale of health and harmony. The stressed individuals are perhaps high and falling, the debilitated are lower on the health scale and trying to rise. But despite their various diagnoses, they all suffer from a fundamental distortion in the harmonious generation of vitality and resistance, which the Oriental healer sees as the major fault and the Western doctor as the minor fault. The harmonizers get on and do something about it. Indeed, the fact that the remedies act on both stressed and debilitated people is an indication of similarity. The drugs themselves do not distinguish one kind of disease manifestation from another, but act according to the degree of debility or distortion.

A dynamic interaction exists between the state of health of the individual and the effectiveness of these remedies. If we understand this, it will be clear how to examine the remedies and to use them.

In the last chapter we discussed the Russian studies in which unfortunate experimental animals were subjected to a number of serious biological threats such as injected bacteria. The animals were much more resistant if they had been given harmony drugs.[9] But it is doubtful if super-rats were created thereby. More probably, as laboratory animals, they were already in a state of considerable stress, and relatively unhealthy. Resistance was restored, not amplified.

It is no accident that workers in a car factory and lorry-drivers who drive for very long hours were chosen for the longest and most careful study of eleutherococcus. Such workers suffer notoriously from stress. We might cast our mind back to Frankenhauser's studies on stress. She used workers who had to keep up with the furious pace of a saw-mill conveyor as her stress archetypes. The inability to relax, to work at a pace and in a manner suiting each individual's character and rhythms, and the constant assault of powerful and often dangerous stimuli produce a stress syndrome which leads to psychological and physical vulnerability. Disease is rife among such workers, and they are bound to reveal the prophylactic effects of harmony medicines.

On the other hand, stress is a very individual affair. Each constitution has its own weak spots. The mass prophylaxis of normal healthy people is suitable for experiment but not for real life. These are restoratives, not vaccines. For best effect, each person needs to have a health strategy worked out on an individual basis, in which the harmony remedies are only one part of a healing regime.

The idea of *state-specific medicines*, medicines whose effectiveness depends on the state you are in, is new. There are no precedents among modern drugs, nor among the means of searching for drugs. Only with the greatest difficulty can the clinical trial be adapted to search for agents which improve health, and it has hardly ever been done.[10] If we are not aware of the influence of the state of the individual or the result of the treatment, the same mistakes will be made with the harmonizers as with all the other traditional remedies that have been thrown out of the window because subtlety has been confused with ineffectiveness. The Russian trials are of value. They are a compromise between the ultra-sophisticated but myopic testing of the West, and the casual attitude to verification in traditional Oriental medicine.

The Russians have wide experience in the use of these restoratives. In 1962 pantocrine was given the rubber stamp for general sale in the USSR by the Ministry of Health. The approval for rantarin was granted in 1971. Since these times it has been widely prescribed and there has been a careful watch on its effects. Eleutherococcus was granted a clinical permit in 1962 and has been consumed in large quantities in the USSR since then, to help those in stress, convalescents, the anaemic, debilitated or aged. Russian doctors prescribe it regularly, dispensing about 75 per cent of all eleutherococcus made, usually in the form of an extract. Most doctors know of it: it is not the special idiosyncrasy of a set of cosmopolitan city doctors. It is available in a number of forms; for example, the Primovsky sugar refinery makes sugar cubes impregnated with eleutherococcus or schizandra extracts, which, as the Soviets put it, 'is very convenient for mass prophylaxis'. Or one can buy eleutherococcus in the form of a soft drink called Bodrost (good health), a kind of health-giving Coca-Cola. The Red Army officers on the Chinese border share the taking of eleutherococcus with the old ladies of Moscow. Workers use it widely to cope with stressful working conditions. The same is true of dibazol, which was used as a general prophylactic before eleutherococcus, and is taken by many people all over the USSR even now from preference or force of habit, despite eleutherococcus's superiority. Professor Brekhman's wife, Dr Grinevitch, has taken dibazol all her life and fully intends to keep up the practice. Brekhman himself prefers to take eleutherococcus.

Actually one product is used in the West for the kind of purposes that eleutherococcus would be used for in the USSR, as a tonic for weak or convalescent patients. This is glucose; which is sugar. It is given in drinks and as powder to the sick and the debilitated, and after operations. It is quickly absorbed and produces a surge of blood glucose which makes more calorific energy available to the tissues. Whether the tissues actually need it or will be able to use it is another question. If the organs are functioning weakly, swamping them with glucose will not restore them. It is like using high-octane fuel to revive a seized engine. While it may sometimes provide a certain temporary energy to the body, there is no evidence that feeding sugar increases resistance or health. Indeed, in the long term it is likely to do the reverse, for a sudden surge of glucose in the blood is itself a stress which the body has to deal with. It is a physiological disharmony. The clearest example of the shabbiness of the modern attitude to health is that one finds packets of devitalizing glucose with 'For vitality' all over them, licensed by the Health Ministry. Yet the thought of allowing any claims whatsoever for the harmony remedies which are uniquely for vitality produces knee-tremble in the same ministries.

In the West, tranquillizers are used in severe stress. But tranquillizers reduce performance rather than increase it, reduce the joy and activity of life and compromise health. Instead of increasing our ability to cope with stress, they increase our ability to ignore it. Instead of improving resistance, they stupefy it. A completely different approach to stress reduction and the prevention of stress-related diseases is needed. Since stress is the tragedy of metropolitan existence, we should at least ask very serious questions about the possibility of the use of harmony remedies as a shield for health.

ON THE ROAD TO RECOVERY

What role can the harmony remedies play when disease has already taken hold? In Oriental traditional medicine, they are used as much to aid the care of disease as in its prevention. Most of the therapeutic mixtures have one or other harmony remedy included in them. It is important to understand how they help the sick despite the fact that they are not curative.

The harmony drugs should help when the strength and vitality of the patient are involved in recovery. If this fact were realized, it would save much confusion concerning these drugs.

Disease itself is a stress. Once an infectious disease has taken hold, there is a life and death struggle in which the immune system attempts to rid itself of the intruders. The immune system proliferates and so do the alien organisms, and a race is established. Hormones, the stress mechanisms and general vitality are involved in this race, for they influence immune capacity. The harmony remedies may therefore weight the scales towards recovery by giving the body extra resources in its fight. However, the harmony remedies are unlikely to affect the progress of quick acute diseases. They are effective only when the stress of disease undermines the body's resistance and energy.

A Korean study has shown that ginseng had no effect on the recovery from acute tuberculosis in animals.[11] Independently, a Russian professor found that pantocrine was very useful in restoring health and strength and aiding the recovery of tuberculosis patients. However, he found that it only helped chronic or secondary forms of the disease, particularly in the elderly. It had no effect on acute episodes.[12]

It is possible that a restorative effect could be so strong that it established spectacular cures of previously intractable diseases. But these cures could be reserved for special occasions. Some people, for example, may be sick because of a severe distortion in homeostasis, their life on a knife-edge. A harmony remedy judiciously applied may be able to add crucial resistance, and a cure rapidly follows. There must have been many examples of this before modern medicine introduced antibiotics. The patient would lie for a long period at the point of death with his immune system and all the body defences fighting a last-ditch battle to dislodge well-entrenched infecting organisms. At this critical stage any gain in vitality, i.e. in access to energy, could make a very large difference.

This must have happened to Lazarus the Second, '. . . who was much emaciated, and reduced unto a perfect skeleton, a mere bag of Bones, by a long Hectick Feaver, joyned with an ulcer of the Lungs; being despaired of by all Friends, I was resolved to try what the Tincture of this Root would doe, which I gave every Morning in Red Cows Milk. And I found his Flesh to come again like that of a child, and his lost Appetite restored, and his natural Ruddy complexion revived in his Cheeks, to the Amazement of his desponding Relations, that he was called Lazarus the second.'[13] Even with antibiotics we can think of similar knife-edge situations: infections in the elderly, heart failure or the degenerative diseases in late stages.

Perhaps the wild root, when obtainable, is strong enough to achieve apparently miraculous cures, giving rise to some notorious legends. A Korean traditional doctor I spoke to ran a clinic which occasionally purchased and used the extremely rare wild ginseng. He reported that rich sick patients occasionally undergo the cure, which costs $10,000 at least. They eat the huge dose of from thirty to fifty grammes of the wild root at one sitting, after which they lurch and fall 'as if drunk'. They go to bed for three days, and then arise renewed and cured. We know that the wild root is much more powerful than the cultivated one, but is it that powerful? The question of occasional miracle cures is still open. It shouldn't disturb our appreciation of the essential adjustive and restorative features of these remedies. We must get used to that before we go for the therapeutic jackpots.

The harmonizers may aid recovery during the latter portion of a disease, when the body is beginning to throw it off anyway, or alternatively when the body is too weakened to fight the disease and is in danger of giving up. It will help where lack of strength delays or prevents the curing of a

disease. It may reduce those draining symptoms which constitute a feeling of being ill. It will be effective in assisting people
to overcome semi-diseases, what the Eastern materia medica
quaintly calls 'removing hypochondrias', and will be of supportive help in the degenerative diseases, which are essentially
a chronic manifestation of previous ill-health.

The Chinese have developed the art of knowing when the
restorative effect of ginseng will hasten recovery and when it
will be useless or even counterproductive. For example, it
should not be used during fever or in the acute phase of an
infection. This is an area of traditional healing skill still unexplored by science.

There are many examples of trials of the use of the harmony
drugs in sickness. For example, in the USSR eleutherococcus
was reported to hasten the recovery of children with recurrent
rheumatic fever being treated at the Khabarovsk Medical
Institute. 'In 1970,' says a Soviet booklet on eleutherococcus,
'Dr L. N. Sobkovich reported the results of studying the
therapeutic effect of eleutherococcus in attenuated forms of
pulmonary tuberculosis in 64 children, 9–15 years old, who
had been ill 2 to 4 years . . . the children were treated with
antibacterial drugs, and also received fish oil, calcium compounds, vitamin complex and eleutherococcus extract . . .
the control group of 30 children received combined treatment
of the same type but without eleutherococcus. The results
indicate that the use of eleutherococcus in combined therapy
contributed to the improvement of the general condition of
the children . . . they felt less tired at the end of the day. . . .
Measured physical exertion revealed a substantial difference in
the two groups . . . the effectiveness of respiration rose.' This
result demonstrates the restorative effect of eleutherococcus.

Likewise, the effectiveness of eleutherococcus is confirmed
in patients who were being treated for chronic pneumonia at
the Pulmonary Institute of the USSR Academy of Medical
Sciences. Eleutherococcus alleviated the debilitating and ener-
vating effects of the protracted disease. A study at the Neurology Institute of the USSR Academy of Sciences also found a
generally faster recovery in patients receiving eleutherococcus
in addition to standard treatments for side-effects of disorders
of the circulation.

Pantocrine has for years been regularly administered to

promote patient recovery in Soviet hospitals and clinics, the earliest clinical reports appearing in the 1930s. It too is found useful in promoting recovery and a restoration of health in convalescents, undernourished and tubercular children, and those weakened by chronic diseases.[14] Professor Albov, for example, has tested it extensively in patients who were one degree under for some time after diseases such as viral infections or dysentery. He notes a restoration of blood pressure, improved mood, digestion, stamina and body weight. He also recounts his experience of the use of pantocrine in helping soldiers with serious war-wounds to return to health and strength.[15]

Compared to the plethora of studies on eleutherococcus, there are surprisingly few studies on the restorative effects of ginseng. This is probably because the Far Eastern countries have been devoted to animal studies, while in Russia few trials with ginseng were carried out before it was superseded by eleutherococcus. Besides the rare Soviet research, some clinical studies have taken place in European clinics and hospitals. Continental Europe has traditionally been more active in restorative and unconventional modes of treatment than Britain and America. In some ways, German medicine is closer to Russia than America. It still has a strong infrastructure of spas, baths, herbs, homeopathy and health clinics run in an old-fashioned way. German interest in prevention and restorative therapy led them to ginseng as soon as it reappeared in the West. Traditionalist German professors recommended it to their patients and dispensed it in numerous private clinics.

One typical study on chronically ill patients of all ages has been carried out by Süttinger. His patients were mostly suffering from debility and general weakness as a result of chronic diseases, particularly of the circulation. In a somewhat loose single-blind trial, he noticed improvements in their general health, including appetite, sleep, digestion, concentration and mental performance, and other indicators.[16] Early Russian clinical studies of pure ginseng briefly reported that it helped patients with physical debility and general weakness caused by various protracted nervous and internal diseases, but no details of these studies are available.[17] Another possible clinical use was pinpointed by Professor Gianoli of Madrid University, who carried out a double-blind study with a ginseng-vitamin preparation for people who were undergoing intensive diet therapy for obesity. Not unnaturally, many of his overweight charges experienced severe slimmers' depression, confusion and psychosomatic problems. He found that the ginseng-vitamin preparation did not produce any detectable change in the blood picture or the metabolism, but the patients lost more weight, were less hungry, were in better moods, felt more capable and were more successfully cured.[18]

We can all visualize situations where the restorative abilities of the harmony remedies would be useful: jaundice, depression, anaemia, prolonged dysentery – in fact, any disease where malfunction of the inner machinery results in tiredness and weakness, and in reduced vitality, resistance and health. One situation is of considerable importance: surgery. If you have ever had an operation it will be obvious to you that the recovery period is one of depression, weakness, tiredness, and susceptibility to infections and complications. Without reducing one iota the care and protection of post-operative patients, one could also supply medicines which will give them strength, increase their resistance, bring back their appetites and reduce the risk of secondary disease.

A careful clinical trial in Korea reported in 1978 has examined the recovery of 120 female patients who underwent a severe internal operation. Sixty of them were given ginseng glycoside active principles and sixty a placebo. The patients treated with ginseng had improved liver function, felt better and put on more weight.[19] Similar studies have been reported in the USSR on patients given eleutherococcus and panto-crine.[20] They were especially useful if the patients were weak, old or chronically sick and there was a real danger that they might not have the strength to pull through. Should we not try these medicines in this way in the West? When serious operations are performed, what drugs are currently available to help the patient recover afterwards?

Despite this twentieth century and its sophisticated curative practice, will doctors continue to treat the diseases of chronically ill patients and leave the patient himself to pray for his own strength and resistance?

We shall now see how the harmony remedies might fit into the treatment of three kinds of disease that cause immense harm and suffering, are widespread in the West, and yet are extremely hard to treat. These are cancer, heart disease and diabetes.

ON CANCER

This desperately feared disease has led to an almost panic-stricken pharmacological search for a cure. Any new medicine of any type is immediately thrust into the laboratory to be endlessly tested for cancer-killing activity. The feverishness of the search has led to senselessness, unintelligence and waste of which the National Cancer Institute's random screening programme is an example. Seventy-five thousand plants have been ground, extracted and applied to cancer cells in the laboratory over a period of twelve years. But they were selected and applied without reference to traditional medicine, in a grossly oversimplified test system designed to detect only those plants which have an antibiotic-like killing effect on a certain kind of cancer cell. Naturally, the trial was an expensive flop.[21]

Unfortunately, the harmony remedies have also been through the same fashionable mill. A number of studies purport to show that ginseng kills cancer cells; two were read at a recent conference in Seoul.[22] These studies are not useful. If you slop carrot juice into a cell culture, the cells will die from contamination. This doesn't mean that the carrot is an anti-cancer drug. The same goes for certain studies in which a large quantity of ginseng extract is injected into animals with cancer to see if the cancer is killed. Clearly one cannot expect the harmonizers, which treat the person not the diseases, to be curative in this way. The results have usually been negative.[23] In one study carried out by scientists in California in which the cancers did get smaller, it turned out that such high doses were used that the animals almost died from overdosage and the results are meaningless.[24] In fact, Russian scientists have reported that very, very high doses of ginseng given to mice could increase the chances of cancer,[25] as can very high doses of almost any kind of medicine. However, this doesn't mean to say that the harmonizers are useless to a cancer patient, it means that we must find the right use for them.

Treatment of cancer is immensely stressful. The cutting, burning and poisoning of cancer patients is almost as frightening as the disease. In a bizarre twist typical of modern medicine, treatment with radiation and chemicals tends to destroy the body's natural resistance to the cancer in the process of destroying the cancer itself. The cancer specialist's dilemma is always whether the accumulation of drastic cures is hastening death rather than delaying it. One example of the result of lowered resistance is that the cancer can spread. Surgery has been shown to encourage reseeding of cancer.

The harmonizers will not attack the cancer, but they will strengthen resistance and energy. This is unlikely to result in a cure, but it may buy more time. It should make the patient feel better and help him to lead a normal life. The fact that the harmonizers improve stress-resistance will have maximum impact in surgery, where they may reduce the risk of reseeding of the tumour. The Russian researcher Dr Yaremenko has investigated this. When animals with cancer underwent an abdominal operation, the percentage of animals whose cancer seeded in other parts of the body increased from 49 per cent to 78 per cent. If they were given eleutherococcus beforehand, there was no increase in reseeding as a result of the operation. Eleutherococcus stopped amounts of the glucocorticoid stress hormone in the body from shooting too high as a result of the operation.[26] Similar results were obtained with rantarin. Professor Lazarev, the man who founded the movement towards prophylactic drugs in the USSR, was able to confirm that the use of eleutherococcus prolonged the life of mice with cancer. The spread of the cancer was inhibited and the general resistance increased, even though the main cancer was unaffected.[27]

Ginseng and eleutherococcus can reduce the general toxic effects of the X-rays, surgery and powerful anti-cancer drugs which are used to attack the growth. (These are, of course, the same noxious agents that were used to stress animals in the Russian survival trials.) Clinical studies have been carried out using the harmonizers to protect patients during drastic treatments. For example, Dr Khatiashvili of the Oncology Department of the Institute of Advanced Medical Training in Tbilisi gave eleutherococcus for fourteen days to thirty-eight patients who had cancer of the lip and mouth. A control group with similar diagnosis and severity were given a placebo. Both groups had the usual X-ray treatment for the cancer. The eleutherococcus patients were not so nauseated and debilitated by the radiation. 'Eleutherococcus substantially improved the

general condition, appetite and sleep, and eliminated devia-
tions in respiration . . . which pointed to the weakening of
the harmful effect of X-ray therapy.' In the eleutherococcus
group the tumours were more rapidly healed, and there was
no reseeding. Similar results of improved tolerance to X-rays
in eighty women with breast cancer were recorded at the
Oncology Institute of the Georgian Health Ministry. At the
famous Petrov Oncological Institute in Leningrad,
eleutherococcus was tested in combination with drugs and
surgery on 107 patients with cancer of the stomach.
Eleutherococcus was given in the comparatively large dose of
five millilitres, which corresponds to five grammes of root per
day. The harmonizer was continued during treatment and
afterwards for at least a year. The use of eleutherococcus
enabled patients to tolerate 50 per cent more anti-cancer drugs
and, since greater doses could be used, the patients lived
longer. Those who had surgery lived for an average of seven-
teen months, as opposed to twelve months in the control
group. Those whose cancer was too advanced to operate lived
an average of eleven months with eleutherococcus and four
months with the placebo. The harmonizers are used quite
widely in the USSR as an adjunct to cancer therapy.

It seems incredible that the West does not use any medicines
at present to protect the patient from the damage of the
treatment. The fundamental health, energy and resistance of
the cancer patient is still neglected, while the doctor engages in
quixotic tilting at the tumour. The use of the harmonizer remedies in the Soviet Union has gone unnoticed for fifteen years!

Cancer is tremendously difficult to cure. I do not maintain
that a traditional doctor with even the best Oriental medical
skills could achieve a very much better cure rate than modern
doctors. However, he probably wouldn't do much worse, and
his patients might live a better life during his treatment. Given
that twenty years' work and billions of dollars have not
generated reliable cures for cancer, is it not about time that
Western doctors and scientists began to look outside their past
failures?

To search for the cure for cancer is like shutting the gate
after the horse has bolted. The major effort should be directed
towards prevention. Cancer prevention is also hard because
the agents which cause it are so pervasive in our environment,

and the reasons for individual susceptibility are so mysterious. Some reduction of body defences against cancer is the result of stress. The harmonizers ought to be able to maintain the shield against cancer-causing agents if used wisely as part of overall health improvement. Cancer and other degenerative diseases will never be conquered without a genuine life-guidance system. Harmonizers will have a role in such a system as part of stress reduction.

Current information concerning susceptibility is expressed only in terms of *probabilities*. You will have x per cent less chance of incurring cancer if. . . . What is missing is a proper theory of prevention taking into account each individual's resistance as well as his constitutional, hormonal and immune 'fingerprint'. Then cancer prevention can be fully *designed*. In this we have much to learn from Oriental traditional skills. An Oriental healer would guide each particular person towards a diet and life-style that maximizes his health at all times. He should be able to understand the failures and weaknesses of organs, metabolism and resistance and specifically promote protection against such subtle degenerative conditions as cancer. If a patient is susceptible to a cancer he should be able to determine this too, and if despite his efforts a cancer begins, he should be able to detect it in an early embryonic stage by means of its effect on neighbouring functions and organ energy states. This will allow him to design a cure at a stage when the cancer is still quite vulnerable.

Tibetan doctors look upon the vast numbers of cancer patients in the West as the price paid for living without insight. They point the finger particularly at modern medicine. They feel that the residues of partly cured diseases accumulate over the years, with cancer as a natural consequence. This has a ring of truth. But science is still chasing viruses with billion-pound butterfly nets and cannot inform us on the matter. If it is true that modern medicine is at all carcinogenic, perhaps we need to look back to the medicine of the Yellow Emperor to protect us from it.

POSTPONING THE CARDIOVASCULAR CATASTROPHE?

'Panax ginseng is a well-known cardiac tonic and widely used in China,' writes Dr Li in a recent US Department of Health study of Chinese herbal medicine.[28] It is used for patients who have just had a heart attack and whose life is threatened by their heart's poor performance. The Chinese doctors found that Western drugs could raise blood pressure but that it soon fell back, while ginseng could maintain the heart pumping for longer. They have also successfully used another plant on our harmonizer list. Salvia multiorrhiza, which has not to my knowledge been the subject of any other research.

A safe medicine which raises blood pressure in such circumstances is of considerable value. But if we search for evidence of the use of ginseng in Europe and Russia in relation to the circulation, we get a surprise, for ginseng and eleutherococcus are used as long-term therapy to *reduce* high blood pressure, with some support from German studies on the chronically sick.

In actual fact, few uses of ginseng appear more confusing than its effect on the circulation. However, few uses are more important. Cardiovascular diseases are the most frequent cause of death in the post-industrial world. They are the archetypal degenerative diseases, which build up insidiously over the life-span as a result of subtle and poorly understood factors in the way of life.

High blood pressure is a precursor of serious damage to the circulation. Some 15 per cent of American adults suffer from it. High blood pressure means that the heart is pumping much harder to overcome extra resistance which, as with any fluid pumped through a pipe, can come from the constriction, obstruction or convolution of the blood vessels. Naturally, this can cause strain and damage to other delicate blood vessels. The damage may act as a focus for arteriosclerosis, the fatty degeneration of the blood vessels. It may help to cause blood clots which block the vessels, and it may combine with various other factors to cause heart failure. People with high blood pressure are roughly four times as likely to suffer a subsequent heart attack.

No drugs cure cardiovascular disease, but a range of substances control its dangerous manifestations and bring down blood pressure, most of them carrying a load of side-effects. Attempts at prevention, as we have discussed, are crude. There is little understanding of how to guide individuals through their life-span so that their arteries remain in pristine condition. Despite jogging and abstention from butter, the arteries of an average middle-aged city American male will probably be like old rope compared to his contemporary in the Himalayan valleys.

In this medical climate, the slightest suspicion of a cardiovascular action by ginseng has sent researchers into the laboratories. They found that if an animal is given small amounts of the active principle of harmony remedies such as ginseng, eleutherococcus or san-chi, there is an instant of lowered blood pressure followed by a period of raised blood pressure and then a return to normal.[29] The nature of this enigmatic effect is further confused by the discovery that large doses tend to have the opposite effect,[30] and if the constituents of ginseng are tested separately some raise blood pressure and others decrease it.[31] The most careful study, carried out at a university in America, came to the conclusion that a steady lowering of blood pressure did occur due to relaxation of the blood vessels in the outer shell of the body.[32] However, there is some disagreement about this.[33] There is also confusion concerning the action of ginseng on the heart. In some laboratory animals it stimulates the heart, in others it slightly slows it.[32] Some studies carried out as early as the turn of the century showed a stronger stimulation of the heart; they may have used better roots than those tested in modern times.[34]

This confusion of observations, so commonplace in ginseng studies, arises from a completely inappropriate manner of looking at the problem – a meaningless answer arising from a meaningless question and years of scientific work down the drain. Most of the studies are trying to demonstrate a new kind of drug action using methods designed for the old. Reference to traditional medicine would make it clear that ginseng and the harmony remedies have a *tuning or adjustive role,* and therefore their effect will always depend on the state of the process being tuned. A snapshot of waves does not tell you about tides. Not one of the above pharmacological studies takes the inner state of the organism into account. Yet blood pressure is the result of a vast web of interrelated homeostatic processes – the actions of adrenaline, stress hormones, the state of the arteries, the salt and water content of the body and the viscosity of the blood, to name a few. The hypothalamus also regulates blood pressure.

Stress is a key to high blood pressure. Continual adrenaline secretion with stress hormones can disturb the internal regulation of the blood pressure. At the same time the activation of the alarm system constricts the blood vessels on the shell of the body. The master stress hormone, ACTH, is also involved. One can create high blood pressure in animals by simply giving ACTH over some time. One of the most recent concepts suggests that salt in the diet interacts in a complex manner with the controls of the *milieu intérieur*, particularly in the adrenal hormones, and together they inhibit the circulation.[35]

Given this dependence of blood pressure on internal harmony, it would be surprising if harmony remedies did *not* affect it. Our knowledge of these remedies leads us to predict that they would tend to adjust blood pressure only if it was abnormally high or abnormally low, which is just what laboratory experiments have shown.[36] I suggest that this occurs because of a restoration of hormonal sensitivity. The reaction to a drastic drop in blood pressure, such as occurs in a heart attack, is therefore stronger, while the day-to-day stress which causes high blood pressure is reduced. Ginseng and eleutherococcus, because of their arousing effect, are more capable of raising drastically lowered blood pressure than lowering high blood pressure. Their effect on low blood pressure would be immediate; and on high blood pressure, long-term and connected with stress resistance and general health.

I have no evidence of ginseng's effectiveness at raising blood pressure apart from the Chinese studies already quoted.[28] However, the logic of the root does support its use in this way to tide a heart-attack patient over a critical period, especially in combination with other remedies that act on the heart itself. One kind of stress, connected with sudden fall in blood pressure, can be deadly: it is called shock. This is encountered in an accident or surgery and arises from loss of fluid combined with the sudden mobilization of stress hormones. Chinese soldiers take ginseng into battle with them in case of the shock of a wound. One could imagine ginseng in use as a component of an accident jab.

When eleutherococcus was given to Russian industrial

workers, episodes of high blood pressure were reduced, but only after four months. Over that lengthy period the effects on blood pressure may well be the secondary result of a.wide variety of changes in the physiological equilibrium. Stress-resistance could bring alterations in the salts, sugars and fats, in diet and mood, all of which would affect the circulation. One would conclude from this that the harmony remedies can adjust raised blood pressure arising from failures in control through stress or hormonal distortion. They will not alter any underlying pathologies such as heart damage.

The other component of the cardiovascular catastrophe is atherosclerosis. This is perhaps the most typical stress-related degenerative disease of today, killing half a million people a year in the United States alone. There is some direct evidence that ginseng treatment can alter one physiological factor which is closely linked with atherosclerosis. This is the cholesterol level. High levels of cholesterol predispose one to sclerotic deterioration of the arteries. Cholesterol is made by the body and is increased both by stress hormones and by consumption of cholesterol in the diet, so it would be a suitable case for adjustment by the harmony remedies. Ginseng was found to reduce the amount of cholesterol in the blood of rats which were given high levels of cholesterol[37] or fats[38] to eat. Their livers destroyed the cholesterol more effectively. The same could be achieved by another harmony remedy, Bupleurum falcatum. Ginseng has no effect when animals are not stressed and their cholesterol levels are normal.[39] There is no question of the harmony remedies curing or reversing the degenerative state. But when combined with other therapies, particularly diet control and exercise, they could delay the onset of the cardiovascular catastrophe.

Uncomfortable side-effects of circulatory disturbances, such as tiredness or impotence, may be reduced by the harmony remedies to a degree unattainable by any current drugs. Professor Albov gave pantocrine to patients with low blood pressure and noticed, along with a rise in blood pressure, reduced tiredness and improved ability to function normally. Japanese clinicians also support the use of pantocrine to bring relief to those incapacitated by low blood pressure.[15] Professor Mankovsky at the Institute of Gerontology in Kiev has tried rantarin with older patients suffering from atherosclerosis in the brain. After twenty days of treatment most of the patients slept better, and had hardly any headaches or dizziness; irritability and depression decreased. Blood pressure was partly returned to normal. The improvements were symptomatic. In the brief period of the trial, no change was noticeable in the course of the atherosclerosis itself.[40] Ginseng and eleutherococcus have also been tested in Soviet patients with high blood pressure, bringing a reduction in headaches, tiredness and depression, as well as improved potency and general functional ability.[41] The effects lasted for some time after the treatment.

The many people suffering from heart and circulatory problems ought to know about the potential of harmony therapy. When combined with changes in diet and when used properly, it represents a revolutionary new approach by which symptoms can be reduced and the body assisted, through its stress-control system. It can blend successfully with other curative practices and, far from generating side-effects, can actually reduce the side-effects arising from more toxic drugs.

But I should add a warning. The use of harmony remedies in circulatory disturbances must be sensitive, careful and under guidance. They should not replace any other medication without expert advice. In some cases alteration of the blood pressure may be an unwanted effect, and the more severe the circulatory problem, the more dangerous is indiscriminate application of these remedies.

DIABETES

Diabetes is in most cases the end result of a deterioration in the maintenance of physiological balance, in this case of energy supply (i.e. blood sugar level). Loss of this homeostasis is known to be the result of a combination of individual susceptibility and life-style. Within the latter we include mainly stress and diet. The stress steroids are especially involved in the complex control of sugar and energy supplies, as are other hormones such as insulin and adrenaline. This makes diabetes a prime candidate for harmony therapy.

As we should expect, research on unstressed animals shows little change. Ginseng, eleutherococcus and schizandra, but not pantocrine, slightly increase the sugar concentration in the blood, as well as causing other metabolic shifts towards increased availability of energy supplies in the body, particularly after exercise.[42] Red ginseng proved to be more effective than white.[43] But if animals have artificially high blood sugar because they are diabetic or have had a sugar diet, or very low bloodsugar, there is then a substantial return to normality.[44] This effect occurs on top of that produced by an injection of insulin.

Diabetes, the final result of disharmony in sugar metabolism, is not cured by harmony remedies. Their use sometimes allows a reduction in the dose of insulin, but as a Chinese author puts it: 'Ginseng is unable to completely correct the metabolic disturbances occurring in . . . the diabetic state. It may be of help if used to produce subsidiary effects in the treatment of the diabetic state, but it cannot be relied upon to act as a substitute for insulin.'[45]

The diabetic would be likely to experience symptomatic improvements in general health which can be prolonged by combining harmony remedies with restrictions on diet and stress. A letter I received from a senior lecturer at a nurses' college gives a hint of the possibilities. He has been a diabetic for sixteen years and suffered from some associated neurological troubles. Much to his distress, he had also become impotent, which 'led me to try a number of regimes in order to counteract the neurological signs, all of which seemed to have a temporary beneficial effect.' He discovered ginseng, took it for a fortnight, and after considering and discounting the possibility of a placebo effect, stated that, 'I am frankly astonished at the results. . . . The improvements include greater capacity for work, better concentration, less lassitude . . . and a general heightening of awareness.'

DRUGS VERSUS DRUGS

The most pervasive stress which we have to deal with is chemical. We live in a sea of poisons, pollutants, toxins and harmful drugs. The average American takes in two and a half kilogrammes a year of food additives, which may be any of 8000 substances. Many poisons exist naturally in food plants or animals. 'Narcotics,' said Sellar and Yeatman cynically, 'were of course intended by Nature for use with a doctor's certificate only.' Modern drugs are very often toxic in subtle or unsubtle ways. Would harmony remedies provide some protection against chemical damage or intoxication?

They are certainly used in this way. The Soviets use eleutherococcus to protect health and where possible vitality of patients receiving powerful drugs. I have some Soviet sugar impregnated with eleutherococcus and schizandra, sold in order to lessen the effects of 'pure, white and deadly' sugar. Eleutherococcus is now being considered for use against pollution, especially air pollution. The Japanese use ginseng in special mixtures to help heroin addicts overcome withdrawal symptoms. Many people, especially the Koreans, find it a great help against hangovers. In the Soviet Union one can buy vodka containing eleutherococcus extract, called *zolotoy rog,* in which the extract is used against hangover. Some claim in addition that it makes you less drunk than normal vodka, others that it gives you a clearer drunkenness of equivalent strength. This question has been the subject of endless disputes between drunken disputants!

There is certainly evidence in support of these uses. The liver is the decontamination site of the body, where chemicals are converted to harmless or useful materials. The liver processes materials much faster in response to stress hormones. There is considerable evidence that ginseng makes the liver more active.[46] The liver manufactures more of the proteins (enzymes) that chop up substances.[47] When animals were given ginseng, Beuplurum falcatum or other harmony remedies, their livers could more easily repair damage to themselves produced by toxic chemicals.[48] There are a few studies going back over the last fifty years in the classical pharmacological mould: drug antagonism. Ginseng was found to reduce the effects of a range of sedatives and narcotics and to restore reflexes of the nervous system more quickly after anaesthesia.[49] Centrophenoxine, too, has been reported to increase the potency of the anti-cancer drug cyclophosphamide, without increasing its harmfulness.[50] Clinical studies have already been mentioned in which the Soviets found that patients who were given eleutherococcus did not become quite so ill as a result of anti-cancer drugs. This suggests that it might be possible to add ginseng to a whole variety of Western drug cocktails in order to help the patient tolerate them and reduce side-effects.

As for alcohol, there is now quite clear proof that ginseng and centrophenoxine cause faster disposal and elimination of alcohol from the blood after drinking.[51] It takes much more alcohol to kill or harm after ginseng or eleutherococcus have been taken.[52] Russian scientists have given vodka to volunteers before submitting them to tests requiring accuracy, speed and co-ordination. The prior ingestion of eleutherococcus improved performance. A similar study is reported from Korea.[53]

A few years ago the *Daily Mail* remarked on the phenomenon of a strange enthusiasm for ginseng among young people in London, and questioned if ginseng was 'an alternative to pot and alcohol'. This was precisely the wrong question. It should have asked whether ginseng did not 'help you recover from pot and alcohol'.

HARMONY THERAPY

Space does not permit analysis of other disharmonies. There is considerable experimental material on the effect of ginseng on the metabolism of fats and proteins, on the production of blood cells and the function of various organ systems. Russian scientists have published two recent books and numerous papers with detailed biochemical explorations of the changes in metabolism arising from the consumption of ginseng and eleutherococcus.[54] All these studies would add volume but not substance to our basic schema of the uses of the harmony remedies. The diseases which the Chinese claim to be affected by ginseng are so varied that they gave rise to myths of a panacea on the one hand, alarm and disbelief on the other. They have now been rationalized. They are ailments with disturbances of homeostasis as their progenitor.

Disease arises in part from our daily life; from the insults, stresses and experiences which accumulate inside us like cracks on a cup, until one little further knock at a weak point breaks the cup into pieces. . . . Medicine should *search out these little cracks and seal them up.* In order to do this it must take into account each individual – his weaknesses, strengths and hormone fingerprint. Hormones are particularly relevant – they determine sex, mould shape, constitution and personality. A sanguine person may have less thyroid and adrenal activity than a choleric person. The humours of Greek medicine are the hormones of today. They can be working together, in harmony, to preserve vitality and resistance, or struggling against themselves to undermine health.

Their pattern is perceived indirectly by the Oriental or indeed the Hippocratic practitioner and healing regimes designed to tune these inner instruments. The harmony remedies are one kind of adjustive therapy, but they should be related to constitution. Different remedies would be more suitable for different kinds of distortions in different people. Ginseng would be more suitable for slothful people but may be too arousing for angry or highly sexed people whom the Chinese would regard as having excessive liver or sexual gland metabolism respectively. Other harmony remedies such as Poria cocos would be used to adjust the content of water in the organs, suitable for wet people.

The hormone-tuning model helps us to understand how ginseng and other remedies should be taken, not as instant cures but as part of a controlled restorative system. The Chinese advise that taking ginseng prior to stress itself will waste its potential. They recommend a period of rest, little food, celibacy and temperance while undergoing therapy. We can see why. It may be impossible to develop long-lasting economies within the glands if they are continually on demand. It would be like putting money into a deposit account while continually withdrawing it from a current account. The result is no interest.

Harmony therapy can be applied to deteriorations on the health ladder which are both before and within the range of diagnosis of Western medicine. However, there are few people in the West who can diagnose disharmonies in reasonably healthy people before sickness. The Oriental skills of subtle pulse reading, iris diagnosis, urine diagnosis and all the other methods of collecting information on the inner state of the organism cannot be found at the local health centre. *Since diagnosis of disease is available but not diagnosis of health, we should rely on the former and do the latter for ourselves.* Health maintenance depends on the self-awareness of each individual. As Illich said: 'Health is a task . . . success in this personal task is in large part the result of the self-awareness, self-discipline, and inner resources by which each person regulates his own daily rhythm and actions, his diet and his sexual activity. Knowledge encompassing desirable activities, competent performance, the commitment to enhance health in others . . . they depend on the spread of responsibility for healthy habits. . . .'[55]

The harmony remedies engender this attitude. They cut across the boundaries set by the descriptive classification of diseases into thousands of separate entities. They spread over the main distinctions of disease and health. They do not obey rules of location in a single organ or tissue. They do not fight the disease itself. Yet they can be shown to be of immense potential value if we adapt to them. They treat the patient, not the disease, which makes them medicines of the New Age as much as the Old Age.

9

The Elusive Elixir

WITHDRAWAL OF THE APHRODISIAC MYTH

A chinese materia medica of the fourth century presented a list of exotic ginseng recipes which, it was claimed, could increase sexual appetite. One remedy combined fresh ginseng with soya, ox-penis and dried human placenta. Ginseng always has been avidly consumed for its supposed aphrodisiac properties. Shen Nung himself recorded that he felt warmth and sexual desire after chewing some root. It was taken in large quantities by Chinese emperors in order to fuel the imperial lust, while ordinary Chinese regard it as the means to father children into their eighties. It has always been present in indulgent regal households, from the French court in the eighteenth century to the Arab potentates of today who consumed $1/4 million-worth last year. It is widely sold in European sex shops. It is often compounded with substances such as vitamin E, a flat contrast to the imaginative ancient Chinese sexual additives; one recipe contains the tongues of a hundred peacocks, spiced with chillies and the sperm of pubescent boys.

Modern Chinese patent medicines, particularly those containing pantocrine, ginseng and sea-horses, are customarily used by the Chinese to increase sexual power. As a science journalist quipped: '. . . The currently most popular form of ingestion to restore vital powers is the ginseng-antler pill in which the vegetable symbolism of the root is combined with the more obvious image of encouragement provided by a deer's horn. This is in keeping with the folklore tradition that the therapeutic benefits of acclaimed aphrodisiacs lie frequently in their outward resemblance to the human organs involved, rather than in their chemical constituents.'

Actually he is almost correct. These substances have collected a reputation as aphrodisiacs which has outstripped their actual potential. The Doctrine of Signatures is partly to blame for this, since both ginseng and pantocrine have a phallic shape, along with a considerable portion of the vegetable world. But despite the enthusiasm of many who have tested ginseng in the laboratory of the bedroom to their satisfaction, ginseng is not an aphrodisiac. An aphrodisiac is an agent specifically affecting sexual activity. The Chinese did not really claim that ginseng did this. They stated that ginseng restored fundamental energy, an energy essential for virility as for health in general. Consequently, they claimed that it was useful in restoring potency, though not in meddling with performance. Indeed, Dr Jeffreys, a wry Victorian doctor, wrote that ginseng seemed to be used 'chiefly in cases of matrimonial unproductivity'. Richard Lucas stated that men use ginseng to avoid completely the male climacteric or menopause and thereby keep hold of their virility as long as they live. He describes his personal experience in Harbin, Manchuria, among refugees from the Russian National Army. Many of these veterans, he records, were nerve-shattered and impotent. They 'stormed the offices of regular doctors' and then turned to the Chinese healers, who cured them with the help of ginseng together with certain other substances. Lucas then continues blithely, '. . . We should think no more of taking a dose of ginseng for sexual impotence than taking a dose of castor oil for constipation . . .'!

It is not so easy. However, there is a very strong case for stating that ginseng and pantocrine can increase sexual energy, and that they would be a considerable help both to those who are potent but sexually exhausted, and to those who are impotent and wish they *could* be sexually exhausted. Sexual power, like other aspects of human performance, depends on health, vitality, motivation, and inner psychological equilibrium. The correct balance of hormones is important for sexual functioning and the difference between the sexual resources of one individual and the next are partly due to hormone finger-prints. Sexual functions are controlled by the hypothalamic brain areas. Any agent, therefore, which can tune body functions hormonally would be expected to improve sexual energy along with other systems that derive their energy from the same deep well. In so far as ginseng and related harmony remedies can increase the energy utilization of organ systems, they would be expected to increase sexual capacity, especially when it is too sluggish and under-used.

There is also a negative relationship between stress and sexual performance. We all know that there is nothing so destructive to sexual arousal as fear or alarm. Consider the instant detumescence that follows a loud bang on the door. In the long term, tension and anxiety inhibit sexual ability and are themselves significant causes of impotence, as a result of the continual stimulation of the 'fight or flight' nerves of the autonomic nervous system, and the stress hormones at the expense of the housekeeping ones. There is a proven incompatibility on the hormone level between stress hormones and sex hormones. As ACTH (the stress master-hormone) goes up, LH (the testosterone master-hormone) goes down. The male sex hormones are therefore reduced in direct relation to the amount of stress hormones in circulation. There is an obvious primal purpose in this. Sex and procreation require peace. The alarm reaction switches body resources to immediate survival. Ginseng and the harmony remedies limit the production of stress hormones, returning ACTH and the glucocorticoids to normal more rapidly and efficiently. Thus they preserve sexual capacity during the stresses of life.

There are suggestions that ginseng actually contains sex hormones. For example, Professor Karzel in his review of ginseng reports Italian chemical studies which showed that various oestrogens (female sex hormones) were present in the root, and states firmly that 'the occurrence of constituents with sex hormone activity in ginseng preparations thus seems to be proven'.[1] 'Seems to be proven' is a contradiction in terms. I would agree more with the 'seems' than the 'proven'. In the absence of sufficient evidence, I don't feel that it is necessary to postulate sex hormones within the root. Any improvements in sexual capacity can be reasonably incorporated into our picture of hormonal tuning by the glycosides.

Small doses of ginseng given to young rats made them raise their tails, which is a frequent but not sufficient indication of sexuality.[2] Increases in the sexual activity of mice which were given ginseng have been reported,[3] but such increases can be observed with different kinds of drugs affecting the nervous system. There is no evidence that ginseng is specifically an aphrodisiac. But if we turn to measurements of sexual capacity rather than sexual activity, there is some positive evidence. When ginseng, eleutherococcus, rantarin or pantocrine were given continuously to young male mice, the weight of their sexual glands increased by up to 50 per cent, depending on the nature of the preparation and the dose.[4-7] However, not everyone has been able to duplicate this effect.[5] When eleutherococcus was given to young female mice, more of them went on heat, the period lasting some 70 per cent longer.[6] Only pantocrine and rantarin had a measurable effect in mature as well as immature animals.[7] These studies suggest that certain harmony remedies affect the balance of hormones so as to increase the sexual master-hormones. We might reasonably suggest that this occurs because of a reduction in the amounts of stress hormones present.

Ginseng and its saponins have been found to improve the egg-laying of hens, and to increase the size of the sexual organs of cocks.[8] Eleutherococcus was given to 240 minks on a Russian mink farm, and their breeding patterns were recorded. There were less than half the number of stillbirths in the eleutherococcus group, and fertility improved. Brekhman records that eleutherococcus is coming into fashion in agriculture in the USSR. It would seem a safer practice than the modern technique of injecting sex hormones into animals to increase productivity, for there are serious worries about the health risk faced by people eating hormone-fed animals.

The harmony remedies, particularly ginseng and pantocrine, may have a use as sexual restoratives, even if they are not aphrodisiacs. This was understood by the Chinese, who described their ability to preserve sexual capacity rather than amplify it. Lih Shin-Chen is quite specific about this in relation to deer antler:

> The spotted dragon
> A pearl on his brow
> Will restore the lower cave
> And portals of the jasper palace.

Improved sexual energy may only be the result of a more general restoration of energy production in the organs. It is one channel for the expression of energy by the body. A friend of mine took a largish dose of ten grams of ginseng and reported back to me that he had an erection that persisted for almost twenty-four hours. But he was devoted to sex at the time. This energy might equally well have been directed towards general health or gardening, depending on the nature of the individual.

Where impotence is due to a lack of sex hormones, stress, and a lack of energy and will, the harmony remedies should be quite effective. But where it is due to advanced degenerative diseases, to infections, to nervous diseases and so on, then therapies need to be within pathology, not beyond it. Sometimes impotence arises as a result of a vicious circle in which poor sexual energy produces inhibiting fears which in turn decrease sexual ability. A brief period of positive sexual activity and inner harmony can often break this cycle.

Or it may simply be the result of poor health. There is a Sufi story in which a physician was consulted by a woman who was infertile. The physician 'took her pulse and said: "I cannot treat you for sterility because I have discovered that you will in any case die within 40 days." When she heard this the woman was so worried that she could eat nothing during the ensuing 40 days. But she did not die. . . . "Now she will be fertile," said the physician. The husband asked how and the doctor replied, "Your wife was too fat and this was interfering with her fertility. I knew that the only thing that would put her off her food would be fear of dying". . . .'

In Japan a team of scientists has found that ginseng constituents can be used to improve sperm production and restore fertility to some individuals with inadequate supplies of sperm.[9] These constituents were found significantly to improve the manufacturing abilities of testis cells in the production of sperm, an effect normally seen with testosterone. In one of the classical psychiatric studies on ginseng, done with mental patients at the Kaschenko Mental Hospital, near Moscow, a number of patients had such an embarrassing resurgence of sexual interest that the discomfited doctors called it a side-effect and discontinued the treatment. Rantarin treatment of arteriosclerotic patients led some to recover sexual functioning and experience a return of potency and libido. Ginseng used to be famous in Russian clinics for sexual problems, and now pantocrine has taken over for this purpose.[10] In one of the few clinical studies on ginseng ever carried out by the Chinese since the revolution, it was found to be effective in treatment of impotence.[11]

The use of harmony remedies to restore libido and sexual capacity is another application in this area of therapies beyond pathology, another case of the pharmacology of harmony. Because of the pathological orientation of modern medicine, there is currently little pharmacological assistance available to modern man in search of potency. Most doctors will be stumped by a request for help in restoring sexual capacity. There are alkaloids such as yohimbine which do have an arousing effect, but it is temporary and the drugs, like all alkaloids, are far more toxic than the glycosides of the harmony remedies. Testosterone, the male hormone, can be injected and this does delay the decline in sexual vigour for many older people. But the effect is also temporary, and can increase the decline of natural production of sex hormone. The harmony remedies would seem preferable because they can be taken repeatedly every year, and they work by improving the long-term hormonal balance, an impossible goal when hormones are injected from outside the body.

HORMONE HELP FOR THE MENOPAUSE

For healthy people, progress through the life-span can take the form of a sedate two-step, but there is one period when health takes a nose-dive: the menopause. Some 85 per cent of women in the UK have distressing symptoms which occur when menstruation ceases. It is also a period of vulnerability and insecurity, when people feel pushed suddenly through a door into old age, and it is an uncomfortable transition.

I began the menopause five years ago. Since then I have suffered not only the usual physical symptoms, particularly backaches and light sweats, but also insomnia, confusion and depression. My doctor says it is 'natural' and 'just my age', and he gives me pain-killers for my back and Librium for what he calls my 'bad nerves'. All his treatment does is make me more tired, so that I get more irritable. I used to enjoy a normal sex life, but now it is something I dread because it is so painful.[12]

Unlike men, whose sexual capacity declines steadily into old age without trauma or sickness, many women face experiences of the utmost unpleasantness during the menopause.

Besides the symptoms described in the letter, the menopause is associated with bone fragility, sagging of the skin and under-lying tissues, cardiovascular disturbances including arterio-sclerosis and heart trouble, and arthritic problems.[12] All too often, women turning for help to the medical profession are told that such symptoms are only a natural part of ageing and as such should be borne with fortitude. It has led to strong support of treatment for the menopause by women's move-ments. They point out with some justification that if men had a menopause the largely male-dominated medical profession would have made sure of therapies for all.

The menopause is the result of a precipitous drop in the level of oestrogen made by the ovaries. Oestrogen is made in response to its own master-hormone from the brain, and hypothalamic areas are in charge. The puppet-master ulti-mately orchestrates the rise and fall of fertility.

If these symptoms are the result of a sudden dramatic drop in oestrogen, then giving oestrogen to women at menopause ought to relieve the symptoms. This is the controversial hormone replacement therapy (HRT for short) pioneered largely in America where it is extremely popular. It is reported to abolish almost all physical symptoms of menopause, restore energy and lift depression. Oestrogen has become known as the 'happy pill' or 'youth pill' among exhilarated women cured of the painful initiations into the change of life. There is evidence that it cuts down the chances of circulatory damage and degenerative diseases that might occur then.[12] Oestrogen treatment is relatively safe, because natural oestrogen can be used in very small doses in a cyclic fashion to reduce depen-dency. But there is a growing anxiety that thrombosis and uterine cancer can be caused by long-term use of oestrogen. After five years of HRT women run fifteen times the normal risk of this form of cancer.

The controversy over HRT has acted as a media vulture, stealing the limelight and obscuring some of the more basic issues at stake. Those who support HRT maintain that the symptoms of menopause are unnecessary, and should be treated. A dentist, they say, does not stop treating bad teeth because their owner was old anyway. They are right, but they do not ask why the symptoms should be present at all. Need this drop in oestrogen occur so precipitously in the first place?

What of those 15 per cent of women in the United Kingdom, what of the women in primitive communities who have none of these effects?

The menopause is necessary. But the side-effects are not, and they can be prevented by good health and by prophylactic measures. The drop in oestrogen sets off chain reactions; it is, like puberty, a time of *hormonal stress* on the body. If resistance is high and health is excellent, the body should be able to cope with the crisis. That being the case, the enchantment with HRT is a typical case of entrapment produced by the claims of modern pharmacology. It encourages dependence on a pill for symptomatic relief, without doing anything for the underlying realities of health. The result is that oestrogen therapy will simply postpone a health crisis, and may precipitate it later on. The increased cancer risk is a warning that therapeutic overkill is occurring.

Oestrogen therapy is certainly useful for relief of severe symptoms, while overall care is needed to maintain hormonal integrity and to fortify health during this time of great psychological stress. This husbandry should begin beforehand, in order to strengthen vitality and avoid the consequences of the impending oestrogen drop altogether.

Some women feel that this is what oestrogen therapy is doing anyway: 'My body . . . needs servicing. HRT is part of that servicing and it keeps my body working properly and, as it were, firing on all cylinders.' But they are misled. HRT does alter hormone levels, but this is not *tuning*; it is *adding*. Accordingly, imbalances are created in the personal hormone pattern which may produce their own health problems later on.

I feel that women should be aware that there are other ways to reduce menopausal symptoms. One of them is the harmony drugs. Despite its traditionally masculine mythology, ginseng is as useful for women as for men, and both benefit equally from its energy. Since ginseng and the harmony remedies act by improving the regulation of hormones (although they are not themselves hormones) it is reasonable that they should be useful in the treatment of much of the debilitating effects of the menopause, and of slight or moderate physical symptoms connected with it. There have been attempts to investigate this possibility. There was a brief flurry of interest in pre-war Germany.[13] A more recent study carried out in Germany involved the treatment of seventy-two women with a ginseng and vitamin preparation and seventy-two with placebos. Symptoms such as flushes, night sweats, nervous tension, headaches and palpitations dropped very quickly during treatment, and improvements were established in depression, insomnia and sexual problems. Symptoms were completely eliminated in forty-three of the patients who were given ginseng as opposed to fourteen of those who were given placebos. The author, a gynaecologist, states that the preparation should be taken by women at an 'early stage, on a purely prophylactic basis . . . in order to increase and maintain their resistance capacity and prevent possible menopausal disorder. If they receive this safe geriatric treatment regularly over a longer time, they will not require hormones. . . .'[14] Pantocrine and rantarin are officially recommended for menopausal problems in the Soviet Union. Pantocrine was found very useful in reduced sexual function and menopausal disorders of circulation, in depression and psychological problems, and pain in the joints. Some of the women treated started menstruating again.

There have not been any studies of ginseng and sexual energy in women . . . but some information has been thrust in front of the medical world nevertheless. 'GINSENG SAID TO INCREASE SEXUAL RESPONSIVENESS,' proclaimed a headline in a UK newspaper. Strangely, it wasn't in the sex press but the staid *Medical News* of 29 June 1978, reporting on two letters in the *British Medical Journal*. The first was from doctors at the Royal Marsden Hospital who stated that they had a case of a seventy-year-old woman who developed swollen, tender breasts after taking ginseng powder regularly for three weeks despite [sic] experiencing a general feeling of 'well-being'. The authors wisely suggested that ginseng had a mild hormonal activity but could only see this as a side-effect of the root. A request for further information resulted in another letter, presenting five more 'cases'.[15] A subsequent letter from Dr Dukes of the Medicines Division in the Netherlands purported to add clarification, but only scrambled the story. He explained ginseng's effects by the presence of small amounts of oestrogen in the root, which is unproved and probably untrue.[16]

None of these doctors suggested any potential uses for such

a preparation. Now if a new substance with 'mild hormonal activity' is discovered there would normally be a considerable flutter of interest in the medical world, because clearly there is a need for such substances in pharmacology. Yet since it was ginseng, and bought without doctor's advice, the doctors in these letters were unable to see these cases as evidence of a therapeutic effect, only of a side-effect. It should be obvious, however, that the differences between a main effect and a side-effect depend on the definition of the therapeutic situation, in the same way as the classification 'weed' depends only on what kind of plants you regard as valuable. I am sure many women would be glad of a side-effect of increased sexual responsiveness.

The time may come when the harmony remedies will be widely prescribed for their hormone-adjusting properties. Women approaching menopause will particularly value these remedies as a milder, safer and healthier version of HRT. However, menopause is only one step on the slippery slope of ageing. Ageing is, after all, the ultimate test of vitality.

'A DECADE TO YOUR LIFE'?

Of all that fantasy can attribute to a drug, nothing can compare with the ability to prolong life. The medieval alchemists had their Philosopher's Stone, the Taoists their Elixir, the Vedic Indo-Europeans had Soma, the nectar of the moon. Beginning with the oldest known myth, the Epic of Gilgamesh, mythology is full of potions for immortality.

Ginseng has collected hopes over the centuries like a snowball, and it has, like the snowball, come to rest in the present all expanded and shapeless. Many journeyers to the East have come back with these hopes, believing them to be realities. Tales are whispered of fabled ginseng roots giving fantastic ages, like the oft-repeated story of the 231-year-old professor who attributed it all to ginseng. The reality is exciting enough, though not so fantastical. Traditional physicians are adamant that ginseng is not the Elixir, but can prolong life somewhat if used carefully. 'If even the herb Chu-sen [ginseng] can make one live longer, try putting the elixir in the mouth,' states a Chinese alchemical book of the second century.

There is no doubt that the aged of China use it, if they can afford to, in attempts to attain a healthy old age and live longer. Often a root is bought for the aged grandparent with the family savings. It will be kept in brandy and eked out slowly. It was not only used by old people in the East: 'Publick Fame saith that the Popes of Rome, who are chosen to that Office when they are very old, doe make great use of this root to preserve their Radical Moysture and natural Heat, that so they may the longer enjoy their Comfortable Preferments,' wrote William Simpson of Yorkshire in a letter to the Royal Society in 1680. The tradition that the emperors of China took good-quality ginseng to retain their energy and youthful powers has been passed on to the mandarins of today: Nehru, Mao, Chiang Kai-shek and many European and Soviet members of the gerontocracy maintained their position with the help of this root.

These legends, and my awareness of the great value placed upon the root by the aged in the Orient, were what first drew me towards ginseng. My first interest was in its possible uses as a Western medicine for the elderly. Having worked through so much material, I can now ask that same question with a little more understanding. Can ginseng add a decade to human life? If not, can it at least improve the last decade?

What is ageing? It is not grey hair, feebleness, wrinkled skin, a bad heart, poor eyesight or any of the characteristics we normally associate with it. We can age with or without them. They are among the effects of ageing; ageing itself is a deep invisible deterioration that occurs throughout life, perhaps from the moment of conception. The best definition is a progressively increasing vulnerability to ever more negative agencies. Ageing is written into the tablets of our genes, but not as step-by-step instructions for dismantling ourselves. Our genes contain details concerning our resistance to the depredations of life, but this resistance has its limits. It keeps man going only for an average of threescore-and-ten years.

We are designed by our genes to course through life for a period long enough to bear children and enjoy a bit more on the other side for good luck! But on top of this design is the effect of our experiences, which can prolong life or shorten it, like a car that is designed to go for 100,000 miles but can be coaxed lovingly through its second 100,000 or brutalized into an early grave. We are given our limits at birth but that leaves a lot of room for manoeuvre.[17]

Disease occurs more often because of the lowered resistance which accompanies ageing, but it is not inevitable and our aim should be to age without it. We want to age slowly and harmoniously. The way to attain the goal is by *husbanding resistance,* cosseting it and strengthening it. Our life-style imprints itself on the body over the years. Stress will make invisible hairline cracks in our resistance, which become visible with the passage of time until the resistance crumbles and degenerative or infectious diseases walk in unopposed.

I asked Don Juan how old is he really, thinking that in order to jump like a mountain goat, as he does, a man has to be young and fit.

'I am as young as I want to be. Because this is a matter of inner strength. If you accumulate inner strength your body will be capable of achieving unbelievable feats. On the other hand if you waste inner strength then you very soon become an old fat man.'

AGEING AND THE HARMONY REMEDIES

There is intriguing support within science for the traditional Chinese remedies. The argument runs as follows. We have defined ageing as lowered resistance – the accumulation of hairline cracks in the cup – which stems from an inability to maintain harmony within. Physiological responses seem to work reasonably well, but when tested by stress their sluggishness becomes clear. A sugar load will not be removed quite so fast, a metabolic or temperature change not executed quite so efficiently, and this applies to all the processes which maintain homeostasis. There is evidence that this is caused, in turn, by failures of hormones, along with other fundamental changes to the molecular machinery of the body.

It starts at the top. The hypothalamus, like other brain areas, loses cells and suffers deterioration. It appears to be less sensitive in organizing the various control systems which maintain inner harmony.[18] The puppet-master becomes sleepy and the puppets disorganized. Chaos scatters all the way down the hormone hierarchy like ninepins, leading in the end to a vulnerable *milieu intérieur.* One of the main problems is that more of the thyroid hormones, insulin, adrenaline or the glucocorticoids are needed to generate a given change in the machinery of the body. This inefficiency generates damage, and obstructs the supply of energy. It reduces vitality and accelerates deterioration of the immune system and body resistance. To cite one piece of evidence: unnecessarily high levels of stress hormones over long periods of life may cause direct deterioration of the cells of the brain.[19]

If hormones can be tuned to maximum sensitivity and equilibrium during earlier life, they will not be so distorted later. Resistance will be maintained and the effects of ageing reduced. An experiment demonstrated that animals which had little exercise during their life had excessive stress steroid in their circulation when they became old. Exercise training, which is the simplest way of improving health, enabled the muscles and tissues to work efficiently while using less steroid, which improved sensitivity and lowered the level of stress hormones in old age.[20] If simple exercise can do it, how much more effective must be the sophisticated methods for strengthening resistance and increasing sensitivity developed by the Taoists. Indeed, the most realistic recipes for longevity put forward throughout the ages tend to describe the key as being a subtle combination of stimulation (activity) and absence of stress (temperance). People who have reached extraordinary ages have had very few illnesses in their lives. They are invariably healthy and active people who are involved and motivated and do not abuse themselves too much. Consider the longest-living people of the world, such as the people of the Hunza valley in North Pakistan and of the Vilcabamba in Ecuador. They have in common a simple diet, rhythmic physical agricultural work, temperate climate, high altitude, seclusion, traditional medicine . . . and absence of stress. The Taoists stated that in order to attain longevity one should live in such a harmonious way that resistance is accumulated during life to be used in old age when it is needed.

Ginseng, we have seen, can increase stress resistance and assist in tuning hormones. It lowers glucocorticoid levels and allows a greater stress response using less hormone. According to our analysis in Chapter 7, ginseng should delay the growth of inner hormonal chaos and therefore produce a healthier old age. It cannot halt the fundamental ageing process; only the mythological elixirs would be able to do that.

But it might be able to help people live out more of their *potential* life-span.

Our analysis tells us something else which is of great importance. Long-term beneficial results will only accrue if ginseng, a Taoist medicine, is used to some degree in the Taoist manner. You don't use a chisel to repair watches. For long-term benefit, ginseng and the harmony drugs must be used periodically by healthy or nearly healthy people undergoing minimal physiological stress.

This makes it quite difficult to investigate scientifically the effects of ginseng on ageing, particularly because the laboratory is stressful. One Russian study did purport to show prolongation of the life-span of rats given ginseng and eleutherococcus. However, insufficient rats were used so that the results should, for the moment, be viewed with caution.[21]

After several false starts I managed to initiate such a trial together with the staff at Chelsea College, London. We obtained a ginseng extract and gave small doses of it to 180 mice with their drinking-water, some for their entire life, and some for the latter portion of their life-span. Ninety mice were left as a control. The ginseng mice died of old age at roughly the same ages as the others. However, there were noticeably fewer deaths in the ginseng group for a couple of months after ginseng was given. Also, certain individuals in the ginseng group considerably outlived all the other mice.[22]

With hindsight, I realize that the study was like a shot in the dark. We should have used larger doses and we should have given it periodically during certain sections of the life-span, rather than continuously during the whole life. The question of using ginseng to maximize life-span thus still awaits scientific verification. It should of course be tried with people, who should take it in the correct manner. Though there would be plenty of volunteers for such an experiment, few scientists would undertake a project which would take threescore-and-ten years (or more?) to complete.

More success in life-span studies has been obtained with centrophenoxine, that putative Western harmony remedy. Studies with mice have indicated that small doses of centrophenoxine can prolong the post-maturity period of the life-span by 30 per cent. Large doses produced a much smaller, almost insignificant, extension of the total life-span.[23] But it is worth noting that, besides the harmony remedies, only one or two substances have ever been shown to increase animal life-span in laboratory trials, and these substances are toxic. Moreover, none of the extensions observed have ever increased the life-span of animals more profoundly than the simple expedient of cutting calories. Life-span extensions of 50 per cent have been achieved by putting animals on a calorie-restricted diet.[24] This supports the view that moderation is a much better method of life-span extension than any drug we know of. Diet and stress control, together with judicious use of harmony remedies, may be the best prolongevity prescription.

GINSENG AS A GERIATRIC TONIC

Much of the Oriental regard for ginseng and its daily usage is for people who have already arrived at old age, not people who want to delay their arrival. It is not difficult to see that the harmonizing and arousing effects of ginseng are almost tailor-made for the aged. Some 60 per cent of old people experience depression. They find it hard to resist physiological stress such as heat or cold, they are highly vulnerable to disease, they are often confused and have reduced brain as well as body function. There is a desperate call for a new drug to stimulate and improve the sluggish mind and body of older people, especially those in institutions. Orthodox medicine has as yet failed to find one. Stimulants are too strong and cause withdrawal reactions, leaving the older person worse off than before. A vitalizing restorative must be safe, non-addictive and effective. The harmony remedies are made for this role. In fact, this is the one use for which even the more sceptical authorities find them acceptable, because it is obvious that there is nothing to compete with them.

Ginseng is in fact already widely used by the elderly of the West. It takes its place among a range of preparations for the so-called non-specific geriatric basic therapy, which means geriatric pick-me-ups. Despite a proliferation of products this group is short on active principles. There is ginseng, procaine – a local-anaesthetic-cum-geriatric preparation pioneered by Ana Aslan and appearing in preparations such as KH3 – and there is centrophenoxine which we have met already. There are vitamins and there are one or two new preparations, such as ergot-derivatives, for increasing the flow of blood and oxygen to the brain in those suffering from brain deterioration. This class of drugs is among the most profitable presently in the world market.

Of all these preparations, ginseng has, in practice, turned out to be the best. The popular demand for it by old people is increasing dramatically and it is now being prescribed in clinics and old-age homes on the continent of Europe. The popularity of ginseng as a geriatric restorative is matched by evidence. While centrophenoxine is undoubtedly effective as a psychological and physical harmony remedy, especially for the aged,[25] its effects are much milder than those of ginseng, and sometimes pale into insignificance beside it. Procaine has been tested clinically but has given only equivocal results – the more impeccable the test, the less chance there has been of showing any result.[26] The largest and most recent study concluded that improvements which occurred were placebo effects.[27] It probably has a slight effect (it is a close chemical relative of centrophenoxine), but much of the success claimed by Aslan for her substance may in fact arise from the strict therapeutic regimen which she uses for her patients.

In contrast, ginseng has been frequently tested among the elderly, especially in old people's homes, often in combination with vitamins and other preparations. Earlier studies are sketchy, anecdotal trials of poor quality; however, later studies are better. There has never been a study which has completely failed to find any effect of ginseng; however, we await a highly sophisticated modern trial of the use of ginseng by old people in daily life.

The best and most recent study is by the top geriatric researchers of East Germany, who gave placebo, ginseng or ginseng plus vitamins to 540 patients. A surprisingly comprehensive battery of tests was used to investigate any improvements in biochemical, physiological, neurological, clinical, psychiatric and psychological functions. An elaborate picture of the health and capability of each old person was built up using some sixty separate tests. Though the results are still being analysed, it seems that the most impressive improvements were in psychological performance, mood, in mental and psychophysical coordination, control of blood pressure, and control of blood sugar. Interestingly, they found that ginseng alone was better than ginseng and vitamins.

In another trial in Italy, ginseng extract was found to produce a significant improvement in the ability of elderly patients to walk and move independently and to find energy for this purpose. There was a reduction in depression and melancholy, and improvements in energy, integration of personality, initiative, concentration, memory and general psychological performance.[28] In Russia, where eleutherococcus and particularly pantocrine/rantarin are given to the elderly, many trials have been reported. In one study using elderly patients with some degree of atherosclerosis, rantarin was found to improve sleep, memory, mood and drive, and to alleviate headaches.[29] If we only had wild ginseng . . . maybe we could see what the ultimate geriatric tonic could do.

The aged are getting a raw deal in industrial cultures. Unless you are fortunate enough to be a politician, professor or patriarch, old age is often a time of endless frustration and despair. No one expects anything from you except nagging dependency. You are probably in an institution, alone, or reluctantly tolerated by a busy family. Often poor, cold and miserable, you have continuous ill health, aggravated by membership of the rubbish dump of society and anxiously dependent on its handouts. Yet the population is getting older as the birth rates fall. By the end of the century there will be twice as many people above 60 as in 1970. Resources need to be shifted towards caring for the elderly, particularly to ensure that they are active and fit.

I believe that using health principles derived from Chinese medicine, it is possible to give the elderly active and fulfilling lives. This involves paying far more attention to diet and exercise, stress reduction and abstention from drugs with cumulative side-effects in favour of relatively harmless drugs which are sensitively applied. It may be that success at that stage in life, when man, 'painted with wrinkles, is ending the comedy which birth began', may send ripples back down the life-span, inducing people to start health husbandry at a time when they are still able to joke about it.

10

Somatensics

'ALTHOUGH LIVING CREATURES ARE THE
UTMOST IN PERFECTION THEY CANNOT
OVERCOME EXHAUSTION.' *Nei Ching*

Our life tends to revolve around the need for stimulation.
From the first cup of coffee in the morning to the last cigarette
at night, we take in stimulants of one kind or another. It is a
universal side-effect of the modern way of life. From London
to Tokyo, our connurbations are throbbing with self-
stimulation. Successful people are often those with an internal
power-house, the effect of which is a continual and intense
arousal as well as veins full of adrenaline. The greatest human
endeavours have usually been performed under the combined
influence of stress hormones and stimulants.

Therefore, if a new stimulant arrives on our doorstep that
has, apparently, more of the advantages and less of the disad-
vantages than any of our socially accepted stimulant drugs, it is
a fact of more than theoretical importance.

We suggested in Chapter 5 that some of the harmony
remedies, particularly ginseng, were able to generate a highly
effective kind of arousal. In Chapter 7 we showed that this
arousal could be balanced because it mimicked the natural
readiness of the mind made alert by stress, will or emotion. We
called it *hormone excitement* to distinguish it from the purely
neuronal excitation.

What are the implications of this? Can these agents actually
extend the powers of healthy people? If so, in what direction? At
what cost? What would the traditional practitioner think of the
millions of young people who use ginseng already to get more
action out of life? The matter needs careful investigation. First
we will ask what an ideal stimulant ought to look like. Then
we will match up the known stimulants and harmony drugs
against these criteria.

THE ART OF AROUSAL

There is an art in stimulation, an almost Epicurean skill in manipulating self-stimulation to reach a desired effect with maximum efficiency and minimum harm.

Firstly, it is important to reach the right level of stimulation. Too little stimulation implies lethargy, apathy and tiredness and is bad for performance. Too much produces overexcitation, jitteriness, agitation and panic. There is an optimum degree of arousal which is different for different people. Some work best at higher levels of arousal than others.

Secondly, stimulation must be of the right type. We need to ask what possibilities result from this stimulation, what functions of the mind are being charged up. Despite the fact that arousal tends to spread over the whole brain, different types of stimulant drugs and different sources of arousal produce different consequences. The arousal should wake up our faculties in concert so that true performance is improved. Concentration, expression, motivation, perception, action, ratiocination, decision and so on should be equally stimulated, otherwise we risk becoming a caricature of ourselves.

A refinement of the art of stimulation would, however, constitute the ability to arouse parts of us which are needed for a specific purpose and relax the rest. But this control is immensely hard to establish, with or without the aid of drugs.

Thirdly, arousal should be easily switched on ('Leave your bed in the morning like throwing away an old shoe') and should fade away easily into deep relaxation. Children have this ability to zoom in and out of states of arousal; they can slip from deep sleep to full wakefulness. It is an ability we tend to lose with age, too often replaced by a state of continuous semi-arousal in which we neither perform efficiently nor rest properly.

Finally, stimulation needs to be in balance with the energy supplies that fuel it. It should not be wasteful of resources. There is a kind of arousal which is out of gear and leads to exhaustion without accomplishment. Alternatively there is arousal which is just sufficient for its purpose.

Economic arousal is a method of minimizing stress, an integration of mind and body in which both run together like a good pair of horses in harness. If we consider the kinds of people whose ineconomy of arousal is leading them to disaster, for example clock-chasers on the slippery slope of degenerative disease, we may agree that economy of arousal is a key to good health.

Oriental medicine can supply new ideas in relation to stimulation and arousal, just as about any other aspect of health; it has the same kinds of statement to make, namely those of balancing states of the body in relation to personality and circumstance. The Yin/Yang concept is useful in understanding the relationship between arousal and energy. Arousal is Yang, which represents action and the burning of energy. Yin is the quiet manufacture and storage of energy. Too much Yang is like a steam-engine with wheels slipping on the track, burning up energy and getting nowhere. With too much Yin arousal is restrained by insufficient energy. The engine is so understoked that there is no steam to run it. If Yin and Yang are balanced, there is economy. Western man, Oriental practitioners state, is already too Yang, and his consumption of stimulating medication increases his Yang nature, to his detriment.

THE NEXT GENERATION OF STIMULANTS?

'Natural high speed' is how it is described among connoisseurs of pharmacological self-administration. By that threefold accolade, they mean a safe natural product which stimulates, with elements of pleasure thrown in for good measure. The Emperor Shen Nung is no less admiring though more sedate with his 'strengthening the soul, brightening the eyes, opening the heart and improving thought'.

The arousal effects of ginseng were the first and easiest of its properties to measure. In Chapter 5 we showed that it improved concentration, co-ordination, endurance and stamina. Its effects on learning, which astonished Petkov, were balanced. In order to ascertain where these remedies lie in the field of stimulation, we should look at their competitors, surveying their quality and nature in relation to the art of arousal.

A stimulant is defined as a drug which increases the level of activity and alertness, by selectively reducing the level of stimulus from the outside world necessary to cause general arousal. In electronic terms, it increases the gain on the brain amplifier so that a smaller signal going in will cause a bigger response. So-called classical stimulants, such as amphetamine, methamphetamine and methyphenidate, act directly on the nerve endings in the higher brain, where they ease the passage of blips from one nerve to the next. They are the strongest of all stimulants.

They increase endurance, general wakefulness and watch-fulness,[1] leading to more rapid movements. But the quality of their arousal is poor. They can disrupt performance of more complex tasks, and do not improve mental agility in concert with mental endurance. Switching from one kind of behaviour to another, solving problems and the exercise of choice become restricted. They also disrupt the sense of time and, at larger doses, of space. The stimulation produced is more of an excitation than an arousal. They tend to promote easily available behaviour patterns, i.e. to amplify whatever behavioural repertoire predominates, at the expense of select-ing which kind of thought or behaviour is appropriate for the situation. As the dose is raised, actions become ever more meaningless, repetitive and inappropriate. A student at my university took amphetamine to stay awake during his exami-nations. He thought he had done well until the examiners recalled him and showed him his paper – on which was his name, scribbled hundreds of times.

Besides imbalance within the mind, their stimulation is also lopsided in relation to the body. The amphetamines have been found to decrease the actual physical performance of athletes,[2] and the same has been noted in animal studies.[3] The higher the dose and the longer such stimulants are taken, the worse is the performance. Athletes find that they may increase stamina when tired, but a person who is fresh and properly moti-vated will not be helped by stimulants. There will often be an illusion of improved ability without any foundation in reality.

Caffeine too is a higher brain stimulant, though safer and weaker than the classical stimulants. It is the most widely used stimulant in the world, contained in coffee, tea, kola and guarana, and used in pick-me-up tablets, tonics and pills to counteract the tiredness produced by other medicines. But the general principles of its action are not different from those of the amphetamines. As a brain amplifier it causes excitation, agitation and insomnia, and it is easy to go over the top into jitteriness, when performance drops drastically. The quality of stimulation is better than that of the amphetamines, but leaves much to be desired. It certainly reduces fatigue and increases activity and learning in trials, but it is doubtful if overall competence is improved above that of a fully awake and motivated person.[4]

Using our guide on the art of stimulation, we can see that the harmony remedies are utterly different. Ginseng, eleutherococcus, pantocrine, etc., greatly increase stamina, and the longer they are given the more they do so. Caffeine increases stamina in the mouse-swimming test. But when caffeine is given over long periods it substantially *reduces* the capacity of the mice to carry out sustained work.[5] Amphetamine also destroys competence if it is taken for long periods. Ginseng does not particularly affect simple spontaneous activity, but it does increase exploration and directed activity. Amphetamine has precisely the opposite effect, increasing mindless activity and reducing interest in the environment.

Many Russian studies have investigated possible stimulatory effects of ginseng. In one case, muscular efficiency was examined in young men on a human physical power tester, the bicycle ergonometer. A certain amount of extract of cultivated ginseng brought a 15 per cent increase in work output. The same amount of extract of wild ginseng produced a 36 per cent increase. Incidentally, this is virtually the only study on wild ginseng I know of, and it does confirm our suppositions concerning the great difference between the wild and cultivated. Then amphetamine was tested and a 16 per cent increase in work efficiency recorded. The authors report that while amphetamine caused both excitement and insomnia, ginseng did not.[6]

An even more profound difference is visible in learning trials. Amphetamine certainly does produce faster responses and quicker learning, as seen in behavioural studies, but it reduces the ability to adapt when the situation alters! This is in absolute contrast to ginseng which, to the excitement of Petkov, not only facilitated learning but also unlearning and relearning. Japanese scientists found that while ginseng active

principles increased learning in a simple maze, methamphetamine actually reduced the speed and competence of the
animals, apparently rendering them indecisive.[7] A similar
Chinese experiment demonstrated that schizandra was better
in these respects than caffeine.[8]

The eyes, windows of the brain, can be used to test stimulants. Ginseng was given to subjects in a controlled trial and an
optician measured the speed at which their eyes adapted to the
dark.[9] Most of the subjects who had been given ginseng were
able to adapt on average one and a half times faster than the
others. Schizandra and eleutherococcus were slightly more
effective than ginseng at the doses given, but caffeine and
amphetamine were weaker. A Russian scientist named Sos-
nova managed to detect significant improvements in the
sensitivity of sight and hearing when harmony remedies were
given. The effect with ginseng began only fifteen minutes after
taking a tincture and continued for some six hours. Schizandra
seeds and eleutherococcus also increased sensitivity which was
still noticeable thirty-six hours later.

Unlike stimulants, the harmony remedies do not produce
an excitation, a jitteriness and tension – the hallmarks of drugs
which amplify the signals in the brain, and drag the rest of the
body into reluctant hyperactivity. They do turn up the volume, but without altering the treble or the bass. The great
reputation enjoyed by ginseng is, we now see, because of the
quality and safety of its arousal, not its strength, although I
suspect that the stimulation of the wild root is unparalleled in
both quality and strength. These remedies affect the mind and
body in concert. Unlike the classic stimulants, the body is
tuned to a state of arousal matching that of the mind. The
hormonal effects make energy available by more efficient
mobilization of resources. It is not produced by the squander-
ing of large quantities of fuel. The boiler is stoked up, and as
the wheels of the engine are fixed on the track the train moves
faster. Vitality is preserved or increased, and without an
energy debt there are no withdrawal symptoms.

By comparison, the cost of taking stimulants is considerable. The excitation leads to a rapid and complete depletion of
energy reserves. Tiredness is a warning of metabolic energy
debts and the accumulation of harmful wastes. Stimulants
ride roughshod over this warning. When dosage ceases,

the increased debt is experienced as withdrawal symptoms.

Stimulants cause stress.[10] They lead to an unnecessary production of the stress hormones, particularly adrenaline, which is exactly the reverse of the kind of arousal compatible with health. They have been found to reduce general resistance rather than increase it, although considering the massive usage of these compounds in various forms, there is remarkably little research on the relationship between stimulants and stress. But it is known that the circulation is put under strain, the kidneys and liver are overtaxed, sleep is prevented and debility results from long-term use.

Studies on the physiology of animals and people after exercise show that if ginseng is taken beforehand there is a more economical burning of carbohydrate fuel stores. Waste products of lactic and pyruvic acids are removed more quickly and there is a greater production of high-energy phosphate compounds, the body's energy currency with which it carries out work.[11]

This would suggest that the harmony remedies increase oxygen consumption to burn up the extra fuel, while other stimulants reduce oxygen consumption since they work by spending energy reserves[12]. Respiration and metabolic rate have indeed been found to increase when ginseng or schizandra was given to animals.[13] More than that, ginseng has been found to increase the respiration of brain cells, while amphetamine depressed it. Ginseng could actually reverse the oxygen need produced by amphetamine in brain tissue.[14]

THE POOR TONICS

Just after the First World War, Professor Embden, Professor of Physiology at Frankfurt, discovered that a dose of about seven grams of acid sodium phosphate increased prolonged muscular work by about 20 per cent. A group of coal-miners subsequently took it for nine months on end, with gains in their output and no apparent harm to their health.

Sodium phosphate belongs to a group of compounds normally present in the body, the phosphates and sugar phosphates, which are intermediates in the metabolic dismemberment of sugar to provide energy. Presumably, taking these compounds in quantity pushes the reactions faster downhill, leading to a surge of energy. This surge is transient and is similar to that produced by taking glucose.

The phosphates have been shown to increase endurance and muscular work in laboratory trials, but have not been adequately demonstrated to extend normal human limits in athletics and such activities. Nevertheless, they are widely taken by people in all walks of life. If you go into a chemist to ask for a tonic, these are the compounds you will be given. They are present in tonic wines, and often used with a certain success in recovery from illness and debility. However, they are weak and, whereas harmonizing remedies encourage the body to make its own energy-phosphate compounds, the tonics simply add them from outside. This allows the body to be as inefficient in the production of energy and as tired as always, apart from the time when the tonic is being absorbed. The tonics give a man a fish, the harmonizers teach him how to catch one.

We should add certain vitamins to this group. One would not normally associate vitamins with stimulation (but see page 250), yet they have certain somatic metabolic effects comparable with the sugar tonics. Perhaps, as Linus Pauling maintains, large quantities of vitamins can push the energy metabolism faster in the direction of energy production, like the tail wagging the dog.

SOMATENSICS

The classification of stimulating drugs is in a terrible mess. There are the classical stimulants, with caffeine and other methylxanthines sometimes appended to them. A number of other compounds can stimulate, including nicotine, strychnine, metrazol, physostigmine and alcohol. They are all toxic and their stimulation at low doses is diverse, e.g. metrazol is a derivative of camphor which particularly stimulates breathing, nicotine stimulates the autonomic nervous system of the body, and physostigmine improves learning ability. There are narcotic stimulants, particularly cocaine. Then there are mild stimulants such as pemoline and piracetam which don't fit in anywhere, and DMAE which is likewise unclassified. Now the harmony remedies appear and upset the applecart. Those harmony remedies which improve human performance do so in such a different way from the other stimulants that I propose to sunder them completely from that category. A new category is needed for those drugs which increase human performance safely and harmoniously without exacting a Faustian toll from health. Only those drugs which preserve resistance while facilitating arousal will be admitted.

I propose that they be called *somatensic* drugs, i.e. drugs which have somatensic effects. The word is a hybrid of *soma* (Greek for 'body') and *tendere* (Latin for 'to stretch'). They are body-stretching or *body-expanding drugs*. It is an apt word, because *tendere* has the same root as 'tune'.

I would like to summarize the relevant properties of the main groups of drugs with effects on arousal in the accompanying Table 6. I stick my neck out, for there is unfortunately so little relevant evidence on many of the drugs that I have had to substitute guesses. Nevertheless it serves to distinguish them on the basis of quality, something which I have never seen attempted before.

Table 5: Drugs with Effects on Arousal

	Side effects	Energy dept	Stress	Insomnia	Strength	Quality of arousal
Amphetamine, classical stimulants	****	****	****	****	****	o
Caffeine and xanthines	***	**	***	**	**	**
Nicotine, strychnine and neurotoxins	****	***	?	***	***	o
Coca	*	*	o	*	**	***
Phosphate tonics, glucose, megavitamins	o	o	*	o	o	o
DMAE, centrophenoxine, pemoline	o	*	?	*	*	**
Somatensic plant remedies	o	o	o	*	***	****

o is minimum; **** is maximum.

The somatensics stand apart from the stimulants, tonics, analeptics (e.g. camphor, metrazole), stimulatory analgesics (e.g. cocaine, novocaine) and neurotoxins (e.g. nicotine). They are also separate from narcotics, and would include the arousing harmony plants, within which there are sufficient types to choose the level of arousal we want. Ginseng is more awakening than eleutherococcus and schizandra, which in turn are stronger than pantocrine or san-chi in this regard. But some of the Araliacaea plants, particularly Aralia manshurica, are even more stimulating than ginseng. There are also harmony remedies which tranquillize, increasing performance where it is hampered by over-excitation. Valerian (Valeriana officinalis) and motherwort (Leonurus quinque) are effective tranquillizers, but so little research has been carried out on them that it is impossible to say if they are harmonizers or not. Rehmannia, China root, liquorice, beuplurum, ginger and many of the other harmony remedies are not at all stimulating.

Centrophenoxine and one of its constituent chemicals, DMAE, have already been tentatively placed in the harmonizer category. These substances are milder and less comprehensive in their stimulatory potential than the saponin harmony remedies, but we can still tentatively call them somatensics. They are used to improve learning and the accomplishment of complex tasks, which are good signs that the arousal is not lopsided in the amphetamine fashion. They are safe; as the manufacturer of DMAE claims, it 'does not depress appetite or cause jitteriness, affect basal metabolic rate, blood pressure or pulse'. But there is too little research on these substances to say much about their quality in relation to the art of stimulation. It is ironic that they are widely licensed, prescribed and officially recognized, on the basis of a dozen or so scientific papers, while the superior harmony remedies with a list of 2000 are ignored. But today a royal birth in the crucible of the laboratory provides rights and privileges unavailable to those commoners born in the crucible of the soil!

We might mention here the safe, mild stimulant magnesium pemoline, for though it is not a harmony remedy it stands apart from the other stimulants because of its gentleness.[14] We await further evidence before assigning it.

One compound which should, perhaps, go into the somatensic category is coca, the leaf from which cocaine is derived. It contains a whole range of chemicals of which cocaine is only one. Coca has fallen from grace in the West only because of the disapprobation of cocaine. But as is clearly evident in the case of ginseng, it is a cardinal mistake to assume that a plant is pharmacologically identical with any single one of its active substances. Cocaine produces a short sharp stimulation somewhat more balanced and useful than amphetamine. Yet in many ways its arousal is a similarly stressful excitation. Tolerance builds up easily and there is a similar drain on energy reserves and vitality. On the other hand, coca is gentler, even more balanced and far safer, and is in the same relation to cocaine as tobacco to pure nicotine.

It is used to increase the performance and endurance of a very large number of Andean peoples, who regard it particularly as an adaptation to the stress of hard work, reduced oxygen and inadequate food. Contrary to popular belief, there have never been any reported side-effects from moderate coca-chewing, apart from those localized to the membranes of the mouth. The quality of coca's stimulation is much better than that of any of the stimulants.[15] As it is a natural product, it provides the added dimension of diversity in the art of stimulation. Antonil, in his penetrating book on coca, describes how the practice of adding lime while chewing generates an alkalinity which affects the rate of absorption of stimulatory alkaloids. Thus coca is chewed with lime for hard work, and without for social and devotional life. 'To this extent the alkaline reagent can be seen as a kind of throttle, an accelerator, used to control and regulate the stimulation resulting from a chew of coca.'[16]

There has recently been a renewal of interest in the possibility of the use of coca (but not cocaine) as a safer alternative to coffee,[17] which actually echoes an earlier report which 'commends it as a tonic, and . . . laments that it is not introduced into Europe instead of tea and coffee as it does not cause so much cerebral excitement'.[18] We might park it in the somatensic category until further evidence emerges. Coca cola contains coca-leaf extract without its active constituents, and kola nut the extract-extract with its caffeine. *Have the wrong constituents been removed?*

Now that we have assessed somatensic remedies, let us consider their use.

HEALTH AND THE ENERGY-VAMPIRE

Before confounding readers with apparently yet another category of uses for the harmony remedies, we should confirm that their use somatensically is *not* a separate type of action. It is the same normalizing and arousing effect that we have been discussing all along. The only difference is the human milieu in which it occurs. Against a background of poor health, the individual will feel an increase in vitality and health. A person who is already in good health will perceive it as an increase in his abilities to carry out demanding tasks. The stresses are likely to be different at the lower end of the health-ladder than at the upper end.

What is the cost of taking these remedies for arousal purposes? Taking harmonizers somatensically wastes the opportunity of using them for the reconstruction of health, because the energy provided by them is not pressed into the service of vitality, but is used up in the demands of the moment. Putting it another way, the experience of stress would prevent sensitization of the stress-hormone system. We do not get something for nothing.

More energy for less hormone gives us a choice to spend the energy or to keep less hormone. Since the effect of these remedies on vitality is cancelled out by their use as stimulants, the tiredness that is the natural sequel to super-performance cannot be avoided. That is not to say that there will be a nasty come-down of the classical stimulant type, but tiredness will be waiting round the corner.

The Chinese understood that ginseng can be used as a stimulant, but they did not revere the root for that reason. Although Chinese soldiers and emperors did make occasional use of the harmony remedies in response to the demands of love or battle, these are the exceptions, not the rule. They regarded the stimulatory effect as a useful spin-off, but relatively unimportant compared to the disciplined use of these medicines for health purposes. After all, a stimulant is useful to some people occasionally, but a drug which increases stress resistance is of fundamental importance to the *well-being of everyone*.

The traditional physician would usually not recommend this manner of using harmony remedies. He would favour restricting their use to purposes of health husbandry, in which case they should be taken without the accompaniment of stress or strain or sleeplessness. Nevertheless, in the real world we all suffer from episodes of stress and exhaustion. We need to complete deadlines, to take exams, to fly aeroplanes and work in steel-mills, to drive lorries and fight in wars. The modern way of life is a giant energy-vampire sucking the vitality out of people and leaving tired shells. Faced with this situation, the traditional physician would rather see ginseng and other harmony drugs used to facilitate arousal and reduce the stress of the moment than face exhaustion and stress, or the use of harmful stimulants and even more stress.

After all, even the Yellow Emperor warned: 'When the forces of Yang are exhausted under the pressure of overwork and tiredness, then the vital essence is cut short, the openings of the body are obstructed and the secretions are retained.' Of course he is very right – there is nothing like overwork to dry up the body. Inhibiting sexual secretions and causing constipation, exhaustion shuts down those peacetime body activities controlled by the housekeeping nervous system, and they stagnate. A little Yang fire provided by a harmony remedy would be quite acceptable. But this is not building health. It is a necessary prophylactic response to avoid the damage of overwork and overstress. It would be better still if the individual stopped the overwork and overstress and took harmony remedies for more positive ends.

DEPRESSION: NEW HOPE?

A new attitude towards the care of the nervous system and the drugs which go with it may pay dividends in the treatment of depression.

Depression is like a black swamp, with the paths of disappointment, frustration and minor failure skirting the edges. The will, which is necessary to retrieve energy from the inner power-house, atrophies. It is difficult to keep a flow of energy from inner resources to thought and action. In biological and Taoist principles, nothing is fixed. If energy cannot be expressed or utilized, the source itself dries up. Lack of will depletes vitality. It has such a debilitating effect on primary energy supply that it leads to reduced movement, reduced expression, sagging tired muscles, reduced breathing, appetite and oxygen intake, reduced metabolism, and often to sickness.

Do the somatensic drugs have any role to play in the treatment of depression? Yes, they do. For depression is a condition which is sometimes easier to treat physically and energetically, since without a return of accessible energy it will be almost impossible to get a depressed person to sustain an interest in anything. His problem may have started with ennui, but it ends with energy. One needs to reverse the procedure. The bioenergetic attitude to treatment of depression is therefore also the Oriental attitude. It begins by strengthening vitality. An effective way to begin treatment is to stoke up energy generation, and this is where ginseng and the harmony remedies have an important use.

Current methods of drug treatment of depression primarily rely on tricyclic antidepressant compounds, which are often combined with tranquillizers to treat anxious or violent depressives. Electroconvulsive therapy (shock treatment) and various other psychiatric procedures are added. Unfortunately, the current drugs have considerable side-effects and, again, do not supply the vitality with which to cope with the world. It is thus especially difficult to treat both debilitated and depressed people, particularly the elderly.

For this kind of patient, the harmony remedies may be profoundly useful by themselves or as an adjunct to other forms of treatment. The millions of people with mild and passing depression, not sufficiently incapacitating to need intervention with powerful and toxic drugs or shock treatment, may find a course of a harmony remedy provides them with a new surge of basic energy and positivity. On the other hand, the remedies would not be useful in serious cases of endogenous depression.

Ginseng and centrophenoxine are now widely used in Europe to treat depressed patients, especially the elderly, with much reported success. Unfortunately doctors in the UK and America have been very slow to catch on, and in these countries most of the depressed old people have to hear of ginseng from their friends and buy it for themselves.

In the Soviet Union ginseng, eleutherococcus and pantocrine are used widely for depression. But as Petkov found, these remedies are useful in people with disturbance of mood, not those with psychoses. For example, Professor Strokina, head of the Neuropathology Department of the Vladivostok Medical Institute, reported favourable therapeutic results with eleutherococcus in eighty asthenic people, including improved mood, ability to concentrate, to sleep and function normally. Ginseng and eleutherococcus are used in mental hospitals, but I have not seen any reports of properly conducted Soviet clinical trials with mental patients.

It may be of interest in understanding depressive illnesses that there is often an excessive production of the stress steroids without the experience of stress. This is not reduced by tranquillizers, and contributes to the debility and fatigue of the depressed person.[19] It is accompanied by a blockage of the production of ACTH-type proteins in the brain, which could be one cause of loss of will, vigilance and general arousal. Since harmony remedies restore the balance of stress hormones, increasing the levels of ACTH in the brain, it would seem rational to use such remedies in the treatment of depression.

Since it has been realized how profoundly and persistently the human mental make-up is influenced by psycho-hormones, some people are considering a move further towards the use of hormones in psycho-therapy. However, psychiatrists and doctors in general know that one cannot use ACTH and steroids as vitalizing and motivating medicines because of the risks, and are desperate for a new drug with a vitalizing action which actually works safely. Fedor-Freyberg imagined that one day a steroid would be found that would have the arousing, vitalizing effect without all the risks and problems. He imagined that one would use it in 'arterio-sclerosis, infections and many other disorders, trauma or surgical operations. . . . Here a drug with a vitalizing psycho-tropic effect would indeed be of considerable value. Even if it could only be applied successfully during a relatively short period of time, it would at least improve the recovery of the curable and relieve the preterminal state of the incurable patients.'[20]

I beg to inform this author and doctors all over the world that this compound is here. Though it isn't a steroid, it is very close to it, and it will work for long periods with complete safety. It has already been in use. For 5000 years.

WORKING WITH SOMATENSIC DRUGS

I have in front of me references to several Russian medical books with titles such as *Man's Work Capacity and Ways of Increasing It* and *The Pharmacology of Motor Activity*. They have all appeared in the last few years, and betray a flurry of Soviet activity on increasing human performance by means of medical manipulation. Distinguished Soviet scientists have been applying their craft to the practical goal of making the body-machine work better. In contrast, I cannot find a single Western book on such subjects, apart from the specialist fields of sport medicine and naval medicine, and even there the Russians seem to be ahead.

Why is this? The Soviet political philosophy embodies a concept derived from Marx and Engels, that all creatures survive only through great labour. Life itself evolves through ceaseless activity and human progress can be assessed by achievements in the sphere of work. This narrow interpretation of biological fitness has made for an intense drive to increase human performance, with the result that it has become politically important for Russia to produce the best athletes, dancers or chess players.

Thus it was to receptive bureaucrat ears that Brekhman preached his unconventional message: that some Far Eastern medical plants had profound stress-resistant properties and were the best agents known to increase human work capacity. What was more logical than to attempt to increase human performance with such remedies, and who more likely candidates than pilots, deep-sea divers and mine-workers? The remedies were quickly tested on people working in poor environmental conditions. For example, eleutherococcus was given to mine-rescuers at the Central Mine Rescue Station, Brandis. Hard work there in hot conditions (40°C or more!) is complicated by the inhalation of gas mixtures containing 50 to 90 per cent oxygen instead of the normal 21 per cent. Eleutherococcus was found to improve work output as well as stabilizing some physiological distortions such as the conservation of water, salts and ascorbic acid. In another study thirty-one out of a group of fifty-one deep-sea divers were given four millilitres of eleutherococcus one hour before their dive to depths of 90 to 160 metres. This group could carry out harder work and showed greater accuracy and co-ordination while carrying out tasks under the sea, and were far less tired on emergence from the decompression chamber.[21]

Soviet sailors and fishermen often experience difficult and dangerous conditions, especially in the north. Russian scientists have paid a great deal of attention to the requirements for adaptation to difficult and lengthy sea voyages.[21] They have recommendations concerning the food, the chemical composition of the drinking water, and the use of prophylactic medicines. Besides vitamins and tonics, the harmony remedies are highly recommended to increase both disease-resistance and performance under these conditions.

When I looked up what the British Government recommends to its captains in the way of such medicines, all I could find in the official medical guide for ships' captains was a recommendation that a metabolic tonic be carried against fatigue. That is a preparation containing strychnine (!), ferric phosphate and sugar. We have already shown that these metabolic tonics are the least effective and interesting of any of the tonic and stimulant medicines known.

Russian workers frequently take eleutherococcus to help them cope. Is this a *Brave New World* action of labour-obsessed Soviet committees who give eleutherococcus and schizandra to car-workers to make them work faster and obscure their unacceptable intention with talk of health?

Not to any extent. The conveyor-belts do not move any faster. It is rather a genuine desire to relieve stress and to increase alertness. As a letter I received stated: 'In Autumn 1973, I was working on the car production line at British Leyland, Cowley. When I transferred to permanent night work I decided to try using ginseng to combat the fatigue I felt in the early hours of the morning. . . . The speed of the belt was not overtaxing, but the relentless repetition was something that everyone developed his own method of fighting. I would take a dose of ginseng powder at about 3 a.m., and the effect was quite marked. It was not that I ceased to feel tired or bored, but that I felt fresh to the situation, as when I had just arrived that night. . . .' I have just heard that the giant German firm of Siemens is giving ginseng to all its workers.

The main way to improve the capacity to work is to start off with sufficient vitality, as a result of a sensitive and intelligent diet and life-style. The jobs themselves should be less stressful, so that there is no need for stress prophylactics or somatensics. But factories from Manchester to Minsk still function in much the same way, and therefore a relief of the psychosomatic assault is welcomed. It seems strange to me that there is usually intense monitoring of the factory environment for harmful chemicals, yet none for stress which produces diseases every bit as dangerous. What overalls can people wear to protect themselves against stress?

Airline pilots are not allowed to take most medicines, including tranquillizers, amphetamine-type stimulants, barbiturates and steroids, before a flight. They are traditionally stimulated by cups of coffee served in flight. But caffeine is a stimulant of only limited usefulness, which can even lower performance rather than increase it, especially when considerable amounts are taken. A tired pilot would be much safer taking a drug with somatensic, not excitant effects. The same is true for lorry-drivers. Many road accidents are the result of drivers taking medication of one kind or another. The Russians recommend eleutherococcus for transport-drivers who need to keep awake.[22]

We can imagine a host of uses for somatensic agents; they could encompass most of the instances for which stimulants or coffee are currently used – exams, marathons, severe climatic conditions, severe training, mountain climbing or expeditions.[22] Indeed, is it not time that a new survival food became generally available? I can easily imagine a suitable one containing somatensic, appetite suppressant, nutritious components. At a time when medicine has designed the most complex therapeutic regimes for disease, with esoteric and expensive chemical formulae, it is extraordinary that a mountaineer has nothing to support him except the glucose in Kendal mint-cake!

SOVIET OLYMPIC ATHLETES TAKE SOMATENSIC DRUGS

Soviet Olympic athletes have taken and still do take eleutherococcus and ginseng before their races! Since this is a rather damning statement I had better say that I have no documentary evidence of this. My source is the academic grapevine. It is possible that I have been misinformed, but unlikely; the use of the harmony remedies in athletics has a long history in Russia, beginning with the earliest studies of the Vladivostok team.

When they discovered that ginseng, and then eleutherococcus, could reduce the times of long-distance races, the athletics directors pricked up their ears. Obviously any drug which could produce the kind of improvements in athletic performance observed in the early trials would not only gain many gold medals for Russia, but might also smash world records.

So they began to test these agents on genuine athletes. Experiments were carried out under the direction of the well-known specialist in sports medicine, Professor Korobkøv. For example, tests with 1500 sportsmen at the Lesgraft Institute of Physical Culture and Sports indicated that eleutherococcus extract could increase stamina and endurance, and improve reflexes and concentration. It was especially effective at increasing the amount of training which athletes could tolerate without harming themselves. In all cases there were no noticeable side-effects, except an occasional transient increase in blood pressure.

A recent book which has appeared in Russia, entitled *Medicinal Preparations with Applications in Sports Medicine*[23] extols the usefulness of harmony remedies for sportsmen. Professor Korobkøv writes in the foreword that, 'The medical substances included in the reference book have nothing in common with doping, and their action is primarily aimed at accelerating the restorative processes after intensive activity and at increasing the body's resistance to unfavourable external influence.'

There is much more here than meets the eye. The harmony remedies have somatensic properties which make them more effective and more efficient at improving human performance than the amphetamines, providing the taker is acting at the limit of his capacity. But they also have other uses, for example disease resistance. It is therefore quite legitimate to state that the harmony drugs are used to increase resistance, as Professor Korobkøv says: 'A sportsman has the same right to pharmacological support and prophylaxis as a winterer in the Antarctic, a mountain rescuer, a scientist during a period of maximum stress, or a cosmonaut.' But is this a red herring to divert public attention away from the use of these preparations somatensically? Is this not like the recent case of a sportsman with fencamfamin in his urine who said he was only using it for hay fever? It is a bit hard to believe that the Russians have improved athletic timings with eleutherococcus in practice runs and then failed to use it in contests, restricting such medicines to use after the race in order to prevent the athletes catching cold.

I believe the situation to be the following. There are strong laws against athletes taking drugs which unfairly improve their performance. The harmony remedies are not on this list at the moment, for the same reason that they cannot be found in any national pharmacopoeia in the West. As long as this situation lasts, the Russians cannot resist the temptation to use these drugs to improve the performance of their athletes. The Russian Sports Committee have banned the use of eleutherococcus during races by their own sportsmen, in order to avoid the scrutiny of sportsmen from other countries and the possibility of international action. However, in practice the ban is not completely effective.

This is the definition of doping agreed in Strasburg in 1962 by a Council of Europe Committee: 'Doping is the administration to, or the use by, a healthy individual of an agent foreign to the organism, by whatsoever route introduced, with the sole object of increasing artificially and in an unfair manner the performance of that subject while participating in a competition. Certain physiological procedures designed to increase the performance of the subject may be regarded as "doping".'[24] This would put the harmony drugs well into the 'doping' category. After all, their somatensic effect is just what the doping definition covers when it refers to 'increasing the performance of the subject'.

However, the doping definition is by no means wholly watertight, for there are many situations which are ambiguous in real life. For example, there are suggestions, again from Russian science, that vitamins in large amounts might be able to increase performance to a limited extent.[25] But one could hardly accuse vitamin-takers of doping, unless one went to the ludicrous lengths of describing it as doping above some arbitrary dose level. This would provide a way out for the somatensic remedies. For example, if athletes say they take the remedies all the year round as part of their natural health-giving diet, it would be difficult to ban them when they are also taken before the race. After all, are garlic, ginger or tea banned because they contain non-physiological substances which may have a medicinal effect? This is, one presumes, what the Soviets' case would be if it came to the crunch. They would point to the 'with the *sole object*' clause, and give the Committee a headache.

How should eleutherococcus, for example, be taken so as to maximize athletic performance? The best way, judging from all the Soviet research mentioned on pages 136–7, is to take it for a minimum of ten days and a maximum of one month before the race, to ensure that a maximum effect had built up. The athlete could actually stop taking it just before the sports event, and he would still benefit. This would not put it outside the doping category. Some of the most famous doping compounds are anabolic steroids which build up strength and 'meat' gradually, and are taken for some time before the race. They are certainly forbidden for sportsmen. On the other hand, if the remedies were not taken for some time before the race, detection would be very difficult. In any case it is impossible to detect the harmony remedies in blood or urine at the present time.

In one sense the somatensic compounds are like the anabolic steroids: they were both Russian introductions. The use of steroids and hormones to increase performance was begun by Russia and later outlawed. The use of somatensic triterpenoidal compounds in sport was also initiated by Russia and is not yet outlawed. They are both the product of the special Soviet concern for understanding and manipulating human capacity for practical purposes, of linking medicine tightly to national goals. Do they both give evidence of Soviet success at improving athletic performance?

This is difficult to answer. One cannot compare countries indirectly, because a small country such as Iceland can hardly be expected to have the same number of exceptional people in the various sports as a country as large as the Soviet Union. It is therefore usual to rate sports competitiveness in relation to the size of the population of different countries. When the number of successes are compared to the population, Europe comes out way on top and Russia is relatively low in the list. But there is a twist to the list. When the number of successes is measured per athlete, in other words the performance of individual athletes is assessed, Russia is indeed on top of the rest of the world by a very healthy margin! This year's Olympics are being held in Moscow. How many gold medals will go to eleutherococcus?

SOMATENSIC DRUGS IN WAR: GENGHIS KHAN AND THE VIETCONG

War is the ultimately stressful situation. Nowhere is it as important to function with maximum power as in combat. The adrenal hormones pour out so torrentially that whole companies of men can exhaust their adaptive energy, use up their fund of stress resistance and have to be hospitalized, without suffering any physical injury. Since the First World War soldiers unable to deal with the extraordinary stresses of fighting have become recognized as legitimate casualties of war.

In the Second World War, the phenomenon of exhaustion was an everyday experience. All psychiatric cases were put into the same bag because of their similar appearance. Extremes of stress manifest in identical fashion, no matter how diverse the cause: 'Their faces were expressionless, their eyes blank and unseeing, and they tended to sleep wherever they were. The sick, injured, lightly wounded, and psychiatric cases were usually indistinguishable on the basis of their appearance. Even a casual observation made it evident that these men were fatigued to the point of exhaustion.'[26] The stress causes degrees of somatic incapacity – poor digestion, ulcers, headaches, palpitations and severe weakness.

Fear is a prime stress, but it is modified or exaggerated, released or suppressed, depending on the conditions of battle and the individuals within it, particularly the presence of a group to share it.

In the desperate situation of warfare, where people clutch at will-o'-the-wisps for help, drugs are inevitably used. War is the ultimate proving ground of drugs for healthy people. The British brew tea in adversity as if it were an ambrosial fluid to calm frayed nerves and stimulate tired ones. The Vietnamese and Chinese soldiers eat ginseng on the battlefields with rather more pharmacological justification. The medieval Islamic sect, the Ashashim, used cannabis so that their perception of reality would be fully subordinated to their aggression. American and Egyptian soldiers have used cannabis extensively in recent years, but the purpose in this case is to make reality less terrible, not more so. What then are the drugs that really help in war? How do ginseng and the somatensic drugs fare in relation to the others, and how much have they been used?

The two stimulants most used in modern war situations are amphetamines and caffeine. But stimulants are dangerous drugs to take into battle, for since they do not remove tiredness itself but only the feelings of tiredness, a long recovery is needed. Neither do they increase the resistance of the fighting man, which is what he needs above all else: resistance not only to psychological and physical exhaustion, but to disease, to death from injury, and to poor conditions. He needs a *survival potion*. Fatigue reduction should be part of a general increase in performance and protection. The Oriental harmony remedies are much closer to the ideal, for they increase resistance in a general sense. Indeed, they work on the mechanism for survival during prolonged fight-or-flight. War is prolonged fight-or-flight. The soldier needs to be indefatigable, and of all known drugs only those with somatensic effects can help him to be so.

Ginseng has always been used by Oriental soldiers. Chinese soldiers in imperial times had ginseng root in their battle packs which they used to increase their resistance in combat. More recently, the Chinese clearly found that ginseng could save life on the battlefield by helping them to resist shock.

The great military success story of modern times is that of the Vietnamese. Their victory over America can be seen on many levels, as the victory of brain over brawn, or of human ability over weaponry. The differences between the attitudes and strategies of the armies is also typified by the drugs they used. The Americans took the amphetamines, the barbiturates, the narcotics and other psychotropic drugs, the pharmacological heavy weaponry.

The Vietnamese relied largely on their own stocks of indigenous plant medicines, and the drug they took with them into battle was, naturally, ginseng. I wouldn't like to speculate how much ginseng contributed to their success – probably not very much by itself, but it was a part and parcel of a way of living and fighting which eventually triumphed. There is an amusing sequel. After the war, during the Paris peace negotiations, the Vietnamese and American negotiators were in session night and day. While the Americans were exhausted after the marathons, the Vietnamese appeared to be as fresh as daisies. When a senior Vietnamese diplomat was asked about it he pulled something out of his pocket by way of an answer – it was a ginseng root.

Genghis Khan and the Mongols came from the best ginseng land in the world. Did they bring ginseng with them? Did it contribute to their amazing fortitude and stamina which enabled them to overrun Asia? I read that forty Russian divisions are stationed along the Russo-Chinese frontier, and hosts of Chinese troops wait on the other side. I find it intriguing that there is eleutherococcus in the Russian camps and ginseng in the Chinese.

GINSENG IN SPACE: NASA'S PROBLEMS

The spaceman's world is one of unbelievable complexity and difficulty. Imagine being suspended weightless in a tiny capsule, the mind anxiously coping with a total reality tolerable only because it is temporary; senses alert to the performance of critical life-support systems, the body receiving unknown amounts of radiation, lungs coping with odd mixtures of bottled air, bones leaking their minerals, all the physiological discordancies of zero gravity, and hormones out of phase through disturbances of normal rhythms.

Both the environmental stress and the prolonged restrictions on mobility will gradually raise the levels of corticosteroids in the body. The astronaut may find himself becoming increasingly anxious as he gets tired. Weightlessness itself produces fatigue. Stress must surely accumulate within the total capsule environment somewhat as heat and moisture will accumulate in a greenhouse. Resistance plummets and the astronaut finds himself increasingly susceptible to diseases and infections. The Skylab crew found that stress amplified seasickness so that nausea built up as time passed. The blood supply shifts at zero gravity and the brain felt 'as if hanging from a tree'. Man can hardly invent an environment more stressful to himself. As one of the spaceflight pioneers recorded: 'It would mean a long imprisonment under the most adverse conditions. The discoverers of new continents performed superhuman tasks in their time, but a trip to Mars would strain the toughest body and mind beyond the breaking point.'[27]

The Russians have applied their expert knowledge of human adaptation and stress to the ultimate stresses experienced by the cosmonauts. They realized that space crews need medicines, not only to treat illnesses, but also to stimulate natural adaptive and resistive mechanisms, enhance performance and eliminate tiredness and stress. In 1967 the Russians reported animal trials using all kinds of possible drugs, including their adaptogenic agents, to test stresses such as that of acceleration. They went on to recommend that stimulant drugs such as amphetamines and caffeine were feasible in restricted circumstances. But ginseng and eleutherococcus were recommended for unlimited use.[28] That was twelve years ago, when ginseng and eleutherococcus were so unknown in the West that the Russians might as well have been talking double-Dutch.

The Soviet teams continued to explore new narcotics and healing agents; they investigated whether their cosmonauts would have altered sensitivity to drugs while in space, and they broadened their unique expertise in the use of drugs to resist stress and increase capacity. Ginseng was taken in earlier space flights. Professor Brekhman writes of this that, 'Some hopes have been pinned on the salts of asparagine and glutamic acid, vitamin B_1 and B_6, pantothenic acid, ATP and particularly the gently acting plant adaptogens of the eleutherococcus kind, which, in contradistinction to substances of the phenamine (amphetamine–SF) group, may be taken for a long time without fear of addiction, sleeplessness or impaired appetite.'[22]

Subsequent research in the cosmodrome into eleutherococcus was successful. The result is that, as I write, Soviet cosmonauts Vladimir Lyakhov and Valery Ryumin, working in the Salyut-6 Soyuz 32 complex, take four millilitres of eleutherococcus every morning.

Western understanding of the medical problems of space crews is highly sophisticated; however, there is a real failure to produce drugs which come up to expectations. For example, a major Western review of drugs in space recognized that all medication must be selected so as not to create aberrations that might lower the astronauts' performance, but no drugs were suggested to reduce them. The concepts of drugs which increase human performance without stress are so foreign to Western pharmacologists that they do not know where to look for them, despite the fact that the Russians have been experimenting and using such drugs in space for over twenty years. Dexamphetamine (dexedrin) was the only drug actually used during the earliest space flights of the Mercury programme. Amphetamine side effects are well known. In the very same reports amphetamine is criticized because it was found to cause a significant deterioration of performance in ground tests.[29]

I pointed this out to NASA staff, who found my ideas 'interesting and provocative'. The Director of Life Sciences of NASA replied that 'NASA have not used any drugs to enhance astronaut performance in space' and described, somewhat tangentially, the extensive varieties of other kinds of medical drugs carried by the space crews. It is not at all clear whether he is denying the scientific reports stating that dexedrin was used, or that he is denying that amphetamines are drugs which can enhance performance. But it is clear that Western astronauts are still not taking the drugs which they need, because they would have to be obtained from sources outside the current pharmacological paradigm.

We have included ginseng, eleutherococcus, some Aralia plants, centrophenoxine and perhaps coca in the lists of somatensic drugs. It is logical that they should at least be tested for use by space crews. Now here we come to a serious medico-political problem. Space crews are heroes, representatives of the people who send them into orbit. American astronauts are models of what Americans would like to be, and the same is true for the Russians. It is therefore unlikely that NASA would risk using medicaments for space crews which the establishment has banned or spurned, since if they did it would be the thin end of the wedge for those drugs.

With space flights becoming longer and longer, the effects of stress become more debilitating. Medical reasons such as loss of bone calcium are given by NASA to explain why they are not contemplating lengthy space flights in the near future. However, the Russians have carried out very lengthy flights recently. While I am not for a moment suggesting that somatensic drugs are completely responsible, I do feel that their more open-minded attitude to the relationship between man and his chemical environment may have helped them to overcome these problems.

PART 4
Conclusions

II
Biomedical Tao

THE LITTLE BRIDGE

A small ginseng root is curled up on my desk as if asleep. It is half-buried under piles of reprints, reports, papers and this book: its book. The root itself, I thought, has shrunk into insignificance in comparison with the vast weight of laboratory analyses, discourses and polemics it has spawned. This disturbed me, for it re-exposed my doubt, that perhaps all this is a storm in a teacup, an unworthy edifice built upon one of the less significant examples of the wealth of the vegetable kingdom. I cleared away the papers, exposing the root, which seemed mockingly to reply that it was no fault of its own that it had generated a snowball of interest in the West of which this book is part. In a different place, it reminded me, it is an object of delighted consumption, not of debate or justification.

Then my mind skimmed over some of the more astonishing manifestations of this wonder of the world. The most expensive plant in human history finds itself chewed in Soviet space capsules. Two hundred and fifty million doses of it are consumed annually in America, despite the assertion of the authorities that it doesn't work. A single medicine is used to sustain the powers of the emperors of China, the Popes of Rome, the sheiks of Arabia, the statesmen of the Far East, the geriatric cases of Europe, cancer patients of the USSR and the heart patients of Shanghai. Active principles, the like of which have never been noticed before, turn up in a host of plants, all of which have strange subtle effects on the body. The Eastern half of our schizophrenic globe is ecstatic in its praises, the Western half is bemused and cynical. Meanwhile, ginseng and its relatives are bringing immediate assistance to people, providing a restorative therapy so far unavailable in Western medicine. My own research began in the darkness of a thousand and one claims and counter-claims, continued with the discovery that ginseng had unique protective effects on cells in the laboratory, on animals and people in stress, and culminated in demonstrating an action on the hormone inter-connections between mind and body. Research which started in the Chinese shop in Soho ended with striking corroboration of the original and most authentic of all statements about the kingly remedies, that of the semi-divine ancestral sage that started it all: Shen Nung. Whatever is its eventual fate, this small root can never be ignored.

Professor Brekhman was invited to lecture in London recently. He began a summary of his experiments on ginseng and eleutherococcus. Slide after slide documented study after study. As he continued, the small auditorium of pharmacolog-ists began to move restlessly. When he finished, one lecturer left with a dark face, muttering, 'You take it if you're sick, you take it if you're healthy; you can't go wrong, can you? It's rubbish.' Hearing him gave me a déjà vu of the time when I first threw up my hands in the face of a thousand scientific papers which seemingly proved everything under the sun.

The question of whether these remedies work or not no longer requires debate. The evidence is overwhelming, and the lack of any appropriate studies in contradiction is a deafen-ing silence. The debate should move to another level, that of relevance to our medicine, our health and our development.

This requires the formulation of the new ideas in a language that everyone understands. The lecturer's dismissal of Profes-sor Brekhman's work occurred because he couldn't relate to the concepts, even though he was supplied with the data. Without proper construction and translation, the novelty of the concepts behind the harmony remedies makes them easier to ridicule than respect. Dr Ignatius Semmelweiss was the first person in the West to understand that disease might be trans-mitted by microscopic agents passed from one person to the next. But since he failed to formulate this discovery in terms that his peers could understand, his suggestion that surgeons should wash their hands before operations seemed as absurd as witchcraft and he was drummed out of town.

Fortunately my job is less hazardous. Not only is Western medicine in a cul-de-sac and ready to listen to suggestions of a way out, but the huge and hitherto unknown mass of scientific material speaks for itself, making an ill-informed dismissal obvious for what it is.

I set out to formulate the case for ginseng and the remarkable Chinese kingly remedies by stepping into the unknown from both Eastern and Western shores. The confusion was cut to size first by selecting the claim of Chinese traditional doctors, since theirs was the system that discovered the roots. This meant a steady journey between the mountains of over-enthusiasm and cynicism, by a pilgrim en route to the East with the classics of Huang Ti and Shen Nung under his arm. In this way it was possible to pick out a group of novel sub-stances, which I termed harmonizers, a range of adjustive and harmonizing medicines. The harmony remedies are the bridge which can transport those ideas over the East–West chasm of ignorance. As remedies claimed by the Chinese to be capable of adjusting inner balance and thus increasing health, they are the embodiment of the harmony approach. As an aggregate of substances they are amenable to scientific investigation. The Eastern stanchion of the bridge was built in Chapters 3 and 4. The Western one is also completed. Some struts have been laid across in Chapter 8. Now we can bring across some ideas.

HARMONY IN A WESTERN FORM

What is harmony? It is a concord in the relation between things. Harmony is only perceivable in the relationship be-tween the organism and its environment against the back-ground of a world-view. If a concept of harmony is to be useful to Westerners in search of health, it must be set against a Western world-view, not against an esoteric Oriental version.

In fact, the concept of a physiological balance has been slowly creeping back into Western thought. Bernard, Cannon and Selye have implanted the notion that outside the body chaos rages, inside all is harmony. The ability to cope and to adapt is health and depends on physiological control systems. This idea of a physiological balance is thoroughly Hippocratic in essence, although little use is made of it in medicine at present. It has outgrown the bare specificity dogma of the revolution in scientific medicine . . . but it is nevertheless still far away from a true harmony view as held by other medical systems.

East and West meet in the stress concept. Unfortunately, the meeting is brief, for the West has stopped at the point of a purely theoretical appreciation of the mechanics of the internal equilibrium. On the other hand, Chinese medicine is a system of vast sophistication beside which our concept of stress is crude. Claude Bernard could possibly have written this: 'When the various forces of the body work in mutual harmony there will be life; when they are associated with each other but do not blend, illness will result.' But he could never have written this: 'In order to bring into harmony the human body one takes as *standard* the laws of the four seasons and the five elements. This method serves as a regulator to man, whether he is obedient or whether he is in opposition to these laws, whether he is successful or whether he suffers failure.' Both quotations are from the *Nei Ching*. Chinese medicine is the logical conclusion of the stress concept; an entire medical system, based on the subtle ebb and flow of agencies in the environment which influence internal harmony. Let us see if we can reinterpret some of its principles.

YIN/YANG

Purple is an individual entity seen by the eye. Yet the mind has the ability to estimate its component primary colours of blueness/redness/greenness and its darkness/lightness. Similarly, the instantaneous energy state of an organ can, through the skill of the Oriental physician, be split up into its component elements – the Yin/Yang polarity, the tendencies towards each of the five elements (heat, dryness, moisture, cold and airiness) and the degree of basic ch'i energy. The organ state is mapped at that moment, taking into account its past and projecting into its future. The healing process adjusts the energy state to bring it in line with that of other organs and within the total picture of an individual's constitution and environment, much as an artist applies his mixed colours to blend into a harmonious and purposeful whole on a canvas.

Ginseng tunes and sensitizes the stress-steroid system. Ginseng's properties are describable in Chinese medicine as reinforcing Yang over the whole body. Therefore we cannot escape the conclusion that Yang energy is in some way influenced by the stress steroids. This conclusion gains support from our knowledge of the actions of these steroids: how they increase the mobilization and usage of energy resources, how they charge up organs, particularly, we might note, the liver, the muscles and the heart, increasing heat, and the secretion of waste. This corresponds to the nature of Yang. The stress steroids are involved in regulating internal combustion along with other factors, such as the thyroid hormones, insulin and adrenaline. One might then suggest that any influences or medicines which shifted the hormone fingerprint towards the burning of energy and the speedier flow of materials through organs would promote Yang, while any influences which encourage quiescence would promote Yin. The exact Yin/Yang balance of energy conversion could subsequently give rise to heat or cold, efficiency or inefficiency, building or destroying.

Everything in life contains elements of both Yin and Yang. In so far as an influence affected the inner state of the organism, it could be incorporated into the advice of the healer, whether it be cabbages or kings. From our knowledge of the sensitivities of the hormone control systems to both inner and outer influences, could we not imagine them as special arbiters of Yin and Yang in the body?

As for ginseng's 'warm' energy, this implies a deep heat visible to the Oriental doctor by a change from cold to warm bodily symptoms. It is not the temporary warmth produced by, say, a hot drink, but rather connected to the *production* of heat. Heat is generated in the body by metabolism, which is controlled by thyroid and, to some extent, adrenal hormones. Both are under the control of the hypothalamic puppetmaster. There is published evidence that ginseng does inhibit the thyroid gland, thereby increasing heat.[1] The extra heat produced in the body could be the natural result of a shift in the hormone balance towards a greater utilization of energy. The boilers are well stoked, and they work hard, churning out biochemical high-energy compounds for the body to burn. On the other hand liquorice, which has Chinese 'cooling' properties, is known to affect the mineralocorticoids which have in many respects opposite effects to the stress steroids.

'Cooling', in Oriental terms, could be in Western language related to shifts in the hormone pattern, damping down the energy state of the organs.

The mineralocorticoids retain salt and water in the body; therefore liquorice should moisten as well as restrain organs. In this way Westerners can understand the use of liquorice to balance stronger remedies which the Oriental healer is using to purify and 'heat' organs. One remedy to purge, the other to protect: a mixture which, the Chinese say, 'walks on two legs'.

Acupuncture too has hormonal effects. Japanese scientists have detected lasting changes in the metabolism after acupuncture. They report a rise in serum cortisol some time after the treatment, and suggest that some of the effects could be due to changes in the hypothalamus as well as other areas of the brain.[2] Recent high-quality American research has demonstrated increases in brain anti-pain hormones, the natural opiates of the body, when acupuncture is used to kill pain. These natural opiates are made in the brain in response to stress. They are similar to ACTH (the master stress hormone – see page 165) and share the same manufacturing process. Can we suggest that acupuncture too alters the energy state of various organs, and reduces pain, by manipulation of the hormone instructions issuing from the lower brain?

Some readers may baulk at all this reductionism. They would consider that such intuitive concepts as Yin and Yang cannot be neatly boxed into a Western biological model. They are right. Polarity is so fundamental that to pin down Yin and Yang, or even 'heating' and 'cooling', to certain sets of body mechanics is like trying to describe the grain in wood in terms of Euclidian geometry. However, I am not trying to explain, but to find points of contact between the two systems. This has an heuristic value. In particular it may help us to appreciate Chinese medicine as a practice arising logically from an alternative metaphysics, not a hotch-potch of absurdities. Science looks at the body, the organs, the biochemicals with its microscope and discovers hormones. The Chinese look at the same biological materials but with a telescope. They discover warming and cooling, Yin and Yang. The two healing systems that arise are both rational and they both work.

BRAIN AND BODY: MEDICINES TO TIGHTEN THE CONNECTION?

One example of how Chinese concepts may be brought over to our benefit concerns mind-body relationships in Western medicine. Since the rise of so-called rational therapeutics, the West has withdrawn the mind into a secure brain-box and viewed it as a distant directorate of the body. The Chinese do not have a distinction of mind/body but see grey matter and red matter as colours on the canvas, making up a picture of a human life as a flux of energy states.

The best model we can find to unravel the mystery of these medicines is that they affect the body's hormonal control systems. Now enough is known about hormones to realize that they integrate psychological and somatic states. The study of hormones (endocrinology) has always been limited by its subversion to the general pathological paradigm of medicine as a whole. Using our bridge, however, we can immediately see that the flux of hormones could be a handle whereby we can visualize the mind and body as a continuum. More than that, there is no reason why this knowledge should not be the basis for a practice of health maintenance, as in China. If we called it body-tuning and thought about hormones adjusting the flow through the various organs, we should have incorporated Chinese concepts into our language and practice, painlessly and to our benefit.

We should have a model to understand how, for instance, a drug could produce both emotional arousal and somatic heat. We may have an intuitive feeling that repression of emotion leads to a sluggish metabolism ('cold fish'), but this could be incorporated into a system of therapy, just as in China, which understands how metabolism and personality are intertwined. Then it would be possible not only to make the suggestion, *'People with repressed emotions may be more likely to incur cancer,'* which is the state of the art at the moment, but to advance to the possible *'Repressed emotions are associated with an imbalanced sluggish metabolism producing carcinogenic wastes. Prophylactic treatment is by heating and purifying remedies.'*

The same goes for the concept of individuality. While Chinese medicine treats the person first and the disease second,

Western medicine does the reverse. Our model would include individuality in Western language by suggesting that moods and constitution are revealed by their hormonal (and possibly neuronal) fingerprint. This would provide an opportunity for diagnosing and realigning biochemical individuality, not only with remedies, but also instruction in the Chinese fashion, in relation to diet and life-style. A restless, excitable, thin person might be advised to eat Yin foods or take moistening medicines before the conditions for disease are created within, possibly, his lungs. Is this inner balancing a juggler's act which need be restricted to Oriental medicine forever?

Chinese medicine and, as we have seen, Hippocratic medicine, is very much concerned with charting the vulnerability of man in relation to constantly changing internal and external worlds. Everything from moods to foods to winds is thought to impinge on health in the long term. Harmony drugs, along with advice and acupuncture, are at the centre of approaches to deal with these constant alterations. But we know that the interactions between man and his environment are controlled by the hormones and nerves of the lower brain areas. Therefore our conclusion that the manipulations of the harmony drugs are located there too fits in well with the Chinese use and understanding of them. As an example we will take the question of biological rhythms.

DEALING WITH BIOLOGICAL TIME

In Oriental medicine, rhythms and seasons were associated with special kinds of susceptibilities. The daily life-patterns of a person are carefully analysed as a cause of disease and regularized as a source of health. Science can certainly confirm that daily rhythms occur in our physiology and in our susceptibility. Secretion of adrenal hormones occurs in a cyclic fashion throughout the day, with a low point normally at the end of the night, and a peak some twelve hours later. Resistance to drugs, surgery, anaesthetics or disease follows faithfully the adrenal beat. This can be easily shown by experiment. In one case a dose of a drug (amphetamine) which killed 6 per cent of a group of mice at their time of maximum resistance killed 78 per cent some hours later.[3] Doctors know that both births and deaths are clustered in the small hours.

The adrenal rhythms give rise to profound changes in body processes – metabolism, blood pressure, salts, activity, sensitivity of the nervous system and appetite are cyclic, and disruption of these patterns inflicts a major stress on the organism. Distortion of the daily clock, such as occurs in shift work or in flying across time zones, reduces performance, health and vitality. It is a serious stress. In a famous experiment the life-span of mice was reduced by 6 per cent compared to a control solely by putting them under jet-lag conditions once a week. G. G. Luce puts her finger on the stress steroids, as we have done in this book: 'Because the glucocorticoids are so important in metabolism and nerve transmission . . . sustained abnormal levels would affect every aspect of a person's functioning, blunting his senses, disturbing the rhythms of food absorption, energy distribution, tissue repair and memory, reverberating throughout the individual like a state of dissonance.'[3]

The harmony remedies should surely be useful in reducing the stressful effects of time distortion. Indeed, their ability to sensitize the adrenal glands might be just what is needed when the glands have gone awry due to discords between their accustomed rhythm and that of a changed world outside the body. Nurses, pilots, plane passengers, those on shift work – few of us can escape the stress of our rhythms. In fact, our entire modern world encourages us to fight our rhythms rather than recognize and adjust to them. Nine-to-five society is run by the clock. The classic response to rhythm disruption is to ignore it with the help of coffee. Harmony remedies ought to be much more useful, although there is as yet no research which would confirm or deny this idea. Maybe we will soon find one or other harmony remedy given free to plane passengers by an enterprising airline.[4]

The harmony drugs interact with hormones which are known to shift with the seasons. Thyroid hormone is secreted most in summer, sexual hormones in the spring. There are seasonal differences in various diseases. Therefore one might expect that there would be seasonal differences in the action of these remedies. Bulgarian scientists who found that ginseng affected the thyroid gland were irritated when they couldn't repeat their finding. It turned out that this was because ginseng (and centrophenoxine) only had this effect in the summer.[1, 5] Russian scientists found that ginseng's effect in the control of diabetes occurred mostly during autumn and winter,[6] and likewise the effect on sexual glands discussed in Chapter 9. Indeed, both pantocrine and ginseng had the reverse effect in the spring.

It is interesting that in Western medicine drugs are regarded as doing the same thing to all people all of the time. Since the drugs are found as a result of one's conception of them, many Western drugs do have equivalent effects over time. In the East, therapies are definitely related to differing susceptibilities with time. Therefore ginseng is a typical Oriental medicine in this regard. Now we can perhaps understand what makes it so – active principles which act on the control systems of the whole organism. If the West, too, accidentally invented a drug which interacted with the control systems of the body, It would presumably turn out like an Oriental medicine: with different effects according to the time it was taken, the constitution of the person taking it, the diet it was taken with . . . and the prevailing attitude and mood.

The hormone matrix is the playground of the Oriental practitioner. How complex it is. He delves into the interior of the body, exploring its susceptibilities, balances, fingerprints and time-prints, all from their different manifestations on the body exterior. Though his symbols are alien, his methods are almost biochemical. Consider the art of urinalysis, where the urine is examined as to colour, taste, consistency, smell, density, and daily variation. The practitioner is his own laboratory and he reads the individual's emotions, stresses, organ states, life-style and so on, using his senses rather than instruments. Naturally, he uses his own system of symbols. Yet we can see his advice on obeying the seasons, or taking different medicines for different times of year, as having effects on the *milieu intérieur* which are scientifically understandable. It would certainly benefit us to do so. Imagine our doctor understanding our cycles and our vulnerability, guiding each one of us through the years with a little hormonal steering now and then to make sure we got the best out of life. In search for medicines for health, we cannot ignore time.

ON VITALITY AND THE CH'I

When the body is worn out and the blood is exhausted is it still possible to achieve good results?

No, because there is no more energy left. . . . Nowadays, vitality and energy are considered the foundation of life. In order to keep them flourishing they must be promoted, and the life force must rule. When this force does not support life, its foundation will dissolve, and how then can a disease be cured when there is no vital energy left within the body?   *Nei Ching*

There is a biological and cybernetic axiom that control systems need energy. The minute and sensitive adjustments that must be made to preserve bodily harmony, or indeed to keep an aeroplane on its course, are absolutely dependent on two factors: an energy supply to make the changes, and a source of information on what changes to make. Energy is needed to make a hormone, a packet of chemical information, and then to destroy it. In situations of stress extra demands are made on this energy + information. The amplification is turned up. It is more demanding to generate a sudden and controlled surge of adrenaline, or any other component of the control system, than to keep it ticking over. Acceleration and deceleration require power. Those people with easier access to energy + information will be able to generate more powerful and accurate surges of their hormones and responses to alarm. I regard vitality as this power (energy) and accuracy (information). Vitality produces a more finely tuned control of the *milieu intérieur* and thus keeps stress-related diseases at bay.

But the converse must also be true. The amount of resistance is limited by the amount of vitality available. This is exhaustion in the deep sense, the sense of the *Nei Ching*. It is the end of the vital essence, at which point disease is inevitable and unstoppable.

Scientific support for the concept of exhaustion of resistance comes from Professor Hans Selye, who both originated the concept of stress and discovered the steroid stress hormones. While exploring the stress system, he found that animals in situations of physiological stress, such as low temperature, went through three stages. First comes an alarm stage. Bells jangle; the ship's captain, the hypothalamus, shouts immediate urgent orders to the hormone crew, and all the physiological defence mechanisms begin. Then the responses settle down to a steady load on the physiology, until after some time they reach a final stage of exhaustion. Mobilization has been too long and too destructive. The animal gives up and succumbs. Professor Selye writes: '. . . Adaptability can be well trained to serve a special purpose, but eventually it runs out; its amount is finite. . . . It is as though we had hidden reserves of adaptability, or adaptation energy in ourselves throughout the body.' Selye's *adaptation energy* can be regarded as the total reserves of energy + information. Could this correspond to vitality, could this be a way of looking at the ch'i?

The ch'i has esoteric and exoteric meaning. The esoteric is the life-force. The exoteric could be the quality of the energy resource, which accurately and efficiently powers the body's control-systems. Ch'i diseases in Oriental medicine are deadly and well-nigh incurable. They often manifest as insanity.

When the ch'i is exhausted, resistance drops right down and Chinese medical methods which aim to help the body heal itself can no longer operate. This is the point which is made to the Yellow Emperor: 'How can a disease be cured if there is no vital energy left within the body?' Or more specifically, 'If one cures the disease by draining the body and vigorous constitution becomes weakened without being supplemented. The evil [infection] will then enter the body of the patient again and the original disease will flare up.'

Resistance requires vitality is a statement which is on the one hand so glaringly obvious that it is hardly worth saying. On the other hand, it is a profound statement about the human body and how it remains healthy. It forms the mainspring of Chinese medical thought. The Chinese doctor seeks first to reinforce vitality, the ch'i, so that the disease can be eliminated by the body's own defences, which need every available bit of energy + information. Almost the entire problem with current Western medical thinking and techniques is that this essential axiom of health, that resistance requires vitality, has been forgotten. Imagine how your doctor would treat you if he relied on that basic principle. Like his Chinese counterpart, he would be ever concerned for your energy. If your ability dropped or you felt one degree under, he would be round like a shot suggesting diets, regimens and medicines to restore vitality and build resistance. The doctor would be a manager of his patient's deep energy + information.

The harmony remedies are used to reinforce the ch'i, especially when it faces serious depletion in long diseases. But they must be used delicately, in the Chinese fashion. If they are taken by the wrong type of person at the wrong time or in the wrong way, the potential ch'i is wasted. Yet drugs are generally not a good way of increasing ch'i. The best methods are those Taoist and Yogic methods which collect ch'i. Practices such as Tai ch'i are the primary means to preserve vitality and are the first steps to harmony and self-transcendence. Needless to say, they affect the hormone balance,[7] but this is *en passant* from the exoteric to the esoteric.

This ch'i is the inner strength, that power that enabled the aged Don Juan to jump like a mountain goat, that power that the Taoists used in pursuit of longevity. The Taoists in ancient China were the masters of longevity, which they saw as a *symptom* of success on their spiritual journey towards fusion with the Tao. They developed methods for attainment of longevity which were a pinnacle of sophistication in stress reduction and the raising of ch'i. Breath control, sexual practices, diet control, herbs, postures, devotional practices and above all quietism were their unique prescription. They understood that to attain longevity stress reduction needs to be subtle. It does not mean to be shut from experience in a monastic cotton-wool box, for that leads to atrophy, not longevity. It means converting the experiences that meet you – whether a change of weather, an assault by another organism, or a plate of food – into ch'i-strengthening experiences. Economic arousal is a way of increasing ch'i. Like the rats that lived twice as long as their partners on half the calories, longevity will result from adaptation to economy.

Subtle and deep, like the Yantse River, the ch'i is not amenable to facile phenomenological interpretation. Whatever aspect of a living entity one examines – there ch'i is found, and yet it is as impossible to grasp as to capture water with a fork.

THE LAYERS OF GURVICH'S ONION

The techniques of science allow us to peep through into yet

another, deeper, level that lies obscured beneath the delicate physiology. This glimpse is sufficient to suggest some of the questions which we should ask in the future, though not to give us answers. We haven't yet approached the question of where this energy that is vitality originates. In biochemical terms, we can describe the phenomenon of a more efficient energy source (in terms of substances like ATP, the mysterious X~P, enzymes, co-factors, etc.), but these do not tell us about its origins. Nor are the body's control-systems more than a superficial answer, for where does their extra energy come from? When these answers run out we could look deeper, to subtle patterns of the distribution of energy throughout the body.

In 1923 the Russian histologist A. G. Gurvich found that the growing cells of an onion root could influence the growth of cells in a nearby root-tip. He put forward the notion of mitogenic rays.[8] Despite onerous efforts to duplicate his results, they could not be properly repeated until quite recently. It has now been confirmed that growing cells issue a very weak electromagnetic radiation in the ultraviolet waveband.[9] Some Russian scientists even suggest that this radiation can carry information from one cell to another, but that it only works if it is very weak.[10] This is of interest to us for two reasons. Firstly, acupuncture, like the harmony remedies, is used by the Chinese to alter energy states in organs. Research has now indicated that electromagnetic phenomena are also involved.[11] Secondly, Gurvich himself tried ginseng in his plant system. He found such a strong effect that he felt mitogenic radiation to be the source of ginseng's vitalizing action. This reminds us of the fact that the Chinese sometimes used to keep ginseng in lead boxes in order to preserve radiation emitted from the root, and of the tales of ginseng melting the snow around it in the mountains.

Now I do not believe that radiation is the source of ginseng's action. There is no evidence for it, and plenty of evidence to support the control-systems ideas discussed in this book. Yet there may be phenomena occurring which, in our Western fashion, we fail to notice since we lack the instruments with which to perceive them. Perhaps there are fields or potentials set up by life which interact positively or negatively with fields in nature. Perhaps the energy of life, the ch'i, is augmented if it is in phase with currents of energy in nature. It may be of a form which we can only visualize given highly tuned intelligence or new forms of instrumentation. It would be well to leave our minds open on the question of deeper, more subtle levels of operation of Chinese medicines.

The promise and yet the mystery of this was brought home to me when I was leafing through a Russian book of Kirllian photographs. These photographs are the result of imprinting the human electron aura on to photographic film. The book was full of richly coloured pictures showing the effects of drugs, foods or diseases on this aura.[12] The most-magnificent human aura of them all was undoubtedly that of a man who had just eaten a Korean ginseng root.

BEYOND THE FRINGE

Some doctors believe that modern medicine is the only genuine medical system ever to appear on the face of this planet. 'Jabbering, obscurantist mysticism,' declaimed Dr Jonathan Miller recently, putting this view with a touch of fey outrage. 'Yins and yangs and astrology and alchemy. They're awful. Most of fringe medicine today is simply a survival of techniques used in antiquity because there was nothing better. They're pathological stages in human development, grotesque failures to understand. To go back to them now is like striking flints to light the gas fire.'[13]

On the other side are those who feel that the protagonists of modern technological medicine are the ones who are jabbering and obscurantist. The problem is partly one of language, for each side jabbers in its own tongue. The traditional practitioners use a more metaphorical code with words like 'natural', 'energies', 'adjustment', 'balance', while the doctors use words like 'carcinoma', 'hyperfunctional', or 'metabolic'. There is a sad lack of intelligent exploration of the other side of the fence in both cases. Critics of fringe medicine have some of my sympathy because there is a certain amount of utter rubbish preached in its name. But as Aldous Huxley genteelly said: 'All sorts of cultists and queer fish teach all kinds of techniques for achieving health . . . many of these techniques are demonstrably effective. But do we see respectable psychologists, philosophers and clergymen boldly descending into those odd and sometimes malodorous wells, at the bottom of which poor truth is so often condemned to sit?' It little credits medical experts if they use fear of quackery as an excuse to avoid taking radical new ideas seriously. If all doctors believed as Dr Miller, half the medicines we have now wouldn't exist, acupuncture would be outlawed, osteopaths would be ostracized, and sufferers of diseases ranging from low back pain and migraine to insomnia and depression would be as poorly treated in the future as they are now.

I hope that I have shown that Chinese traditional medicine is a system so elegantly logical, so complex and yet obvious, so ancient and yet advanced, that in several important areas this system is way ahead of us today. Yins and Yangs have a sense behind them, and it is mainly our own grotesque failure to understand which has kept them hidden. The problem is that such concepts are severely under-represented. Yins and Yangs do not have sufficient spokesmen who can communicate them in the language of science. They are left to be formulated only in the language of Western dreamers and transcultural adventures. But with a clear and open mind, other medical systems can be understood, while to pronounce them 'awful' from the beginning will leave us forever woefully tasting our own medicine.

The arguments and speculations in this chapter show bridge-building is at least possible. As to whether it is advisable, I believe that there can be no question of it. A situation where Eastern and Western medicine stand on opposite banks of the river and shout incomprehensible slogans at each other is utterly unhealthy. There are vital lessons to be learnt from Oriental medicine which could complement our own system and plug its gaps. This isn't fringe medicine. It is beyond the fringe.

12
Dreams of the Future

HIPPOCRATES' NEW FACE

Scientific medicine is a colossus with tremendous power. Its methods have been highly successful in the treatment of many serious diseases. Vaccinations are an example of modern medical thought at its best. But its very success at the apparent instant cure of many specific diseases has driven it headlong down a one-way street. In its haste, historically and culturally conceived views of the health of man and his relationship with the world around him have been abandoned. The price has been paid in the sacrifice of long-term health.

Time tests us. Life's stresses make invisible hairline cracks in our resistance which accumulate like a hieroglyph of our being. Unfortunately these marks are left below the threshold of our normal awareness. We may be aware of feeling low or off colour or sick, but we usually cannot observe how daily life has caused this disharmony. Medicine faithfully reflects this interior blindness, and is therefore incapable of designing regimes for resistance. Rarely can it follow the future trajectories of its present manipulations. Indeed, the current crisis in medicine is partly due to a reluctant recognition that the derelictions of yesteryear have produced the degenerative diseases of today, while no one is quite sure how the derelictions of today will affect our health in the future.

Medical treatment is a seriously stressful experience. It pays so little regard to health that not only do its medicines result in chemical stress but its treatment produces psycho-physical stress. Hospitals and doctors' surgeries are anxiety-ridden places. From the moment a child is born, a white coat represents the principles of cold intrusion by strangers into its innermost world. Stress hormones flood at the sight of a hypodermic needle. One researcher found that the very injection he was using to sample cholesterol in the blood *created* cholesterol in the blood as a stress response! Now medical treatment is not a piece of cake wherever you are. But in the Oriental system the practitioners were much more concerned that their activities would not cause further harm. They did not, for example, use invasive methods of diagnosis: poking catheters up penises and needles into tissues. Instead, they looked at external signs with a finely tuned sensitivity. Their inquiries into life habits were a mandatory part of diagnosis and brought them closer to the patient. They almost never used surgery, their herbs didn't make you feel bad. Techniques such as acupuncture were relatively painless and restricted to the superficial tissues of the body.

There is a deep cultural basis to the stressfulness of medicine. A society freer of stress and angst will create and use a medical system that doesn't cause stress, while a society like ours which is imbued with stress invents a medical system that gives it.

If a physician reverses and spoils the natural condition of a body, health can never again be recovered. Those who use fullness in order to create emptiness, who use evil in order to bring out normalcy . . . will only bring about a contrary reaction and hurt the patient's health. Instead of bringing about compliance, they bring about conflict. Blood and vital substances become scattered and spoiled, the normal constitution becomes completely lost . . . this interrupts man's long life and brings disaster over the patient.

Health is a delicate business. The Yellow Emperor warns gloomily that the meddling of doctors can produce a lifetime of trouble. In the same breath he whispers the secrets of a true physician: to strengthen vitality and resistance at all times so that the body heals itself, to balance the various qualities and functions of the organs, intuitively to guide each individual within the whirlpools of his environment so as to achieve his full potential in mind, body and life-span.

The Yellow Emperor was right concerning the horrific results of the destruction of harmony. Long-term stress will cause resistance to drop, the blood vessels to become sclerosed, the mind to lose its powers, the body cells to turn against each other, the metabolism to become deranged and the body to be afflicted with irreversible deteriorations. These are not due to the strong stress that bursts out in acne or migraines, but the invisible unconscious stresses of overstimulation, diet and toxins. This is well understood in Chinese medicine. The *Nei Ching* stated that: 'When the body is frequently startled and frightened, the circulation in the arteries and veins ceases.' They understood that in order to deal with this subtle damage one needed insight. Even if the battle scars of life are too subtle to be clearly seen by each individual, it is the doctor's job to point out this process to the patient. The doctor, the guide, *must* have this wisdom if he is to encourage the husbandry of health.

Modern medicine has gone in the opposite direction. Instead of encouraging self-awareness of the inner causes of disease, it attempts to remove the responsibility for health from the individual altogether. It promises in return a safety-net in case a person gets ill. But the more you rely on a safety-net, the less chance there is of learning how to balance. People are falling into the medical safety-net in such numbers that the health care system can no longer bear the burden. The result is, of course, that holes are appearing in this net and it is no longer as safe.

We shouldn't do without our safety-net. It is the miracle of modern medicine, and no medical system in the history of the planet has such good curative techniques for those seriously ill. But it should be combined with life-long and sensitive prophylactic medicine so that the safety-net and the hospital are only places of last resort.

Medicine has been see-sawing between the specificity and the harmony models long enough in the history of Western culture. Now that it has come to rest at Homo Librium we all realize the predicament we are in. Whether we choose Aristotle, the Renaissance, the Church, Faraday, the Reductionists or the drug companies as our scapegoats, it is time to start out on a return journey to Homo Equilibrium, with the hope that for once medicine will be stabilized equally between the two.

There is no need to turn the clock back. This would be making the same mistake as medicine itself during its erratic history. The power of science needs to be harnessed and wedded to a teaching of the maintenance of health into old age.

The resultant synthesis will look like Hippocratic medicine with a scientific face. Rational therapeutics can be rescued from its cul-de-sac, where it is still ramming itself against the barrier of the diseases of later life, and set lumbering in a new direction.

In my view, this offers the only realistic possibility of a serious extension of the life-span of those in industrial societies. There are no elixirs round the corner. In the long run only the gamut of techniques of health husbandry will be capable of beating the degenerative diseases. This would add some fifteen years to our average life-span.

The cultivation of vitality and resistance implies not only a longer life, but also a better one. 'Exuberance is beauty,' cried William Blake. There is no real dividing line between the development of the body and its preservation, between development of the body and development of the spirit. Health is fulfilment of our potential.

PHARMACOLOGY COMES OF AGE

Drug companies are stymied by the monstrous cost of producing fewer and fewer remedies, nervous health directorates see side-effects wherever they look, and an emerging health-conscious generation has begun again with herbs and health products. Pharmacology is stuck. It doesn't have a broad new theoretical foundation with which it can progress beyond the old cure, pure and sure. Pharmacology is floundering in an outdated pathological paradigm, whereas it should have developed into an independent science. It should deal with the entire relationship between man and the substance of his environment. Pharmacology's current crisis spells a Kuhnian turning-point, from which the only way out is a drastic rethinking of pharmacology's fundamental conceptual basis. It needs a new theory for the use, detection and testing of the substances of the environment which affect man. Part of this theory is, I believe, carried on the back of the small root that goes . . . goes . . . from East to West. It bears a novel form of pharmacological wisdom and, more importantly, a unique collection of scientific investigations with which to translate this wisdom.

Current pharmacology is blessed for its pains with a fundamental belief that genuinely restorative remedies do not exist. Any that may occasionally come to notice are quickly labelled 'tonics' (whatever that means!) and discarded as insignificant, or fraudulent. They cannot be acceptable to a pharmacological tradition which judges medicines by the one disease – one cure criterion. Since they would be invisible by the usual methods of drug-testing, everyone agrees that they are worthless except some who actually try them carefully and notice their effects. Then, like the little boy and the emperor's new clothes, they point and cry, 'But there *is* something!' at which point the crowd turns on them with, 'Have you never heard of the placebo effect?' What follows is a great controversy with one side failing to see the purpose of taking medicines that cannot cure a specific disease and the other side powerless to prove their awareness that these medicines do improve health.

This situation is a modern-day version of the old see-saw conflict between the humoralists and the empiricists in the eighteenth century. We have again the woolliness of the former and blindness of the latter. Neither have been aware that this is the *first time* since the heady rise of scientific medicine two centuries ago that adequate scientific evidence exists for the value of restorative medicines used specifically to increase health.

The value of such an example is considerable. It is hard to focus on health maintenance in the midst of a world full of practices which squander health. But one clear example is a rallying point.

It is fascinating that these restorative remedies are useful at all levels of health, from the dying who take it on their deathbed to the Olympic super-healthy who squeeze out the last ounce from their performance. It is a unique concept for Westerners previously used to the disease-doctor-pill-hospital notion of a drug. It fits well with the Eastern view of health as a continuous unbroken scale, like Jacob's ladder, upon which one travels up or down according to the level of ch'i, of resistance energy with which the individual responds to his environment.

Ginseng is more arousing, eleutherococcus more related to metabolism, pantocrine more ruttish and liquorice more hydrating, although their effects overlap. The pharmacology of the future will be able to employ a wide range of mild restorative and protective medicines. They will be the vocabulary of a medical system that reads the person like a book, and detects developments in the early chapters before they move to a disease dénouement. Health is relative to constitution, and therefore a wide range of restorative and adjustive remedies will be needed to fill out the specific gaps in each person's resistance.

Pharmacology must in one way or another turn to adjustive therapies if it is to evolve beyond pathology into preventive medicine. However, none of these developments will be possible unless sanity returns to the methods of discovering drugs, which currently ensure the rejection of medicines that are mild, restorative or prophylactic. Because of the mouse-disease test model and the clinical trial, those very agents would be missed in the search for new drugs, since they do not show up their properties in short-term statistical examinations of their effects on populations of diseased and mindless laboratory animals.

Scientific testing is not useless. It has brought us the life-saving medicines of today – vaccines, antibiotics, anti-malarials, insulin, antimycotics, antihistamines, analgesics and a multitude more. It has, in the end, confirmed Shen Nung. But it has also brought us toxic medicines where safe ones could have been used. Many of our common medicines began as poisons, while large numbers of well-tried, safe remedies are abandoned without proper trial.

I will never forget the shock I received when I opened an issue of the *New England Journal of Medicine* a few years ago and saw there an account of an experiment in a New York hospital in which cortisone was given to hepatitis patients. More of them died than those not given cortisone. Trying out strong preparations in this way is problematic to say the least, but am I going too far to suggest that it is negligent to choose such a compound for testing on patients when there are medicines already in use for thousands of years in the East specifically for this disease, medicines which are known to be completely safe and yet remain untested?

New drug laws are still being made which are well-meaning but which systematically exclude reliable, mild and harmless drugs because their effects are not easily testable. As Louis Lasagna, a leading figure in the pharmacological establishment, stated, the 'ultimate surrealism will be the demand that the safety and efficacy of over-the-counter drugs be tested by formal control trials. Surely the performance of drugs used in the process of self-diagnosis and self-treatment is best gauged as such. Primary criteria should be the patient's satisfaction, not the doctors in double blind.'

Only with the greatest difficulty can clinical trials be adapted to search for non-specific medicines that improve general health. Firstly, there are no guidelines in Western medicine to decide who is perfectly healthy and who not quite so healthy. Is a person who has three colds a year more or less healthy than someone with flatulence, or someone else with an allergy to cats? Secondly, the effects would anyway be so subtle, and individual variation so great, that it would need a cast of thousands. Thirdly, the goal one is measuring is a long-term one. Who can carry out a clinical trial lasting for the human life-span?

The animal-testing and classic clinical trial should be left for the segment of pharmacology for which they are appropriate, namely the testing of strong curative drugs. They are useful models within that sphere. However, where the health and potential of an individual human being are concerned, such methods are as irrelevant as a clinical trial to test the efficacy of a perfume, a wine or fresh air. Where doctors need trials in order to establish or confirm the action of a certain remedy for health, they would need to carry out a very large study, taking into account the constitutions, mind-body states and life-styles of the individuals tested. This would be essentially a test for healthy people in daily life. Medicines for climbing the health ladder can only be tested in this way.

THE SAGE *IS* THE LABORATORY

One valuable method of detecting drugs, which might pick up subtle remedies more effectively than any other, is the intro-spective self-testing of pharmacological agents by highly sen-sitive individuals. We know that it is possible, given training, to be aware of subtle phenomena within the body, e.g. the peristaltic motion of the intestines, the patterns of the heart beat and, particularly, the changes wrought by small quan-tities of drugs. Early physicians were trained from childhood to amplify their powers of observation and intuition. They were often also shamans and magicians who frequently made use of altered states of consciousness. They then turned the extra insight obtained while in trances to the healing of the members of their tribes and the discovery of medicines. Although this thesis is rarely put forward by medical historians, early medical discoveries were partly revelational in character. One can see this process in practice today in some primitive communities, where the witch-doctor uses his powers of sensitive insight to discover medicines. Often he is inspired by 'dreams' in which a plant appears to him and tells him of its powers.

Could it not be true that the kind of drugs arrived at by testing in the laboratory of the body are different from those found through the testing in the laboratory of the experimental animal? For one thing, self-testing and deep observation of the effects of drugs is likely to generate mild drugs that produce minimal changes to the internal chemistry. These are the drugs likely to be missed by testing with rats. Intuitionally-discovered drugs are likely to be safer, for any harmful effects would be immediately apparent. Even in modern times, the side-effects of drugs often only appear after they have been taken by members of the public who complain.

More interestingly, self-testing is likely to discover drugs which have a beneficial effect on the healthy, not just on the sick. Would not remedies for health be more easily discovered by giving them to wise men rather than stupid guinea pigs?

Traditional knowledge of remedies is a compendium of both lists of useful substances and principles for their preparation and application. This was arrived at by the three intertwined strands of empiricism, logic and revelation. The Chinese do not doubt that their subtle remedies were discovered by insight, not by some kind of empirical testing on thousands of diseased people by means of monstrous and unending clinical trials. Shen Nung was assumed to have a 'grace'. In the folk tradition he is reported to have discovered seventy new remedies in one single remarkable day.

The pharmacology of the future should not be afraid of utilizing 'specialists in high intensity introspection', as Charlotte Bach calls them, modern-day shamans with a profound pharmacological intuition, to discover new drugs and suggest principles for their use. We are delicate beings, and drugs we take today can affect health half a century away. How then can one trust even ten thousand rats to give us the answers?

FROM DRUG TO DROGUE

'Drug' comes from the medieval German word '*drogue*', meaning a dry herb. Modern pharmacy has been in existence f r only 1 per cent of the time that man has been preparing medicines for himself. During this brief period man has redefined this thing we call a drug as a refined or synthetic chemical, concentrated and identified.

The two most common reasons used to defend the practice of extracting from a plant a more toxic and therapeutically narrow substance are that such a substance is easier to take and easier to standardize and control exactly. But it is questionable to what extent this control is to the benefit of the patient as opposed to the benefit of principles of scientific exactitude. For it often means that a plant with a rich variety of constituents is converted to a pill containing, say, exactly 200mg of a single compound, which is then prescribed in the same manner to everyone ('three a day after meals'). In this case control has been lost, not gained. Therapeutic diversity is wasted and the wealth of possibilities for treating each individual with a matching synthesis of constituents is gone. While in some cases it is undoubtedly of benefit to know exactly how much of a certain constituent you are giving to a patient, the game is often not worth the candle.

The processing and synthesis of remedies is often unnecessary on therapeutic grounds and is carried out only for commercial reasons. In Russia, for example, which has modern medicine but a state pharmaceutical industry, drugs are synthesized or processed rather more where necessary than where profitable. Many preparations are left in plant or extract form. In the ninth edition of the *State Pharmacopoeia* about 20 per cent of the specifications were for plants in one form or another.

There is plenty of evidence now that this purification habit has the inevitable sequel of deriving a pure toxic drug from a harmless medicinal plant. For example, reserpine was isolated from rauwolfia, and used extensively as a psychoactive drug in the West until severe side-effects were recognized. Now pharmaceutical companies are considering going back to selling a cruder mixture of components from the plant.

The analysis of the ginseng root told us that it contains a highly complex mixture of components, much more effective therapeutically than any single component. We described the music of the root, the arousal of the panaxatriols, balanced by the panaxadiols. Ginseng therefore adds to the growing body of data, now accepted by many pharmacologists, that on therapeutic grounds it is often better to leave the components as a balanced mixture than indulge in fruitless and costly attempts at purification. The folly of equating a plant with any of its active principles is clearly expressed by the chemical analysis in Chapter 6. We showed that the chemical fish you pull out of a natural product depends only on the bait you use to catch and identify it. There are always fish left uncaught.

Many of the drugs in use today are originally derived from plants, and some are still cheaper to extract from the plant and purify rather than synthesize. Of the 1.532 billion prescriptions dispensed in the US during 1973, a quarter contained active constituents derived from plants, but only 2.5 per cent contained extracts from crude plant drugs.[1]

The huge resources devoted to synthesis and purification are an irrational indulgence of the chemists' world-view. This is especially galling to Third World countries, who have been trading their medicinal plants rich in active constituents to the industrial countries, who return them in expensive pills denuded of pharmacological diversity. Of course, economic pressures also force the synthesis of active principles, and these may one day include the saponins of the ginseng root. There may not be enough root to go around. But if in the long run Western medicine accepted that a large part of the purification and processing of natural products is irrelevant or detrimental to the practice of healing, the huge funds diverted to drug companies for this purpose could be directed to the growers instead, to everyone's benefit.

It should be a principle of the pharmacology of the future that a natural product be used unless there are sound and sensible therapeutic reasons why the pure active principles would be better.

The first step should be to re-examine the older drugs cast

out of the pharmacopoeia and the medicines of the traditional healers. There are half a million plants growing on this planet, and some people state that less than 5 per cent of plants have been investigated for pharmacological active principles. Even here, since the current testing models have been used, the plants have only been tested against certain diseases. There is tremendous opportunity for the detection of new medicines using improved theory. It is already common to find completely new activities in old well-tried plants. For example, oils of onion and garlic were recently studied and found to assist the body in reducing fat and cholesterol levels.[2] This study was carried out without huge resources; in fact the few new drugs which have been discovered from plants in recent years have involved something like a tenth of the cost of the discovery of an average synthetic drug.[1]

The potential is illustrated by the National Cancer Institute plant screening programme which we have already mentioned. Seventy-five thousand different plants were tested; however, they were only tested against one or two animal tumours (compared to the several hundred known), they were only extracted in a single fashion, and they were not tested for activity against any other disease. 'This single example clearly points out that in the most extensive pharmacological investigation of plants in the history of the world, only a fraction (1 per cent) of the total available plants have been evaluated for a *single* type of activity. Thus even plants from this study can be considered "uninvestigated".'[1]

Professor Farnsworth has called this unexplored world of potential medicines a 'sleeping giant'. There are signs that the giant has opened an eye. A new World Health Organization drive has been announced to investigate and preserve traditional medicine around the world as a cheap, reliable and widely available method of health care. 'The effectiveness of much of traditional medicine is now an accepted fact,' says the WHO Regional Director of Western Pacific. 'Nevertheless there has been over the years a relative lack of attention to the use of medicinal plants in health care. . . . While many synthetic drugs have side-effects which can be worse than the signs, symptoms and pathology of the condition itself . . . traditional preparations which have been used for many years are generally free from side-effects if properly prepared and used.'[3] WHO has started a cold war against the drug salesmen, but we still have a long way to go.

THE 'IMMACULATE CONCOCTION'

What a bounty there is waiting for us if we could apply our vast technical awareness to a *wise* search for new remedies. For example, an enlightened pharmacology will have a wide range of sophisticated substances for stress reduction. Mixtures could be designed to match the kind of stresses to be experienced: one for the flight controller, one for the racing cyclist and one for the GI. Who knows what stresses are waiting for us in the year 2001? What about the stress of novel forms of pollution, including the possibilities of nuclear fallout?

There exist extraordinary substances for the treatment of our sicknesses, and others, the hallucinogens, for the alteration of mental states. One can imagine a further series of remedies concerned with our abilities. The theoretical foundations for this may have been laid by the discoveries concerning the hormones that act within the brain, altering awareness, perception and mood. The harmony remedies may be harbingers of new substances that influence various psychohormones in ways that can hardly be imagined now. One consequence of this has already been pointed out by the great and imaginative biologist, J. B. S. Haldane, over fifty years ago:

We already know however that many of our spiritual faculties can only be manifested if certain glands, notably the thyroid and sex glands, are functioning properly, and that very minute changes in such glands affect the character greatly. As our knowledge of this subject increases we may, for example, be able to control our passions by some more direct method than fasting and flagellation, to stimulate our imagination by some agent with less after-effects than alcohol. . . . Conversely there will inevitably arise possibilities of new vices similar but even more profound than those opened up by the pharmacological discoveries of the nineteenth century.[4]

There is a promise of mild mood-altering substances, that might counter episodes of depression, or perhaps amplify desirable states such as enthusiasm. They might uniquely increase our behavioural options, in a finely tuned and Epicurean manner, more like the taste organ in *À Rebours* than the mental hammers in *The Naked Lunch*. When one considers that the reward centre of the mind is located in the hypothalamus, the possibility of some future 'immaculate concoction', in the words of J. B. Ford, is real enough.

Like any drug which affects the human psyche, there will be opportunities for abuse of these remedies as well as use. They may be abused as surrogates for emotional experience. It is perhaps disturbing to contemplate a society where people could manipulate their levels of emotional tone using roots rather than rock music. It conjures up images of *Brave New World*. But the abuse would actually be more like that of the somatensic over-use of ginseng today – wasteful rather than destructive. It would be almost welcome compared to the debilitating abuses of today's tranquillizers, stimulants and sedatives, which bring oblivion rather than surrogation.

Although all these remedies would be exciting innovations, they are all tools, and only as beneficial as the skills with which they are used. They are born of a philosophy of harmony and that is the way to use them. The greatest possible abuse is therefore nothing to do with the drugs at all but with the situation in which they are taken, for the drugs are only part of an entire way of looking at medicine, health and life. If these harmony remedies were adopted but taken purely somatensically, as a 'cure' for tiredness: if they were taken with the same old curative principles, it would be a tragic abuse.

THE BEST OF THE OLD AND THE NEW – OR THE WORST?

All the ideas in this book have flowed from the meeting of the concepts of Oriental medicine and the practice of science. This marriage has already occurred in China. Is it a fruitful or a sterile union?

Superficially it seems to be successful. 'The integration of traditional medicine into Western medicine . . . is a long and difficult task, but it is of the highest importance for China and for the world, and an achievement greatly to be desired. . . .' So wrote Professor Huard.[5] Many Western doctors have visited China recently and returned astonished. A recent World Health Organization meeting on traditional medicine stated that, 'The tremendous success of the Chinese experience in the integration of Western medicine and Chinese traditional medicine continues to provide the shining example of the potential which lies in integration for the promotion and development of systems of traditional medicine.'⁶ However, the commentators are often rightly amazed at the extraordinary success of the Chinese in improving the health of their people, but wrongly ascribe this to the fusion of the old and new. In actual fact, the health of the people is largely due to their training in hygiene and improved quality of life, while the two medical systems have not fused – they coexist.

Traditional medicine has been successfully preserved and is now a living system in China. It stands separate from Western medicine. Patients are given a choice. The attempts at unification are only now beginning at an academic level. Part of the difficulty lies in the fundamentally opposed ways that the two systems looks at the world. It must be stressed that the paraphernalia of healing, whether they be a million-dollar neutron-beam irradiation machine or chameleon extract, arise from the concepts of medicine, and these from the basic world-view. There is conflict between the two languages of healing, which prevents the construction of a common therapy as if it were the tower of Babel.

Early attempts to wed the *Nei Ching* with Western anatomy failed miserably, even after the Chinese began to practise a little dissection. It was impossible because, as we have pointed out, anatomy deals with structures observable to the eye, while the *Nei Ching*'s 'viscera' are invisible patterns of function and energy. For example, the 'kidney' in the *Nei Ching* is not the same kidney that a Western doctor knows. Chinese scientists have suggested that the traditional 'kidney' is in fact the testes! But they still cannot understand it. A recent visiting team of Western pharmacologists to China admitted, 'We were not so well versed as we might have been in the principles and theory of Chinese medicine,' but added, 'And it was but small consolation to learn that Western-trained Chinese physicians also do not find it easy to master traditional concepts . . . the bulk of traditional texts remain untranslated.' They also noted that, 'Western and Chinese medical structures exist side by side but are theoretically compartmented.'⁷

The danger exists that in the race for curative solutions the more subtle aspects of Chinese traditional medicine may be lost, particularly those of health husbandry and preservation

of the ch'i. Traditional medicine has become more empirical
and materialistic. Much of the early teaching has been turned
on its head. 'In their prolonged struggle against Nature the
working people of our country established the art of healing as
well as acupuncture therapy,' writes a recent editorial. On
hearing of the *struggle against* Nature, Lao Tzu would turn in his
grave. It is a fundamental error according to the traditional
medical philosophy. The modern Chinese also clearly bring
down the ancient sages: 'The Confucianists wilfully assert that
Shen Nung composed the Pen Tshao. . . . Even the author-
ship of the Nei Ching was ascribed to Huang Ti. . . . This of
course is a reversal of history . . . acupuncture came into
existence and was gradually improved as a result of the
development of social production. Medical work requires a
collective effort of a large number of people . . . by no means
can this be achieved by those "born with innate genius".'[8]
There could be no more obvious statement of the distance
between modern and traditional thinking.

This may not have mattered to the Chinese overmuch while
they were attempting to halt plagues and keep infants alive
during their first year. But now Chinese medicine has
achieved that and is creeping ahead into the difficult phase:
preserving health further into old age. That means generating
such a high standard of health care that it pushes the life-span
slowly up and up, beyond the point at which the West has now
become firmly bogged down in a morass of chronic diseases. It
is in this difficult phase that the unification of old and new may
have the greatest impact. My impression is that the Chinese
have a great potential knowledge of the two medicines, which
could push their life-expectancy way beyond any other country in the world, but that the Chinese have not yet learnt to
take the best of the old and the new. They are at the beginning.

The difficulties inherent in the linkage of the two is illustrated by the attitude of the South Koreans, who are also
experimenting with the two systems. They feel strongly that
they are the true guardians of traditional medicine, because the
Maoist dialectic materialism is fundamentally incompatible
with the traditional way of thinking. They are partly right.
But the pot is calling the kettle black, for the runaway com-
mercialism of South Korea is also contrary to the interests of
traditional healing. The Yellow Emperor would hardly

approve of the Korean manner of selling medicaments like candies.

The Chinese adaptation of traditional medicine has, paradoxically, made it more acceptable to Westerners, and hastened its passage out of China. As traditional medicine continues to mate with its modern grandchild, it takes on a youthful form. But this youthful form is beguiling. It looks attractive but may be no more than our own form clad in new clothes. In other words, if we try to bring back some Chinese medicine, we may find ourselves bringing our *own* medicine back again. There is a much discussed recent example of this. The People's Republic announced the discovery of some new substances that were thought to attack cancer. Western experts investigating them were disappointed, for nothing radical seemed to have been discovered. Yet they missed the real sublime power of traditional drugs. Those scientists were going shopping for some Oriental wisdom and coming back with tape recorders.

How long will it be before we can buy harmony remedies in the chemist, before the National Health dispenses deer antler extract, and before our doctors begin to prescribe subtle medicines to keep us healthy? Perhaps sooner than people think. After all, the Chinese pharmacologists have been doing all the hard work for us: standardizing preparations, selecting the effective plants, determining the correct way of using them, and learning to manufacture them. Even more than that, the Chinese have removed the psychological and conceptual barrier to traditional medicine which has been such an unworthy part of the Western heritage. We must not forget also the extent to which Chinese medicinal plants have relatives on our doorsteps. The plants are always there, though intelligent human interaction with the plant world is often lacking. It may also be true that such medicines will arrive in the West through the back door – through the will of the people and their commercial leverage, rather than through the explorations of pharmacists and pharmacologists. This has already happened in the case of ginseng, which was discovered by people experimenting with novel forms of healing.

Another advantage which will hasten the change is the

current climate of self-questioning. There has always been criticism both within and outside the medical stockade. The limitations of medicine are becoming clear, if not to doctors whose faculty for self-criticism has atrophied after years of medical schools and hospitals, at least to those on the fringe and to an aware proportion of the recipients of Western healing skills.

We can sum up the position using the metaphors of the *Nei Ching*. Chinese therapy is concerned with breaking hairs, the Western with wielding hammers. There is a time when both are needed. The Chinese have recently learnt how to wield curative hammers. The West still needs to learn how to break hairs.

Medicine is only a component part of a social psyche, just like music or architecture. Change in one segment of our perception affects others. As we look round, we see the see-saw swinging right across our culture. We are discovering that the outer environment has been treated with as much disdain as our inner environment, resulting in a momentum towards ecology. A feeling for harmony begins to diffuse through all areas of cultural consciousness.

Many of these changes in values have come from the East. The Oriental concepts of harmony in healing are only a section of a broad stream of ideas and techniques, taken up by the scouts on the edge of the Western pack, and gradually filtering through to the rest. There is a veritable torrent of Western culture in the opposite direction. These flows are part of progress. This is particularly the case with attitudes to health, which are the means whereby man guides his own evolution.

I hope this book will encourage a beneficial exchange, not only between Eastern and Western attitudes to health, but also between the fringe who are forced to extremes by uncertainty, and the professionals who would rather hide within the cul-de-sac. More than that, I hope it encourages everyone to think more deeply on the meaning as well as the means of health. The crystallization of Oriental concepts of health lies in the understanding that health can only be bought with wisdom:

When the minds of people are closed and wisdom is locked out, they remain tied to disease.

In that case their feelings and desires should be investigated and exposed and their ideas explored. It will soon become obvious in what way those who have vitality flourish.

Appendix
Ginseng and You

SAFETY FIRST

The very first requirement of kingly plants is harmlessness. How safe are the harmony remedies? Science has confirmed that ginseng is absolutely safe. The lethal dose of the whole root has been independently determined by almost every researcher who has seriously studied ginseng and has been found to be so far above the usual dose that it is not worthy of concern. Brekhman, for example, found that experimental animals would have to take about 30g of Russian root per kg body weight to die. That is equivalent to over 2kg at one go for a man. A scientist at the University of Milan gave 10g per kg to mice (equivalent to 700g to a man), and there were no noticeable ill effects,[1] while Professor Savel at Paris University has calculated that the lethal dose of ginseng extract to mice was 2g/kg, something like 1000 to 5000 times the effective dose. When he tried feeding the actual root to mice to test its harmfulness he was stumped, for he couldn't physically give them sufficient ginseng to cause serious harm. The mice suffered from enlarged stomachs due to overeating, but were otherwise well.[2]

Long-term trials with large amounts have never shown any harmful effects and we have given ginseng to 180 mice at the University of London from birth to death without any sign of detriment.[3] Naturally, a man may not need to take a lethal dose to be harmed by a drug. Drugs can cause all kinds of side-effects. They may be harmful when taken by people who have certain diseases or weaknesses or they may be incompatible with other drugs.

Are we not to be concerned at the discovery, reported in Chapter 5, that ginseng components make animals dopey?

The answer is no. The sedation is a part of the action of ginseng, but the evidence shows that, at least in Korean ginseng, it is normally neutralized and balanced by components which work in opposite directions to give an end result which is more stimulatory than sedatory. The sedatory effects will only be apparent if humans take the pure Rb_1 glycosides. The pure constituent Rb_1 is out of context, and does not represent the root. This is, of course, a powerful argument against the Western practice of isolating a single active constituent from a plant, putting it in a pill, and discarding the rest.

The lethal doses of the pure active principles are anyway very high. They vary from 300mg per kg for Rb_2 to 1300 for Rg_1 when injected, and several times this amount when eaten. A man would have to take 50g or so of the pure Rg_1 crystals, if such a quantity could be produced somehow, in order to have a reasonable chance of committing suicide with it. Currently, this is more than the *entire* world supply of this precious material.

Eleutherococcus is also extremely safe. The lethal dose, like that of ginseng, has been repeatedly shown to be in the region of 30g/kg body weight. Animals given eleutherococcus for many months in large doses look very well. Their appetite is good, they put on weight and seem to increase in strength.[4] Some animals have been given eleutherococcus from birth to death with anything but ill-effects. There are no known major side-effects.

The toxicity of all the other tonic remedies is also very low. The lethal dose of the mixed saponins of platycodon, for example, was even more than ginseng. The lethal dose of Polygala tenuifolia mixed saponins was ten times less than ginseng. Although this is still safe (a man would have to eat about 1/4k of the root at one go for a toxic dose) this puts it outside the kingly class, confirming Shen Nung's classification.[5] The Araliaceae plants studied by the Russians are all quite safe, a man needing to eat roughly 1k of most of these plants to receive a toxic dose, and naturally this harmlessness also applies to the triterpenoidal saponins within them.

Every health ministry in the Western world that has met ginseng has accepted that it is safe, even though most are yet to be convinced of its efficacy. Britain and most other Western countries allow it on unrestricted sale without claims, while the United States Food and Drug Authority considers ginseng when used as a tea to be generally recognized as safe (GRAS), but mentions that, 'This status of ginseng tea is based solely on human experience.'[6] Eleutherococcus was classified in the same way. They cannot be sold as a medicine, they cannot be sold with any claims, and they cannot be sold as a food additive since they have not passed the relevant regulations. The FDA takes the strange position that they are 'unaware of any adequate scientific evidence or controlled scientific studies that demonstrate medical properties for Panax ginseng'.[6]

In Israel, however, the ministry does not allow ginseng on open sale. When I challenged a top official of the Health Ministry who readily admitted his support for the ban, he said that ginseng was not safe, for 'people like ginseng too much, so it must be addictive'. He acknowledged that indeed he did not have any evidence to back up this extraordinary statement, but that it was the responsibility of commercial interests to provide it. More rational medical opinion around the world acknowledges that 4000 years of continuous and wide usage of ginseng is evidence of its harmlessness in reasonable doses, if not its effectiveness.

On the other hand, all this does not mean that ginseng cannot produce any side-effects. It can. There is no medicine known that does not have any side-effects at any dose. Ginseng's possible side-effects are subtle and do not constitute toxicity. They can occur when ginseng is taken in the wrong way, particularly when ginseng is taken in large amounts by people who do not need it for reasons of health. There may be side-effects arising from the over-arousal, which may occur particularly with people who are naturally excited, nervous and highly strung. The side-effects might take the form of irritability, sleeplessness and raised blood pressure. These side-effects were well known to traditional doctors who specified which harmony remedies should be taken by which kind of people. When in doubt it is better to err on the safe side and take a remedy, such as eleutherococcus, which is less stimulatory.

There is more chance of side-effects appearing if somatensic drugs are taken together with stimulants. It is so common to take tea and coffee at all times that it is likely that many people who take ginseng will take caffeine too. This cannot be recommended and may promote over-stimulation. The hormonal and neuronal stimulation are then piled on top of each other to excessive effect.

A recent report has been published by Dr Siegel, at the University of California, who studied 133 ginseng users and reported that 14 of them had certain side-effects, including nervousness, insomnia and raised blood pressure. The author suggests these side-effects were the result of interference with corticosteroid levels. This is an unconvincing study since it was not in any way double-blind. These side-effects could have been due to many other factors in the life-style of these people. My view, however, is that while Siegel's paper is not proof, it is still probably correct, and these side-effects can occur in certain kinds of people if ginseng is wrongly used. Most of the people who reported side-effects were taking ginseng in large quantities for a year continuously, together with caffeinated drinks. This is, as Siegel noted, ginseng abuse, not ginseng use.[7]

TAKING GINSENG

Ginseng and the harmony remedies should be taken as part of a regime of health restoration, preferably guided by an Oriental practitioner or skilled healer. However, this is not always possible. I have therefore put together some guidelines, culled from traditional sources, scientific material and personal experience. They are not hard and fast rules, but general principles, and should not be considered medical recommendations.

1 Ginseng should be taken in courses of approximately one month's duration. After each course, leave a period of at least two months. The exceptions to this are the aged and chronically sick, who may take ginseng continuously.

2 Courses of ginseng should be arranged for the autumn and winter.

3 Occasional use may be made at any time of the somatensic (arousal) effects of ginseng in order to counter periods of particular stress or challenge. But this should not be too frequent and preferably not for more than two days at a time.

4 In general, people who are highly energetic, nervous, tense, hysteric, manic or schizophrenic should not take ginseng. Young and vital people will not gain much from taking

ginseng except under Note 3 above. It should *not* be taken during acute illnesses, fevers or any disease with 'heating' symptoms.

5 It should not be taken with stimulants (including coffee) or antipsychotic drugs or during treatment with hormones. It has never been shown to have any negative interactions with other drugs, but it is always wise to consult a therapist if in doubt.

THE ROOT PILE

There are many different grades and types of ginseng and they all fetch different prices and are prized by different sections of the ginseng-eating Eastern cultures. The best ginseng is the old, perfectly formed wild ginseng of Manchuria, Korea and the Ussuri. These roots never reach the public eye. They are not for sale. Go into a Chinese pharmacy and ask for one and see what happens. It is like going into a local jewellers and asking for a piece of the Koh-i-Noor diamond. The six armed Manchus that came to Lubin were guarding a single, smallish wild root. The same situation prevails with the Korean san-sam, wild mountain ginseng. Few have seen it and it is so expensive that it has never been submitted to proper investigation. It is also impossible to state which of the wild ginsengs is better.

On the other hand, the best that is commonly available today is still rather special. This is partly cultivated ginseng. The ginseng grown in the royal parks by the emperors and still growing there now is known as kirin or imperial ginseng. It is distinguishable from the best mountain wild ginseng by careful examination. It is expensive – Chairman Mao is known to have taken this ginseng and its usual cost is $200 per ounce. The Korean version is the ginseng planted where wild ginseng was plucked. In the present-day Chinese materia medica this grade is known as Tassel wild. Next on the list is the Pa-huo Tassel which is cultivated ginseng left behind in the field after its last transplantation for more than sixteen years. Following this is the Tassel cultivated, ordinary farm-cultivated roots. They correspond to the Korean standard cultivated. Finally there is the Pond Bottom Tassel which is ginseng grown from leftover roots in abandoned fields. These neglected roots often look gnarled and deformed.[8]

As far as cultivated roots are concerned, the Chinese white is possibly slightly better than the Korean and the Japanese is the least good. The Koreans have made a sturdy attempt at standardization of growth conditions and processing. Batches of ginseng of the same age, grade and method of curing are surprisingly uniform.

Curing does make a difference to the quality. The red ginseng is normally regarded as slightly better than the white ginseng, provided the curing is done properly. Red ginseng is certainly invulnerable to decay, whereas the white root is still subject to the attack of one or two pests even when dried. But the difference goes deeper. The steaming process immediately stops any chemical reactions from occurring within the root. Therefore the red ginseng is probably fresher and may have more medicinal constituents within it. There is some chemical evidence that red ginseng contains greater amounts of certain minor constituents. It is certainly the case that only the better quality roots end up as red ginseng. Mind you, I have experienced rotten red roots with the consistency of chewing gum, the colour of mud and the taste of putrid olives.

As far as the commercial brands are concerned, my suggestions are:

1 Look for the whole root where possible, which is usually better than powdered root, which is better than extracts, which are better than instant teas, which are better than cosmetics.[9]

2 Red is better than white.

3 The larger and older the better.

4 Capsules have on analysis generally yielded more active constituents than tablets. Some tablets seem to have lost their active principle completely during manufacture.[10]

5 When buying Korean red roots, make sure that they originate from Korea and the container has the seal of the Korean Office of Monopoly. There are imitation Korean roots on the market grown in Japan.

6 Where Korean or Chinese ginseng is unavailable, eleutherococcus should be used. It ranks higher than American cultivated root, which ranks higher than the Japanese root.

7 Wild American ginseng is of good quality. Cultivated American or Canadian roots should be bought according to the same principles described above.

Notes

The notes are constructed in standard format. The author's name is followed by the title of book or journal, volume number, page number, publisher and date. (R) = Russian, (K) = Korean, (J) = Japanese, (Ch) = Chinese, (G) = German, (B) = Bulgarian, (F) = French.

Where references are not followed by one of these letters they are in English. A single language abbreviation at the end of more than one reference indicates that they are all in that language.

CHAPTER 1

1 Yuan, G. C., and Chang, R. S., *J. Gerontology*, *24* 82–85 (1969)
2 Fulder, S. J., *Experimental Gerontology*, *12* 125–131 (1977)
3 Kreig, M., *Green Medicine*, Harrap & Co. (1965)
4 Lucas, R., *Nature's Medicines*, Neville Spearman, London (1969)
5 Hansard, London, 22 October 1975

CHAPTER 2

1 Howe, G. M., *Man, Environment and Disease in Britain*, Pelican Books, Harmondsworth (1976)
2 Illich, I., *Limits to Medicine*, Marion Boyars, London (1976)
3 McKeown, T., and Record, R. G., *Population Studies*, *16* 94–122 (1962)
4 Kristien, M. M., Arnold, C. B., and Wynder, E. L., *Science*, *195* 457 (1977)
5 Forbes, W. H., *New Eng. J. Med.*, *277* 71 (1967)
6 Mahler, H., *WHO Chronicle*, *31* 60–62 (1977)
7 Mather, H. G., *et al.*, *Brit. Med. J.*, *3* 334 (1971)
8 Eustrom, J. E., and Austin, D. F., *Science*, *195* 847–851 (1977)
9 Gould, D., *New Scientist*, 2 December 1976

10 *WHO Technical Report*, No. 615, Geneva (1977); *WHO Chronicle*, *32* 154–155 (1978)
11 Reports summarized in *New Scientist*, 6 April 1978
12 Coleman, V., *The Medicine Men*, Arrow, London (1977)
13 Turner, G., and Collins, E., *Lancet*, August 1977
14 Bharati in Brough, J. (ed.), *Poems from the Sanskrit*, Penguin Books, Harmondsworth (1968)
15 Brock, A. J., *Greek Medicine*, Dent & Sons, 1929
16 Quoted in Rosenberg, C. E., *Perspectives in Biology and Medicine*, *20* 485–506 (1977)
17 Chapman, J. S., *Arch. Env. Health*, *28* 356–357 (1974)
18 Claridge, G., *Drugs and Human Behaviour*, Allen Lane, London (1970)
19 Melmon, K. L., and Morrelli, H. F. (eds.), *Clinical Pharmacology*, Macmillan, New York (1972)

CHAPTER 3

1 a) Auricularia auricula, an astringent related to the European mouse-ear hawkweed which has, interestingly, also been used since medieval times for haemorrhoids
   b) A relative of the common fritillary
   c) Sophora flavescens, a relative of indigo, much used as an antiseptic
2 Palos, S., *The Chinese Art of Healing*, Herder & Herder Inc., NY (1971)
3 Huang Ti, *Nei Ching Su Wen: The Yellow Emperor's Classic of Internal Medicine* (trans. Veith, I.), Williams and Wilkins, Baltimore (1949)
4 Huard, P., and Ming, W., *Chinese Medicine*, World University Library, Weidenfeld & Nicolson (1968)
5 *The Way of Life, According to Lao Tzu* (trans. Brinner, W.), Capricorn Books, NY (1962). All quotations of the *Tao Te Ching* are from this source, which makes up in simple appeal what it lacks in scholarship. But then, Lao Tzu despised scholarship: 'Rid of formalized wisdom and learning, people would be a hundredfold happier.'
6 Taken from translator's introduction to the *Nei Ching*
7 Li Lun, *Scientica Sinica*, *28* 581 (1975)
8 Tao Tsang, quoted in Maspero, H., *Le Taoisme*, Paris (1950)
9 Brekhman, I. I., Grinevitch, M. A., and Zarva, L. A., *IXth Congress International de médécine néo-hippocratique, Genes*, 213–225, 8–11 October 1972; Brekhman, I. I., Grinevitch, M. A., ibid., 231

10 Jeffreys, W. H., and Maxwell, J. L., *Diseases of China*, John Bale, London (1910)
11 Yao Chai Hsueh, *Study of Medicinal Substances*, Nanking Pharmacological Institute (1972)
12 Actually, tonic could have been a good word if it had been left with its original meaning, namely 'tune'. Both come from the same Indo-European root t–n. However, the word has changed and lost itself in gin-and-tonic associations

CHAPTER 4

1 Pryshwyn, M., *Zen Shen*, Moscovskiet-vo Pisatelsi, Moscow (1934)
2 Embolden, W. A., *Bizarre Plants*, Studio Vista, London (1974)
3 Lucas, R., *Nature's Medicines*, Neville Spearman, London (1969)
4 Stuart, G., *Chinese Materia Medica*, Shanghai (1911)
5 Grushvitzky, I. V., 'A Contribution to the Knowledge of Biology of the Wild Growing Ginseng (Panax ginseng CAM)', *Jour. Bot. USSR*, *44* 1694–1793 (1959; R)
6 Lee, C. Y., and Lim, S. U., *Kor. J. Ginseng Sci.*, *1* 51–58 (1976); Chung, H-S., and Kim, C-H., in *2nd International Ginseng Symposium*, Seoul, Korea (1978)
7 Foulk, G. C., in *Papers Relating to the Foreign Relations of the United States*, Washington, Government Printing Office (1886)
8 Hu, S. Y., 'The Genus Panax (Ginseng) in Chinese Medicine', *Economic Botany*, *30* 11–28, (1976)
9 Lucas, R., *Ginseng: The Chinese Wonder Root*, R & M Books, Spokane, Washington (1972)
10 Baranov, A., 'Recent Advances in our Knowledge of the Morphology, Cultivation and Uses of Ginseng (Panax ginseng C. A. Meyer)', *Economic Botany*, *20* 403–406 (1966)
11 Jartoux, Père, 'The Description of a Tartarian Plant called Ginseng', *Phil. Trans. Roy. Soc. London*, *28* 237–247 (1714)
12 Lafiteau, J. F., *Concernant la précieuse plante du gin seng la Tartarie découverte en Canada*, Paris (1858; F)
13 Schorger, A. W., *Ginseng: A Pioneer Resource*, Wisconsin Academy of Science, Art and Letters, *57* 65–74 (1969)
14 Harding, A. R., *Ginseng and Other Medicinal Plants*, Columbus, Ohio (1908)
15 Dymock, *Pharmacographica Indica*, Hamdard National Foundation, Pakistan
16 Hara, H., *J. Jap. Bot.*, *45* 197–212 (1970); *Flora Eastern Himalayas* (1966)
17 Ainshie, W., *Materia Indica*, Longmans (1826)

18 Translated by Dr S. Y. Hu (c.f. Note 8)
19 See, for example, *A Barefoot Doctor's Manual*, Running Press, Philadelphia (1977), and RKP, London (1978)
20 Hong, M. W., *Korean J. Pharmacognoscy, 3* 187 (1972; K)
21 Vogel, V. J., *American Indian Medicine*, University of Oklahoma Press (1970)

CHAPTER 5

1 Brekhman, I. I., *Zen-shen*, State Publishing House for Medical Literature, Leningrad (1957; R)
2 a) Medvedev, M. A., 'The Effect of Ginseng on the Working Performance of Radio Operators', *Papers on the Study of Ginseng and Other Medicinal Plants of the Far East, 5*, Primorskoe knizhnoe izdatelsvo, Vladivostok (1963; R)
   b) Koryakovchev, V. S., 'Influence of Single Dose of Ginseng Root Extracts on Absolute Eye-sight Sensitivity in the Process of Dark Adaptation', *Papers on the Study of Stimulant and Tonic Remedies: Ginseng and Schizandra chinensis*, Vladivostok (1951; R)
3 Sandberg, F., in *Proceedings of the International Symposium on Ginseng*, Seoul, Korea (1974). The method used is that of Frøberg.
   Karlsson, C. G., *et al.*, in *Coffein und andere Methylxanthine, International Symposium at Erlangen-Nuernberg, October 1968* (eds. Heim, F., and Ammon, H. P. T.), F. K. Schattauer, Stuttgart and New York (1969; G)
4 Rückert, K. H., in *Proceedings of the 2nd International Ginseng Symposium*, 85–92, Korea Ginseng Research Institute, Seoul (1979)
5 Brekhman, I. I., *Med. Sci. Serv.*, 4 17–26 (1967)
6 Brekhman, I. I., in *Papers On the Study of Stimulant and Tonic Remedies* (q.v.)
7 Pharmacological test with ginseng extract G115, Consultox Laboratories, London (1974; submitted)
8 Brekhman, I. I., and Grinevitch, M. A., *Apt. Delo, 6* 34–38 (1959; R)
9 Estler, C. J., Ammon, H. P. T., and Herzog, C., *Psychopharm., 58* 161–166 (1978)
10 Porsolt, R. D., Le Pichou, M., and Jalfre, M., *Nature, 266* 730–732 (1977); Porsolt, R. D., and Jalfre, M., *Nature, 274* 512–513 (1978)
11 Petkov, W., in *XXth International Physiological Congress, Brussels*, 721–722 (1956)
12 Petkov, W., *Drug Res., 5* 305–311 (1959); ibid., *11* 288–296 (1961); ibid., *11* 418–423 (1961; G)

13 Petkov, W., Shivatcheva, Su, *Dissertations of the Research Institute for Neurology and Psychiatry*, 3 99–114 (1957; B)

14 Petkov, W., *Pharmaz. Zeit*, 113 599–605 (1968; G)

15 Brekhman, I. I., in *Material for the Study of Ginseng and Luzea*, 2 124–131 (1955; R)

16 Luria, A. R., *The Working Brain*, Allen Lane, London (1973)

17 Petkov, W., Azev, Em., Ovcharov, R., *Proc. of Postgrad. Med. Institute*, 8 1–19 (1961; B)

18 Thompson, R. F., *Foundations of Physiological Psychology*, Harper & Row, New York (1967)

19 For an understanding of these drug behavioural studies, see Iversen, S. P., and Iversen, L. L., *Behavioural Pharmacology*, OUP (1975)

20 Takagi, K., Saito, H., Tsuchiya, M., *Jap. J. Pharmacology*, 22 339–346 (1972); ibid., 23 43–56 (1973); ibid., 23 29–41 (1973)

21 Hong, S. A., Oh, J. S., Park, C. W., Chang, H. K., and Kim, E. C., *Korean J. Pharmacol.*, 6 1–9 (1970); Hong, S. A., *Ch'oesin Uihak*, 15 87–91 (1972; K)

22 Hong, S. A., Park, C. W., Kim, J. H., Chang, H. K., Hong, S. K., and Kim, M. S., *Korean J. Pharmacol.*, 101–11 (1974; K): and in English in *Proceedings International Ginseng Symposium,* Central Research Institute, Office of Monopoly, Seoul (1974)

23 Takagi, K., Saito, H., Tsuchiya, M., *Jap. J. Pharmacology,* 24 41–48 (1974); Lee, D. J., Choi, H., *Choongang Vihak*, 9 591–595 (1965; K). This paper reported that ginseng had no effects on the speed of spinal reflexes in rats.

24 Saito, H., Morita, M., and Takagi, K., *Jap. J. Pharmacology*, 23 49 (1973); ibid., 24 119 (1974); Kaku, T., Miyata, T., Uruno, T., Sako, I., and Kinoshita, A., *Drug Res.*, 25 539–547 (1975)

25 Saito, H., Tschuiya, M., Naka, S., Takugi, K., *Jap. J. Pharmacol.*, 27 509–516 (1977)

26 Brekhman, I. I., and Dardymov, I. V., *Ann. Rev. Pharmacol.*, 9 419–430 (1969)

27 Efrinova, V. I., Glebova, N. F., and Orlova, M. I., *Zhur. Vish. Nerv. Deyat*, 5 741–746 (1955; R)

28 Brekhman, I. I., in *The Pharmacology of Oriental Plants* (eds. Chen and Mukherji), 97–102, Pergamon Press, Oxford (1963); idem, *Eleutherococcus*, Nauka Publishing House, Leningrad (1968; R)

29 Rusin, V., *Ya. Mater Izuch. Zhen'shenya Drugikh Lek. Sredstv. Da'n Vost.*, 7 27–31 (1966; R)

30 Brekhman, I. I., and Dardymov, I. V., *11th Pacific Science Congress, Tokyo*, 8 11 (1966); Brekhman, I. I., and Dardymov, I. V., *Lloydia*, 32 46–51 (1969); idem, *Farmakol. Toksikol*, 29 167–171 (1966). The latter is in Russian.

306   NOTES

31 Brekhman, I. I., Dobryakov, J. I., Taneyeva, A. I., *New Data on the Pharmacology of Spotted Deer Antlers* (Medicinal Remedies of the Far East Series, No. 9), Vladivostok (1968); Pavlenko, S. M. (ed.), *Pantocrine*, second edition, Parts I–II, Gorno-Altaisk (1969); Dobryakov, J. I., Mirolynbov, I. I., Ryashchenko, L. P., and Sopova, M. S., 'Spotted Deer Bibliography', in *New Data. . . .* (op. cit.; R)

32 Brekhman, I. I., Dobryakov, J. I., and Taneyeva, A. I., *Izvest. Sibirskogo Otdelenia Akademin Nauk. SSSR,* Biol. series, *10* 112–115 (1969; R), p<0.0001 for the extended administration.

33 Brekhman, I. I., Taneyeva, A. I., ibid., *5* 38–45 (1969; R). For ergonometry p<0.01.

35 Brekhman, I. I., *Rantarin (New Medicinal Preparation from Reindeer's Non-ossified Antlers)*, Medexport, Moscow

36 Thullier, G., Rumpf, P., and Thullier, J., *Compt. Rend. Hebd. des Séances, 249* 2081–3 (1959; F). Also at Xme Congrès de la Soc. Neurochirurgie de Langue Française, Lille, 27–28 May 1960. I do not know if this is published.

37 Pfeiffer, C. C., Jenney, E. H., Gallagher, W., Smith, R. P., Bevan, W., Killam, K. F., Killam, E. K., and Blackmore, W., *Science, 126* 610–611 (1957)

38 Murphree, H. B., Pfeiffer, C. C., and Backerman, I. A., *Clinical Pharmacology and Therapeutics, 1* No. 3 303–310 (1960); Lemere, F., and Lasater, J. H., *Am. J. Psychiat., 114* 655–656 (1958); Schorer, C. E., and Lowinger, P., *Dis. Nerv. Syst., 20* 267–269 (1959)

CHAPTER 6

1 Garriques, S. S., *Ann. Chem. Pharm., 90* 231 (1854; G)

2 Shibata, S., Fujita, M., and Itokawa, H., *Tetrahedron Lett., 10* 419–422 (1962); ibid., *11* 1239–1242 (1962); with Tanaka, O., and Ishi, T., *Chem. Pharm. Bull., 11* 959–61 (1963); ibid., 962–966 (1963); Elyakov, G. B., Strigina, L. I., Khorlin, A. Ya, and Kochetev, N. K., *Izv. Akad. Nauk. SSR, 11* 2054–8, (1962; R); Lin, Y. T., *J. Chinese Chemical Society* (Taiwan), *8* 109–113 (1961); Horhämmer, L., Wagner, H., and Lay, B., *Pharm. Ztg, 99* 303 (1959); ibid., *106* 1307–11 (1961; G)

3 Elyakov, G. B., and Strigina, L. I., *Dokl. Akad. Nauk. SSR, 158* 892–895 (1964); Dzizenko, A. K., Ellkin, Yu. N., Strokina, E. V., Strigina, L. I., and Elyakov, G. B., ibid., *173* 1080–2 (1967); ibid., *156* 92–94 (1964); ibid., *162* 569–572 (1965); ibid., *207* 1351–1354

(1972; R). Elyakov, G. B., in *11th Pacific Science Congress, Tokyo*, *8* 10 (1966); Elyakov, G. B., Strigina, L. I., Uvarova, N. I., Vaskovsky, V. E., Dzizenko, A. K., and Kochetkov, N. K., *Tetrahedron Letters*, *48* 3591–3597 (1964); ibid., *51* 4669–4674 (1965); ibid., *52* 141–144 (1966); *Tetrahedron*, *24* 5483–5491 (1968). Kochetkov, N. K., et al., *Izv. Akad. Nauk. SSR, Ser. Khim.*, *8* 1409–1416 (1972; R). Shaposhnikova, G. I., Ferens, N. A., Uvarova, N. I., and Elyakov, G. B., *Carbohydrate Research*, *15* 319–321 (1970)

4 The saponins were first separated and isolated by a technique called thin layer chromatography. This consists of the guided diffusion of a spot of the mixture of substances along an absorbent surface. A series of spots appears which can be separated and chemically analysed. The sugar parts of the saponins were split from the rest by strong acid. Then the non-sugar parts (called the sapogenins) were analysed by converting them to various other compounds until one was found which had characteristics well established by previous investigators. The structures of the sapogenins have also been investigated by all kinds of methods such as mass spectroscopy and, more recently, C^{13} nuclear magnetic resonance. This probes not only the basic structure of the molecules but also their shape, and how all the little appendages on the shape are arranged in three-dimensional relation to each other. Then all the sugars were analysed, and the problematic task of finding out just how and where the sugars are joined to the sapogenin was completed. Finally, some work was carried out on comparison of these saponins to other known saponins, and whether they might have become converted or damaged during the process of extraction and purification.

The designations Ra, Rb, etc., relate to the position of the spots on the chromatogram. The fifteen now discovered include the six found earlier by Elyakov. Besides the protopanaxadiol and protopanaxatriol types, there is one saponin with another core triterpene called oleanolic acid.

The dominant ginsenosides in all the roots of Panax ginseng are Rb_1, Rc, and Rg_1, with slightly less Rd and Re and minor amounts of the others. Then there are special saponins which are found in the leaves and buds. These, called F_1, F_2 and F_3, are not found in the root. They are of the panaxadiol type. The flowers also contain triterpenoids, particularly of the Re type. The top parts of the plant may contain surprisingly large amounts of the saponins. The flowers, for example, contain about 2.5 per cent by weight of Re, and other saponins in such small quantity that Professor Tanaka of Japan was able to obtain quantities of pure Re without any chromatography at all.

308   NOTES

Tanaka, O., Nagai, M., and Shibata, S., *Tetrahedron Letters, 37* 2291–2297 (1964); Tanaka, O., Nagai, M., Ohsawa, T., Nanaka, N., and Shibata, S., ibid., *40* 391–396 (1967); Nagai, M., Ando, T., Tanaka, O., and Shibata, S., ibid., 3579 (1967); Tanaka, O., Tanaka, N., Ohsawa, T., Iitaka, Y., and Shibata, S., ibid., 4235–4238 (1968); Iida, Y., Tanaka. O., and Shibata, S., ibid., 5449–5453 (1968); Shibata, S., Ando, T., and Tanaka, O., *Chem. Pharm. Bull.*, *14* 1157–1161 (1966); Nagai, M., Ando, T., Tanaka, N., Tanaka, O., and Shibata, S., ibid., *20* 1212–1216 (1972); with Ohsawa, T., and Kawai, N., ibid., *20* 1204–1211; ibid., *19* 2349–2453 (1971); ibid., *20* 1890–1897 (1972); ibid., *22* 2407 (1974); ibid., *24* 2204 (1976); Nagai, M., Tanaka, O., Shibata, S., *Tetrahedron, 27* 881–889 (1971); Kaku, T., Miyata, T., Uruno, T., Sako, I., and Kuioshita, T., *Drug Res.*, *25* 343–347, (1975); Asakawa, J., Kasai, R., Yamasaki, K., and Tanaka, O., *Tetrahedron, 33* 1935–1939 (1977). Reviews: Shibata, S., in *Symposium on Gerontology*, *Lugano*, 69–76 (1975); Kim, J. Y., and Staba, E. J., *Korean J. Pharmacognoscy*, *5* 85–101 (1974; K); Shibata, S., in *International Gerontological Symposium*, *Singapore*, 183–198 (1977); Shellard, E. J., and Jolliffe, G. H., ibid. (1977)

5 The American root contains no Ra, Rg_2, Rh, Ro nor Rf, and almost no Rc. Yet there is a very large blob on the chromatogram for Rb_1. Another saponin in American roots is not found in the Asiatic species. Drs Kim and Staba of the University of Minneapolis have also found interesting seasonal and age differences in the saponin profile of the American species. Kim, J. Y., and Staba, F. J., *Korean J. Pharmacognoscy*, *4* 193 (1973); idem, in: *Proceedings of the International Ginseng Symposium*, The Research Institute, Office of Monopoly, Korea, 77–93 (1974)

6 Ando, T., Tanaka, O., Shibata, S., *J. Jap. Soc. Pharmacog.*, *25* 28 (1971; J); Namba, T., Yoshizaki, M., Tomimori, T., Kobashi, K., Mitsui, K., and Hase, J., *J. Pharm. Soc. Japan*, *94* 252–260 (1974; J); idem., *Planta Medica 24* (1974)

7 Kondo, N., Aoki, K., Ogawa, H., Kasai, R., Shoji, J., *Chem. Pharm. Bull.*, *18* 1558 (1970); Kondo, N., Marumoto, Y., and Shoji, J., ibid., *19* 1103 (1971); ibid., *24* 253 (1976); ibid., *25* (1977)

8 Shibata, S., in *Symposium on Gerontology*, *Lugano*, The Research Institute, Office of Monopoly, Seoul, Korea (1976); Kondo, N., Shoji, J., and Tanaka, O., *Chem. Pharm. Bull.*, *21* 2701 (1973); Otsuka, H., Yukio, N., Ogihara, Y., and Shibata, S., *Planta Medica, 32* 9–17 (1977)

9 Chung, B. S., *Korean J. Pharmacog.*, *5* 175–179 (1974; K)

10 Takahashi, M., Isoi, K., Yoshikura, M., and Osugi, T., *J. Pharmacog. Soc. Japan*, *81* 771–773 (1961); ibid., *86* 1053–1056 (1966; J). The structure of panaxynol is 1,9,-cis-hepta-decadine-1,6,-

diyn-3-ol. Many other hydrocarbons have been detected.

11 Wrobel, J. T., Dabrowski, Z., Gielzyuska, M., Merasimuk, K., Ivanov, A., Kabzinska, K., Poplawski, J., and Ruszowska, S. *Thuszcze Srodki Piorace Kosmet., 17* 63–72 (1973; in Polish)
12 Kormatsu, M., Tomimori, T., and Makiguchi, *J. Pharmacog. Soc. Japan, 87* 122–126 (1969; J)
13 Goto, M., *J. Pharmacog. Soc. Japan,* 77 471–4 (1957; J); Kim, Y. E., Juhn, K. S., and Hu, B. J., *Yakhak Hoeji, 8* 80–84 (1964; K) .
14 Lee, C. Y., and Lee, T. Y., *Proceedings of the Symposium on Phytochemistry,* University of Hong Kong, 171 (1964); Solov'eva, T. F., Prundnikova, T. I., Ovodov, Yu S., *Rast. Resur., 4* 497–501 (1968; R); idem, *Carbohydrate Research, 10* 13–18 (1969); Takiura, K., and Nakagawa, I., *J. Pharmacog. Soc. Japan, 83* 298–300 (1963); ibid., *83* 305–308 (1963; J)
15 Gstirner, F., and Vogt, H. J., *Arch. Pharm., 299* 936–944 (1966); ibid., *300* 371–384 (1967; G)
16 Pijk, J., and Kim, J. I., *J. Pharm. Belge, 19* 3–18 (1964; F); Gribovskaya, I., and Grinevich, N. I., *Agrokhimiya, 10* 124–131 (1970; R)
17 Takatori, K., Kato, T., Asano, S., Ozaki, M., and Nakashima, T., *Chem. Pharm. Bull., 11* 1342–1343 (1963)
18 Han, B. H., Park, M. W., Woo, L. K., Woo, W. S., and Han, Y. N., in *Proc. of 2nd Int. Ginseng Symp.,* 13–17, Korea Ginseng Research Institute, Seoul (1979)
19 Butenko, R. B., *Probl. Pharmacog., 21* 184–191 (1967); Butenko, R. B. Grushwitsky, I. V., and Slepyan, L. I., *Bot. Zheit., 7* 906–913 (1968); Slepyan, L. I.; *Rast. Resur.,* 7 175–186 (1971; R)
20 Furuya, T., Kojima, K., Syono, K., Ishi, T., *Chem. Pharm. Bull., 18* 2371–2 (1970); with Uotani, K., and Nishio, M., ibid.. *21* 98–101 (1973)
21 Jhang, J. J., Staba, E. J., and Kim, J. Y., *In Vitro, 9* 253–259 (1974)
22 A recent paper describing the various methods of culture was published by C. Horn, who works for the Korean Atomic Energy Research Institute, in *Proceedings, Int. Ginseng Symp.,* op. cit. See also Kita, K., and Sugi, M., *J. Pharmacog. Soc. of Japan, 89* 1474–1476 (1974; J)
23 Oh, J. S., and Lim, C. K., *Insam Munhum Teukjip (Seoul), 2* 22–26 (1964); Woo, L. K., *Yakhak Hoeji, 17* 123–128 (1973; K); Kasai, R., Shinzo, K., and Tanaka, O., *Chem. Pharm. Bull., 24* 400–406 (1976)
24 Shibata, S., in *New Natural Products and Plant Drugs with Pharmacological, Biological and Therapeutic Activity* (eds. Wagner, H., and Wolff, P.), 177–196, Springer-Verlag, Heidelberg (1977); Saitoh, T., Kinoshita, T., and Shibata, S., *Chem. Pharm. Bull., 24* 1242 (1976)

310 NOTES

25 Kubota, T., Tonami, F., and Hinoh, H., *Tetrahedron*, *23* 3333 (1967); *Tetrahedron Lett.*, *24* 676 (1968); Aimi, N., and Shibata, S., *Tetrahedron Lett.*, *39* 4721–4 (1966)
26 Kubota, T., Kitani, H., *Chem. Comm.*, 1005 (1968); ibid., 190 (1969); ibid., 1313 (1969); Akiyama, T., Tanaka, O., and Shibata, S., *Chem. Pharm. Bull.*, *20* 1945 (1972); ibid., *20* 1952 (1972); ibid., *20* 1957 (1972)
27 Fujita, M., and Itokawa, H., *Chem. Pharm. Bull.*, *9* 1006 (1961); Sakuma, S., Sugiura, N., Tanemoto, H., Amakawa, H., and Shoji, J., *Abstr. 95th Meeting Pharm. Soc. Japan*, 247 (1975; J)
28 Shimizu, Y., and Pelletier, S. W., *J. Am. Chem. Soc.*, *88* 1544 (1966); Tsutikani, Y., Kawanashi, S., and Shoji, J., *Chem. Pharm. Bull.*, *21* 791, (1973); ibid., *21* 1564 (1973)
29 Kawai, K., Akiyama, T., Ogihara, Y., and Shibata, S., *Phytochemistry*, *13* 2829 (1974)
30 Kulshoestha, D. K., and Rastogi, R. P., *Phytochemistry*, *12* 887 (1973)
31 Sandberg, F., *Planta Medica*, *24* 392–396 (1973); Ovodov, Yu S., Frolova, G. M., Nefedova, M. Yu, and Elyakov, G. B., *Khimin Prirodnik Soedinenii*, *1* 63–64 (1967) (latter R); see also note 10 above
32 Elyakov, G. B., Cherezova, R. V., in *Chemistry of Natural Compounds 1* 47 (1968); Elyakov, G. B., Chetyrina, N. S., and Dobyakov, J. I., *Khimico-Farm. Zhurnal*, *11* 21–24 (1971) (latter R)
33 Govanov, I. A., Libizov, N. J., and Gladkikh, A. S., *Farmatsiya*, *19* 23 (1970; R), summarized in *Chem. Abst.*, *73* 95408 (1973)
34 Refer to any standard textbook of pharmacognoscy.

CHAPTER 7

1 Bernard, C., *Le cons sur les phénomenes de la vie* (1879), quoted in Jacob, F., *The Logic of Living Systems*, Allen Lane, London (1974)
2 Cannon, W. B., *The Wisdom of the Body*, Norton & Co. New York (1939)
3 Selye, H., in *Society, Stress and Disease* (ed. Levi, L.), 299, OUP, London (1971)
4 Cannon, W. B., *Bodily Changes in Pain, Hunger, Fear and Rage*, C. T. Brandford & Co. (1953)
5 Bittles, A. M., Fulder, S. J., Grant, E. C., and Nicholls, W., *Gerontology*, *25* 125–131 (1979); Chin, H. W., *Seoul Uidae Chapchi*, *15*, 1–6 (1974; K)
6 Kim, E. C., Cho, H. Y., and Kim, J. M., *Korean J. Pharmacognoscy*, *2* 23–28 (1971; K); Hong, S. A., Park, C. W., Kim, J. H.,

Chang, H. K., Hong, S. K. and Kim, M. S., ibid., *10* 1–11 (1974; K). An English translation of this last paper can be found in the *Proceedings of the International Ginseng Symposium*, Office of Monopoly, Seoul (1974)

7 Hong, S. A., Oh, J. S., Park, C. W., Chang, H. K., and Kim, E. C., *Korean J. Pharmacology*, *6* 1–9 (1970; K)

8 Carson, S. A., in *Society, Stress and Disease* (ed. Levi, L.), OUP London (1971)

9 Brekhman, I. I., and Dardymov, I. V., *Ann. Reviews Pharmacol.*, *9* 419 (1969)

10 Brekhman, I. I., and Kirillov, O. I., *Life Sciences*, *8* 113–121 (1969)

11 When they also received antibiotics, their lifetime could be increased threefold. Brekhman, I. I., Majanskiy, G. M., *Izv. Akad. Nauk SSSR, Ser, Biol.*, *5* 762–765 (R); Brekhman, I. I., *Eleutherococcus, Izdatestvo 'Nauka'*, Leningrad (1968; R)

12 Anon., *Chinese Med. J.*, 77 296 (1959); Chang, P. H., *Acta Pharm. Sinica*, *13* 106–111 (1966; Ch); Tsung, S. I., Chen, C., Tang, S., *Acta Physiol Sinica*, 27 324–8 (1964; Ch)

13 Park, D. L., *Insam Munhun Teukjip*, *2* 55–65 (1964; K)

14 Freidman, S. L., Khlebnikov, H. N., in *Biol. Akt. Veshchestva Rastenievod* (ed. Balin, Ya.), 113–116, Zhivotnovod Med., S-kh. Institute, Saratov, USSR (1975; R)

15 For reference to this endocrine control see, for example, Thompson, R. F., *Foundations of Physiological Psychology*, Harper and Row, New York (1967)

16 Tsung, S. I., Chen, C., and Tang, S., *Acta Physiol. Sinica*, 27 324–8 (1964; Ch); Rosin, M. A., in *Materials for the Study of Panax ginseng and Other Medicinal Plants of the Far East*, 123–8, Vladivostok (1963; R). There are also reports that ginseng does have an effect in assisting animals to overcome general stress even after removal of the adrenals; see, for example, Kim, C. C., *Katorik Taehak Uihakpu, Nonmunjip, 9* 29–44; Yoon, H. S., Kim, C., ibid., *21* 25–35 (1971; K). However the effect is slight, and I believe can be satisfactorily accounted for by small amounts of stress steroids which are still present, particularly from the ovaries, after the adrenal glands are surgically removed.

17 Choi, C. K., *Ch'oesin Uihak*, *14* 109–112 (1971); Cho, S. E., ibid., *14* 135–8 (1971); Choi, C. K., and Kim, C., *Katorik Taehak Uihakpu, Nonmunjip, 21* 211–225 (1971; K)

18 Petkov, W., and Staneva, D., in *The Pharmacology of Oriental Plants* (eds. Chen, K. K., and Mukherji, B.), 139–45, Pergamon Press, Oxford (1963); Petkov, W., and Staneva, D., *Arz. Forschung (Drug Research)*, *13* 1078–1081 (1963: G). The parameters used are the levels of ascorbic acid and cholesterol in adrenal cortical tissue.

19 Anon., *Chinese Med. J.*, 77 296 (1959; Ch); Hu, C. Y., and Kim, C., *Katorik Uihakpu, Nonmunjip*, 12 49–60 (1967); Hu, C. Y., Kim, C. C., and Kim, J. K., *Choesin Uihak*, 10 73–77 (1967); Sunwoo, C., and Kim, C., ibid., 8 77–89 (1965); Kim, C. C., Kim, J. K., and Hu, C. Y., ibid., 10 57–63 (1967; K); Avakian, E. V., and Evonuk, E., *Planta Medica*, 36 43–48 (1979)

20 Brekhman, I. I., and Dardymov, I. V., *Lloydia*, 32 46–51 (1969); Brekhman, I. I., in *Pharmacology of Oriental Plants*, 97–102; Wang, P. H., Chang, S. C., and Chu, S. Y., *Acta Pharm. Sinica*, 12 446–452 (1965), on san-chi (Ch)

21 Kim, C., Kim, C. C., Kim, M. S., Hu, C. Y., and Rhe, J. S., *Lloydia*, 33 43–48 (1970)

22 Mr Lee Harris invented this as an advertising jingle.

23 Kim, H. R., and Kim, W. B., *Ch'oesin Uihak*, 15 87–90 (1972); Kim, W. B., and Chung, H. Y., ibid., 15 83–86 (1972); Park, W. H., and Moon, Y. B., ibid., 13 81–84 (1970; K)

24 Choi, C. K., *Ch'oesin Uihak*, 14 109–112 (1971); Choi, C. K., and Kim, C., *Katorik Taehak Uihakpu, Nonmunjip*, 21 211–215 (1971; K)

25 Oura, H., and Hiai, S., in *Proceedings Int. Gins. Symp.*, 23–32, The Central Research Institute, Office of Monopoly, Seoul, Korea (1974). Hiai, S., Sasaki, S., and Oura, H., *Planta Medica*, 37 15–19 (1979)

26 Nagasawa, T., Oura, H., Hiai, S., and Nishinaga, K., *Chem. Pharm. Bull.*, 25 1665–1670 (1977)

27 Shori, D., PhD Thesis, Department of Pharmacology, Chelsea College, London; Fulder, S., in *Proc. 2nd Int. Ginseng Symposium*, 25–28, Seoul, Korea (1969)

28 De Wied, D., *Hospital Practice*, 123–131 (1976)

29 De Wied, D., in *Symposium on Developments in Endocrinology*, 9–18, Organon International, OSS, Netherlands (1976); de Wied, D., Bohus, B., Gispen, W. H., Urban, I., and Greidanus, Tj. B. R. W., 'Hormonal Influences on Motivational, Learning and Memory Processes', in *Hormones, Behaviour and Psychopathology* (ed. Sachar, E. J.), 1–14, Raven Press, New York (1976); McEwen, B. S, Gerlach, J. L., Luine, V. N., and Lieberberg, I., *Psychoneuroendocrinology*, 2 249–255 (1977)

30 Zerssen, D. von, in *Psychotropic Actions of Hormones* (eds. Itil, T. M., *et al.*), Spectrum Press, New York (1976); Fedor-Freybergh, P., ibid., 1–51.

31 Professor Peter Forsham, quoted in Selye, H., *The Stress of Life*, McGraw Hill, New York (1956)

32 Wolthius, O.'L., and de Wied, D., *Pharmacol., Biochem. and Behaviour*, 4 273–278 (1976)

33 Kim, J. M., Hong, S. A., and Park, C. W., *Ch'oesin Uihak, 16* 57–63 (1973; K)

34 Chen, S-E., Sawchuck, R. J., and Staba, E. J., in *Proc. 2nd. Int. Ginseng Symposium*, 55–66, Korean Ginseng Research Institute, Seoul (1979). Staba notes that the heart stimulants digoxin (a triol) and digitoxin (a diol) show exactly the same phenomenon. They are steroidal glycosides.

35 Brekhman, I. I., and Dardymov, I. V., *Sb, Rab. Inst. Tsitol. Akad, Nauk SSSR, 14* 82–88 (1971; R). Actinomycin D., a protein-synthesis inhibitor, stopped improvements in perform-ance of mice in stamina tests when they had been given eleutherococcus or dibazol, but not if they had received amphetamine.

36 See Chapter 6, Note 24.

37 Lazarev, N. V., in *7th All-Union Congress of Physiology, Biochemis-try and Pharmacology*, 579, Medgiz, Moscow (1947; R); Rozin, M. A., *Medicinal Remedies for Restoration Therapy and Prophylaxis of Diseases of the Nervous System*, Izdamie Voenno-morskoy Medicinskoy Acad., Leningrad (1951; R)

38 Thullier, J., in *Regional Neurochemistry* (eds. Kety, S. S., and Elkes, J.), 481–488, Pergamon Press (1961); Meszaros, J., Gajewska, S., *Drug Res., 22* 1923–1926 (1972)

39 Petkov, V., *Minerva Medica, 58* 516–525 (1967; Ital)

40 Tanner, O., *Stress*. Time-Life International (Nederland) B.V. (1977)

41 These examples quoted from Reynolds, V., *The Biology of Human Action*, W. H. Freeman & Co., Reading and San Francisco (1976)

42 Bourne, P. G. (ed.), *The Psychology and Physiology of Stress*, Academic Press (1969)

43 Frankenhauser, M., *J. Psychosomatic Res., 21* 313–321 (1977)

44 Johansson, G., *Biological Psychology, 4* 157–172 (1976)

45 Pelletier, K., *Mind as Healer, Mind as Slayer*, Dell Publishing Co., New York (1977)

46 For details see Stein, M., Shiavi, R. C., and Camerino, M., *Science 191* 435–440 (1976)

47 Rabkin, J. G., and Struening, E. L., *Science 194* 1013–1020 (1976)

48 Riley, V., *Science 189* 465–467 (1975). Quoted in Pelletier, op. cit.

49 Monjan, A. A., and Collector, M. I., *Science, 196* 307–308 (1976)

50 Kang, H. R., *Katorik Taehak Uihakpu, Nonmunjip, 19* 130–152 (1970); Kang, J. W., and Chung, I. E., ibid., *18* 1–14 (1970); Suk, B. H., and Chung, I. C., ibid., *17* 17–30 (1969); Chung, H. Y., and Kim, C., ibid., *22* 13–23 (1972); Choi, S. N., and Kim, C., ibid., *25* 143–51 (1973); Kim, C., Choi, H., Kim, C. C., Kim, J. K., Kim, M. S., and Kim, M. K., *Korean J. Physio., 5* 23–42 (1971; K)

51 Chun, C. S., *Katorik Taehak Uihakpu, Nonmunjip, 19* 317–331 (1970; K). This would explain the Russian observation that there is less spreading of tumours during surgery when ginseng is given.

52 Murata, I., and Hirono, F., *Daisha, 10* 601 (1973; J)

53 Yaremenko, K. V., in Brekhman, I. I., *Eleutherococc.*, Meditsina, Moscow (1978; R)

CHAPTER 8

1 Shurgaya, Sh. I., Turchinskig, V. I., and Gagarin, I. A., in *Climatic/Medical Problems and Medical Geography in Siberia*, 111–113, Tomsk (1974; R)

2 Galanova, G. K., in *Adaptation and Adaptogens* (ed. Brekhman, I. I., 126–127, Vladivostok (1977); idem in *Reports of the 2nd All-Union Conference on Man's Adaptation to Different Geographical, Climatic and Working Conditions, 2* 44–46, Novosibirsk (1977; R). The total figure of 60,000 is personal communication from Professor Brekhman.

3 Lebedev, A. A., in *Medicinal Substances of the Far East*, tenth series, 107–114 and 115–119, Khabarovsk (1970; R)

4 Kapitanenko, A. M., *Voyenno-meditsinskiy zhurnal, 2* 84 (1958; R)

5 Mans, J., and Robert, J., *Médécine et collectivité, 12* 1–3 (1965; F)

6 Ebert, L. Ya., Bucharin, O. V., and Motovskiy, I. M., *Medical Prophylaxis of Influenza*, Chelyabinsk (1969; R)

7 Gramenitskaya, V. G., and Grushvitskii, I. V., *Mikrobiologiya, 25* 221–226 (1956; R)

8 Krylov, A. V., Kostin, V. D., and Chuyan, A. M., *Acta Virol.* (Prague), *10* 75–76 (1972); Wardrope, A. J. B., Belgian Patent No. 666, 877, 16 Nov. 1965

9 Brekhman, I. I., and Dardymov, I. V., *Ann. Rev. Pharmacol., 9* 419 (1969)

10 Practically the only time this has been done in the UK in recent years is the lengthy and expensive trials to test the advantage of using vitamin C to prevent the common cold. The results are still in dispute.

11 Pyun, H. W., and Lee, C. J., *Katorik Taehak Uihakpu, Nonmunjip. 17* 109–116 (1969; K)

12 Shmelev, N. A., Korovina, Yu. P., and Odnoletova, F. F., in *Pantocrine,* Part 2, 101–104, Gorno Altaisk (1969; R); Gavrilenko, V. S., ibid., 105–112.

13 Simpson, W., *Some Observations Made upon the Root Called Nean, or Ninsing*, letter to Royal Society, London (1680)

14 Reshetnikova, A. D., *Sovetskaya Meditsina*, *2* 23–26 (1954; R)

15 Albov, N. N., in *Pantocrine*, Part 2, 53–72, Gorno Altaisk (1969; R)

16 Süttinger, H. von, *Erfahrungsheilkunde*, *18* 259–263 (1969); Schmidt, *Prophylaxie*, 280 (1968; G)

17 Discussed in Turova, A. D., *Medicinal Plants of the USSR and their Application*, 27–36, Moscow (1967; R)

18 Gianoli, A. C., Cabello, M., and Schertenleib, F. E., in *Proc..Int. Geront. Symposium, Singapore*, 207–221, Pharmaton S. A., Lugano, Switzerland (1977)

19 Chang, Y-S., Lee, J-Y., and Kim, C-W., in *Proceedings of the 2nd Int. Ginseng Symposium, Seoul* (1978)

20 Arapov, D. A., in *Pantocrine*, Part 2, 92–98, Gorno Altaisk (1969; R)

21 Schepartz, S. A., *Cancer Treatment Reports*, *60* 975–977 (1976)

22 Arichi, S., *Proceedings of the 2nd International Ginseng Symposium, Seoul* (1978); Hirang, W. I., and Cha, S., ibid.

23 Kim, I. J., and Kim, M. M., *Katorik Taehak Uihakpu, Nonmunjip*, *16* 161–186 (1969; K); Mironova, A. I., *Vopr. Onkol.*, *9* 42–44 (1963; R)

24 Lee, K-D., and Huemer, R. P., *Jap. J. Pharmacol.*, *21* 299–302 (1971)

25 Ronichevskaya, G. M., *Vopr. Onkol.*, *13* 67–71 (1967; R)

26 Yaremenko, K. V., *Mater. Izuch. Zhenskenya Drugiskh Lek. Sred. Dal'n. Vostoka*, 7 109–116 (1966; R)

27 Lazarev, N. V., and Brekhman, M. D., *Med. Science & Serv.*, 9–13 (1967); Stukov, A. N., *Problems of Oncology*, *12* 57–60 (1966); ibid., *12* 126 (1966); ibid., *13* 94–95 (1967; R)

28 Li, C. P., *Chinese Herbal Medicine*, US Dept. Health, Education and Welfare, Pub No. (NIH) 75–732 (1974)

29 Petkov, W., *Arch. Exp. Path. Pharmak.*, *236* 298 (1959; G); Burkat, M. E., and Saksanov, P., *Farmakol. Toksikol.*, *10* 7–15 (1947; R); Ching, L. P., *Chinese Reports of the Research Institute of Peiping*, *4* 1–12 (1937; Ch); Zakutinski, *Farmakol. Toksikol.*, *1* 13–16 (1944; R)

30 Kaku, T., Miyata, T., Uruno, T., Sako, I., and Kinoshita, A., *Drug. Res.*, *25* 539–546 (1975); Turova, A. D., op. cit. in Note 17

31 Kitagawa, H., and Iwaki, R., *Fol. Pharmacol. Japan.*, *57* 348–354 (1963; J); Takagi, K., Saito, H., Tsuchiya, M., *Jap. J. Pharmacol.*, *24* 41–48 (1974)

32 Wood, W. B., Rok, B. L., and White, R. P., *Jap. J. Pharmacol.*, *14*, 284–294 (1964); Lee, K-S., in *Proc. Int. Ginseng Symposium*, Office of Monopoly, Korea (1974)

33 Kim, C., *Insam Munhum Teukjïp (Seoul)*, *1* 29–38 (1962); Rhim, J. O., *Korean Intern. Med. J.*, *10* 401 (1967; K)

34 Watanabe, S., *Chuo Igakkai Zasshi, 274* 1225 (1918); Yonekawa, h. *Keio Igaku Zasshi, 6* 633–657 (1926; J)

35 Genest, J., Nowaczynski, W., Boucher, R., Kuchel, O., *Canadian Med. Assoc. J., 118* 538–549 (1978)

36 Lee, S. B., and Cho, K. C., *Katorik Taehak Uihakpu, Nonmunjip, 20* 89–99 (1971); Oh, J. S., Lim, J. K., Park, C. W., Han, M. J., *Korean J. Pharmacol., 4* 27–31 (1968; K)

37 Nahm, C. C., *Korean J. Int. Med., 3* 49–67 (1961); Kim, H. C., *Insam Munhum Teukjip, 1* 129–149 (1962); Johng, H. W., ibid., *2* 38–50 (1964; K)

38 Ikehara, M., Shibata, Y., Higashi, T., Sanada, S., Shoji, J., *Chem. Pharm. Bull., 26* 2844 (1978); Yamamoto, M., *Metabolism, 10* 645 (1973; J)

39 Cho, H. W., and Oh, J. S., *Yakhak. Hoeji, 6* 19–20 (1962); Park, J. W., *Insam Munhum Teukjip, 4* 83–108 (1971; K); Sakakibara, K., Shibata, Y., Migashi, J., Sanada, S., and Shoji, J., *Chem. Pharm. Bull., 23* 1009–1016 (1975); ibid., *24* 2985–2987 (1976)

40 Mankovsky, N. B., and Belonog, R. P., 'The Effect of Rantarin on Old People', in Brekhman, I. I., and Grinevich, M. A. (eds.), *Biological Resources from the East and South East*, 110–123, Vladivostok (1979; R)

41 Turova, A. P., and Aleshkina, *Sov. Med., 17* 168–169 (1953); Matukhim, V. A., and Mayanshkii, G. M., *Materials*, etc. op. cit. in Note 2, Chapter 5.

42 Bykhovisova, T. L., *Izv. Akad. Nauk SSSR Ser. Bid., 35* 915–918 (1970; R)

43 Kondo, J., *Fol. Pharmacol. Jap., 5* 389–416 (1927; J)

44 Ibid., Petkov, W., op cit. in Note 29; Brekhman, I. I., and Oleinikova, T. P., *Materials for the Study of Ginseng and Far Eastern Medicinal Plants, 5* 249–251 (1963; R); Pegel, N. B., *Tomsk, 3* 137–138 (1964; R); Tsuao, C., Yen, C. C., and Lei, H. P., *Yao Hsiao Hsiao Pao, 7* 208–212 (1959; Ch); Tank, L. I., *Farmakol Toksikol., 18* 64 (1955; R)

45 Wang, C. K., and Lei, H. P., *Chinese J. Intern. Med., 5* 861–865 (1957; Ch)

46 Oura, H., *et al., Planta medica, 28* 76–81 (1975); Oura, H., Hiaia, S., Odaka, Y., and Yokozawa, T., *J. Biochem.,* 77 1057–1065 (1975); Oura, H., Nakashima, J., Tsugada, K., and Ohta, Y., *Chem. Pharm. Bull., 20,* 980 (1972)

47 Hahn, D. R., *J. Pharmaceut. Soc. Korea, 20* 119 (1976); Hahn, D. R., in *Proc. 2nd Int. Ginseng Symposium*, 135–140, Korea Ginseng Research Institute, Seoul (1979)

48 Bupleurum: Archi, S., Konishi, H., and Abe, H., *Liver, 19* 430–435 (1978). Ginseng: Juhn, S. K., *Ch'oesin Uihak, 5* 631–634

(1962; K). Other Oriental drugs: Haginawa, J., and Harada, M., *Yakugaku Zasshi, 86* 231–235 (1966; J)
49 Min, P. K., *Fol. Pharmacol. Jap.*, *9* 310–326 (1930); ibid., *2* 238–255 (1931; J); Woo, L. K., Hong, M. W., Lee, C. K., Oh, J. S., and Woo, C. H., *Kwahak Kisulchuh*, Seoul (1968); Oh, J. S., Park, C. W., and Moon, D. Y., *Korean J. Pharmacol.*, *5* 23–28 (1969; K)
50 Kanzawa, F., Hoshi, A., Tsuda, S., and Kuretani, K., *GANN, 63* 409–413 (1972; J)
51 Petkov, W., in *Proc. Int. Geront. Symposium*, Pharmaton, Lugano (1974); Petkov, W., Koushev, V., and Panova, Y., *Acta Physiol. Pharmacol. Bulg., 3* 46–50 (1977; B)
52 Shin, M. R., *Koryo Taekakkyo Uikwa Taehak Chapchi, 13* 231–246 (1976; K); Brekhman, I. I., *Eleutherococc*, Nauka, Leningrad (1968)
53 Shin, M. R., *Kor. J. Gins. Sci.*, *1* 59–78 (1976)
54 See for example Dardymov, I. V., *Zenshen and Eleutherococcus*, Nauka, Moscow (1976; R)
55 See Chapter 2, Note 2

CHAPTER 9
1 Karzel, K., in *Proceedings of the International Ginseng Symposium*, 49–56, The Research Institute, Office of Monopoly, Seoul (1974)
2 Yonekawa, M., *Keio Igaku Zasshi, 6* 633–657 (1926; J)
3 Kwon, Y. J., and Kim, C., *Katorik Taehak Uihakpu, Nonmunjip, 26* 135–141 (1974; K)
4 Shibata, K., *et al.*, *Kita Kauto Medical J.*, *14* 243 (1964; J); Moon, Y. B., and Park, M. H., *Korean J. Physiol.*, *4* 103–106 (1970; K)
5 Shibata, K., Tadakoro, S., Kurihaa, Y., Ogawa, H., and Miyashita, K., *Insam Munhum Teukjip, 4* 253–269 (1971; K)
6 Brekhman, I. I., op. cit. in Chapter 5, Note 29
7 Brekhman, I. I., *et al.*, op. cit. in Chapter 5, Notes 32 and 33
8 Hong, S. A., Hau, D. S., and Lee, C. H., *Hyunddae Uihak, 1* 43–45 (1964); Hong, B. J., *et al.*, *Hanguk Chiuksau Hakhoechi, 18* 355–361 (1976; K)
9 Shida, K., Shimazaki, J., and Urano, E., *Jap. J. Fert. Sterility, 16* 166–173 (1971); Ishigami, J., *Metabolism and Disease, 10* 590 (1973; J); Yamamoto, M., in *Proc. Int. Ginseng Symposium*, 129, Office of Monopoly, Seoul (1974)
10 Gottleib, J. G., in *Pantocrine*, Part 2, 99–104, Gorno Altaisk (1969; R); Ginsberg, Yu. Z., in Materials &c. 137–144 (1951; R), *see* Chapter 5, Note 29.

11 Kuzminsk, P. A., *Chien K'ang Pao*, *204*, 22 November 1951 (Ch)
12 Cooper, W., *No Change*, Arrow Books, London (1976); Seaman, B., and Seaman, G., *Women and the Crisis in Sex Hormones*, Rawson Assoc. Publishers Inc., New York (1977)
13 Sun, I. S., *Arch. Exp. Path. u. Pharmakol*, *170* 443–457 (1933); Weber, U., *Süddent. Apotheker Ztg*, *78* 645–648, 657–658 (1938; G)
14 Warnecke, G., *Zeit. fur Therapie*, *2* 90–95 (1974; G)
15 Palmer, B. V., *et al.*, *BMJ*, *1* 1284 (1978); Koriech, O. M., *BMJ*, *1* 1556 (1978)
16 Dukes, M. N. G., *BMJ*, *1* 1621 (1978)
17 Comfort, A., *The Biology of Ageing*, Freeman, UK (1979)
18 Dilman, V. M., *The Lancet*, *1* 1211–1219 (1971); Everett, A. V., and Burgess, J. A. (eds.), *Hypothalamus, Pituitary and Ageing*, Charles C. Thomas (1976)
19 Landfield, P. W., Waymire, J. C., and Lynch, G., *Science*, *202*, 1098–1102 (1978); Landfield, P. H., Lindsey, J. D., and Lynch, G., *Neuroscience Abst.*, *4* (1978)
20 Severson, J. A., Fell, R. D., Vander Tuig, J. G., and Griffith, D. R., *J. Applied Physio.*, *43* 839–843 (1977); Thorp, G. D., *Med. Sci. Sports*, *7* 6–11 (1975)
21 Golotin, V. G., Berdyshev, G. D., and Brekhman, I. I., in *Medicament Treatment in Advanced and Old Age*, 94–96, USSR Academy of Medical Sciences, Kiev (1968; R); also in *Forschritte der Medizin*, *24* 957–958 (1970)
22 Bittles, A. H., Fulder, S. J., Grant, E. C., and Nicholls, M. R., *Gerontology*, *25* 125–131 (1979)
23 Hochschild, R., *Exp. Geront.*, *8* 177–183 (1973); Hochschild, R., *Gerontologia*, *19* 271–280 (1973)
24 McKay, C. M., Sperling, G., and Barnes, L. L., *Arch. Bioch.*, *2* 469 (1943); Ross, M. H., Lustbader, E., and Bras, G., *Nature*, *262* 548–553 (1976)
25 Destrem, H., *La presse medicale*, *69* 1999–2006 (1961); Gedye, J. L., Exton-Smith, A. N., and Wedgwood, J., *Age and Ageing*, *1* 74–80 (1972)
26 Aslan, A., *Gerontologia Clinica*, *3* 148–176 (1960); Zung, W. W., Gianturco, D., Pfeiffer, E., Wong, H. S., Whanger, A., Bridge, T. P., and Potkin, S. G., *Psychosomatics*, *15* 127–131 (1974); Ostfield, A., Smith, C. M., and Strotsky, B. A., *J. Am. Geriatric Soc.*, *25* 1–19 (1977)
27 Oslon, E. J., Bank, L., and Jarvik, L. F., *J. Geront.* *33* 514–530 (1978)
28 Poggi, E., Sforzini, D., and Lazzati-Crespi, G. L., *Rivista di Neuropsichiatria e Scienze Affini*, *18* 93–107 (1972; Italian)
29 See Chapter 8, Note 45

CHAPTER 10

1 Costa, E., Garattini, S. (eds.), *Amphetamines and Related Compounds*, Raven Press, New York (1970); Robbins, T., and Iversen, S. D., *Nature: New Biology*, *245* 191 (1973)

2 Blum, *Psychopharmacologia, 6* 173–177 (1964); Smith, G. M., and Beecher, H. K., *JAMA, 172* 1623–1629 (1960)

3 Iversen, S. D., and Iversen, L. L., *Behavioural Pharmacology*, OUP, London (1975)

4 Eichler, O., *Kaffee und Coffein*, 2 Aufl. Springer, Berlin (1976; G)

5 Estler, C. J., Ammon, H. P. T., and Herzog, C., *Psychopharm.*, *58* 161–166 (1978)

6 Chernen'kii, I. K., in *Materials for the Study of Ginseng and Luzea*, *2* 171–173, (1955; R)

7 Saito, H., Tschuiya, M., Naka, S., Takagi, K., *Jap. J. Pharmacol.*, 27 509–516 (1977)

8 Chou, C. H., and Chang, H. M., *First Conference of the Society of Chinese Physiological Science, Yao,* 61–62 (1956); Ku, Y U., and Cheng, K. Y., ibid., 59–61 (Ch)

9 Shchichenkov, M. V., in Materials &c. see Chapter 5, Note 4(i) 241–244; Koryakovchev, V. S., see Chapter 5, Note 4(ii)

10 Clark, W. G., Blackman, H. J., and Preston, J. E., *Arch. Int. Pharmacodynam.*, *170* 350–363 (1967)

11 Dardymov, I. V., *Sb. Rab. Inst. Tsitol.*, *Akad. Nauk. SSSR*, *14* 76–81 (1971); see also Chapter 8, Note 54 (R)

12 Park, C. W., *Korean J. Pharmacol.*, *5* 28–33 (1969); Chung, Y. W., *Soul Uidae Chapchi, 12* 24–30 (1971; K)

13 Belanosov, I. S., Konstantinov, A. A., Krasilnikova, A. P., Makarevich, N. I., *Tr. Khabarovsk Med. Inst. Sb.*, *16* 34–44 (1959; R)

14 Meadley, R. G. S., *The Practitioner, 195* 680–683 (1965); Gelfand, S. Clark, L. D., Herbert, E. W., Cameron, D. E., Gelfand, D. N., and Holmes, E. D., *Clin. Pharmacol. Therap.*, *9* 56 (1968)

15 Andrews, G., and Solomon, D., *The Coca Leaf and Cocain Papers*, Harcourt, Brace and Jovanovich, London and New York (1975)

16 Antonil, *Mama Coca*, Hassle Free Press, London (1979)

17 Weil, A., *Am. J. Drug and Alcohol Abuse, 5* 75–86 (1978)

18 Johnston, J. F. W., *The Chemistry of Common Life, 2,* Blackwood, London (1840)

19 Lader, M., *The Psychophysiology of Mental Illness*, Churchill, London (1974); Gregoire, F., Brauman, H., de Buck, R., Corvilain, J., *Psychoneurendocrinology*, *2* 303–312 (1977)

20 Fedor-Freybergh, P., in Itil, T. M., Laudahn, G., and Herrman, W. M., *Psychotropic Action of Hormones*, Spectrum, New York (1976)

21 Strakhov, A. P., *Adaptation of Sailors on Prolonged Ocean Voyages*, Meditzina, Leningrad (1976)

22 Brekhman, I. I., *Man and Biologically Active Substances*, Pergamon Press, Oxford (1980)

23 Belenkiy, Ye. B., and Gotovtsev, P. I. (eds.), *Medicinal Preparations with Applications in Sports Medicine*, Meditsina, Moscow (1974; R)

24 'Doping of Athletes', special report by the Council of Cultural Co-operation of the Council of Europe (1968)

25 Ushakov, A. S., Myasnikov, V. I., Shestkov, B. P., Agureev, A. N., Belakovsky, M. S., and Rumyantseva, M. P., *Aviat., Space, Environ., Med.*, *49* 1184–1187 (1978)

26 Hanson, F. R., quoted in Bourne, P. G. (ed.), *The Psychology and Physiology of Stress*, xvii, Academic Press, New York (1969)

27 Quoted in Clamedson, C.-J., in Levi, L. (ed.), *Society, Stress and Disease*, 232, OUP (1971)

28 Belai, V. F., *Problems Farmakologii v. Kosmicheskoi Meditsine*, technical translation published by School of Aerospace Medicine, Brooks, Texas (1967)

29 Schmidt, C. F., Lambersten, C. J., *Annual Rev Pharmacology*, *5* 383–404 (1965)

CHAPTER 11

1 Petkov, V., and Koushev, V., *Bull. Inst. Physiol. Bulg. Acad. Sci.*, *10* 139–147 (1966; B)

2 Omura, Y., *Int. J. Acupunct. and Electrotherapeutic Res.*, *2* 1–31 (1976)

3 References to all of this work will be found in the extensive bibliography of Luce, G. G., *Body Time*, Paladin, St Albans (1973)

4 Sabena was nearly persuaded to serve ginseng tea to passengers, but backed out at the last minute

5 Petkov, V., *Experimentalna Medizina i Morphologia*, *4* 166–175 (1965; B)

6 Shass, E. Yu., *Fedsh. i Akush.*, *11* (1952; R)

7 Udupa, K. N., Singh, R. H., Dividevi, K. N., Pandey, H. P., and Rai, V., *Ind. J. Med. Res.*, *63* 1676–1679 (1975)

8 Gurvich, A. A., *Problems of Mitogenic Radiation as an Aspect of Molecular Biology*, Meditsina, Leningrad (1968; R)

9 Quickenden, T. J., and Hee, Q. S. S., *Biochem. Biophys. Res. Comm.*, *60* 764 (1974)

10 Kaznachayev, V. P., *et al.*, *Psychoenergetic Systems*, *1* 37 (1974)

11 Playfair, G. L., and Hill, S., *The Cycles of Heaven*, Souvenir Press, UK (1978)
12 Lane, E., *Electrophotography*, And/Or Press, San Francisco (1975)
13 Jonathan Miller, interview in *Vogue*, London, November 1978

CHAPTER 12

1 Farnsworth, N. R., and Morris, R. M., *Amer. J. Pharmacy*, *148* 46 (1976)
2 Bordia, A., Bausal, H. C., and Arora, S. K., *Atherosclerosis*, *21* 15–19 (1975)
3 World Health Organization Seminar on the Use of Medicinal Plants in Health Care, Manila (1977)
4 Haldane, J. B. S., *Daedalus, or Science and the Future*, Kegan, Paul, Trench and Trubner, London (1924)
5 See Chapter 3, Note 4
6 *The Promotion and Development of Traditional Medicine*, WHO Technical Report No. 622 (1978)
7 Lasagna, L., *Am. J. Int. Med.*, *83* 887 (1975)
8 Li Lun, *Scientica Sinica*, *28* 581 (1975)

APPENDIX

1 Trabucchi, E., *Forschungsrapport*, Pharmakol Institute, University of Milan (1969; G)
2 Savel, J., *Rapport d'expertise sur la toxicuté du gériatrie pharmaton*, Faculté de Pharmacie de Paris (1971; F)
3 Bittles, A. H., Fulder, S. J., Grant, E. C., and Nicholls, M. R., *Gerontology*, *25* 125–131 (1979)
4 See Chapter 5, Note 29
5 Hong, S. A., Kim, J. H., Kim, O. S., Lee, H. J., Lee, Y. R., Lee, C. H., Han, D. S., Song, W. K., Kim, Y. S., and Ko, C. S., *Tusam Munhum Teukjip*, *2* 51–54 (1964; K)
6 Letter from FDA to me, 16 May 1979
7 Siegel, R. K., *J. Am. Med. Ass.*, *241* 1614–1615 (1979)
8 One paper has been published on this question (Chang, J. C., *Cosmetics and Toiletries*, *92* 50–57, 1977), in which the author confirms that there is no evidence that ginseng works as a cosmetic
9 Hu, S. Y., op. cit. in Chapter 4, Note 8
10 Liberti, L. E., and Der Marderosian, H., *J. Pharm. Sci.*, *67* 1487–1489 (1978)

Index